# PET-Based Molecular Imaging in Evolving Personalized Management Design

*Editors*

SANDIP BASU
ABASS ALAVI

# PET CLINICS

www.pet.theclinics.com

*Consulting Editor*
ABASS ALAVI

July 2016 • Volume 11 • Number 3

**ELSEVIER**

1600 John F. Kennedy Boulevard • Suite 1800 • Philadelphia, Pennsylvania, 19103-2899

http://www.pet.theclinics.com

**PET CLINICS Volume 11, Number 3**
**July 2016 ISSN 1556-8598, ISBN-13: 978-0-323-44851-2**

Editor: John Vassallo (j.vassallo@elsevier.com)
Developmental Editor: Meredith Clinton



*PET Clinics* (ISSN 1556-8598) is published quarterly by Elsevier Inc., 360 Park Avenue South, New York, NY 10010-1710. Months of issue are January, April, July, and October. Periodicals postage paid at New York, NY, and additional mailing offices. Subscription prices per year are $225.00 (US individuals), $366.00 (US institutions), $100.00 (US students), $255.00 (Canadian individuals), $412.00 (Canadian institutions), $140.00 (Canadian students), $260.00 (foreign individuals), $412.00 (foreign institutions), and $140.00 (foreign students). To receive student and resident rate, orders must be accompanied by name of affiliated institution, date of term, and the signature of program/residency coordinator on institution letterhead. Orders will be billed at individual rate until proof of status is received. Foreign air speed delivery is included in all Clinics subscription prices. All prices are subject to change without notice. POSTMASTER: Send address changes to PET Clinics, Elsevier Health Sciences Division, Subscription Customer Service, 3251 Riverport Lane, Maryland Heights, MO 63043. **Customer Service: 1-800-654-2452 (U.S. and Canada); 314-447-8871 (outside U.S. and Canada). Fax: 314-447-8029. E-mail: journalscustomerservice-usa@elsevier.com (for print support); journalsonlinesupport-usa@elsevier.com (for online support).**

*Reprints*. For copies of 100 or more of articles in this publication, please contact the Commercial Reprints Department, Elsevier Inc., 360 Park Avenue South, New York, NY 10010-1710. Tel.: 212-633-3874; Fax: 212-633-3820; E-mail: reprints@elsevier.com.

PET Clinics is covered in MEDLINE/PubMed (Index Medicus).

# Contributors

## CONSULTING EDITOR

**ABASS ALAVI, MD, MD (Hon), PhD (Hon), DSc (Hon)**
Professor, Division of Nuclear Medicine, Department of Radiology, Hospital of the University of Pennsylvania, University of Pennsylvania Perelman School of Medicine, Philadelphia, Pennsylvania

## EDITORS

**SANDIP BASU, MBBS (Hons), DRM, DNB, MNAMS**
Professor, Radiation Medicine Centre, Bhabha Atomic Research Centre, Tata Memorial Hospital Annexe, Mumbai, Maharashtra, India

**ABASS ALAVI, MD, MD (Hon), PhD (Hon), DSc (Hon)**
Professor, Division of Nuclear Medicine, Department of Radiology, Hospital of the University of Pennsylvania, University of Pennsylvania Perelman School of Medicine, Philadelphia, Pennsylvania

## AUTHORS

**ABASS ALAVI, MD, MD (Hon), PhD (Hon), DSc (Hon)**
Professor, Division of Nuclear Medicine, Department of Radiology, Hospital of the University of Pennsylvania, University of Pennsylvania Perelman School of Medicine, Philadelphia, Pennsylvania

**EMILY C. AYERS, MD**
Internal Medicine Resident, Department of Medicine, Hospital of the University of Pennsylvania, Philadelphia, Pennsylvania

**GURDIP KAUR AZAD, MBBS, MRCP, FRCR**
Clinical Research Fellow, Division of Imaging Sciences and Biomedical Engineering, Cancer Imaging Department, King's College London, St Thomas' Hospital, London, United Kingdom

**SANDIP BASU, MBBS (Hons), DRM, DNB, MNAMS**
Professor, Radiation Medicine Centre, Bhabha Atomic Research Centre, Tata Memorial Hospital Annexe, Mumbai, Maharashtra, India

**OLE STEEN BJERRING, MD**
Department of Gastrointestinal Surgery, Odense University Hospital; Department of Clinical Research, Faculty of Health Sciences, University of Southern Denmark, Odense, Denmark

**GANG CHENG, MD, PhD**
Department of Radiology, Hospital of the University of Pennsylvania, Philadelphia, Pennsylvania

**PATRICK COLLETTI, MD**
Professor of Radiology, Department of Radiation Therapy, LAC-USC Medical Center, Keck Medical School of USC, Los Angeles, California

**GARY J. COOK, MBBS, MSc, MD, FRCR, FRCP**
Professor of PET Imaging, Head of Cancer Imaging, Division of Imaging Sciences and Biomedical Engineering, Cancer Imaging Department, King's College London; Clinical PET Centre, St Thomas' Hospital, London, United Kingdom

**KALPA JYOTI DAS, MD**
Diagnostic Nuclear Medicine Division, Department of Nuclear Medicine, All India Institute of Medical Sciences, New Delhi, India

**GHASSAN EL-HADDAD, MD**
Assistant Member, Division of Interventional Radiology, Department of Radiology, H. Lee Moffitt Cancer Center and Research Institute, Tampa, Florida

**STEFANO FANTI, MD**
Professor, Nuclear Medicine, AOU di Bologna Policlinico S. Orsola-Malpighi, Bologna, Italy

**SARA FARDIN, MD**
Department of Radiology, Hospital of the University of Pennsylvania, Philadelphia, Pennsylvania

**SAEID GHOLAMI, MD**
Department of Radiology, Hospital of the University of Pennsylvania, Philadelphia, Pennsylvania

**POUL FLEMMING HØILUND-CARLSEN, MD, DMSc**
Professor, Department of Nuclear Medicine, Odense University Hospital; Department of Clinical Research, Faculty of Health Sciences, University of Southern Denmark, Odense, Denmark

**NEVINE HANNA, MD**
Resident, Department of Radiation Oncology, Huntsman Cancer Hospital, Salt Lake City, Utah

**SØREN HESS, MD**
Associate Professor, Department of Nuclear Medicine, Odense University Hospital, Odense, Denmark; Division of Nuclear Medicine, Department of Radiology and Nuclear Medicine, Hospital of South West Jutland, Esbjerg, Denmark; Department of Clinical Research, Faculty of Health Sciences, University of Southern Denmark, Odense, Denmark

**SINA HOUSHMAND, MD**
Department of Radiology, Hospital of the University of Pennsylvania, University of Pennsylvania, Philadelphia, Pennsylvania

**ANDREI IAGARU, MD**
Division of Nuclear Medicine and Molecular Imaging, Department of Radiology, Stanford University, Stanford, California

**ANUSHA KALBASI, MD**
Department of Radiation Oncology, Hospital of the University of Pennsylvania, University of Pennsylvania, Philadelphia, Pennsylvania

**RAKESH KUMAR, MD, PhD**
Professor and Head, Diagnostic Nuclear Medicine Division, Department of Nuclear Medicine, All India Institute of Medical Sciences, New Delhi, India

**ABHISHEK MAHAJAN, MBBS, MD, MRes**
Consultant Radiologist, Department of Radiodiagnosis, Tata Memorial Hospital, Mumbai, Maharashtra, India

**ANTHONY R. MATO, MD**
Assistant Professor of Medicine, Department of Hematology/Oncology, Perelman Center for Advanced Medicine, Philadelphia, Pennsylvania

**ESTHER MENA, MD**
Russell H. Morgan Department of Radiology and Radiological Sciences, Johns Hopkins School of Medicine, Baltimore, Maryland

**CRISTINA NANNI, MD**
Nuclear Medicine, AOU di Bologna Policlinico S. Orsola-Malpighi, Bologna, Italy

**VIKAS OSTWAL, MBBS, MD, DM**
Department of Medical Oncology, Tata Memorial Hospital, Mumbai, Maharashtra, India

**PER PFEIFFER, MD, PhD**
Professor, Department of Clinical Oncology, Odense University Hospital; Department of Clinical Research, Faculty of Health Sciences, University of Southern Denmark, Odense, Denmark

**ROHIT RANADE, MBBS, DRM**
Radiation Medicine Centre, Bhabha Atomic Research Centre, Tata Memorial Hospital Annexe, Mumbai, Maharashtra, India

**ALI SALAVATI, MD, MPH**
Department of Radiology, Hospital of the University of Pennsylvania, University of Pennsylvania, Philadelphia, Pennsylvania; Department of Radiology, University of Minnesota, Minneapolis, Minnesota

**SHAILESH V. SHRIKHANDE, MBBS, MS**
Gastrointestinal and Hepato-Pancreato-Biliary Service, Department of Surgical Oncology, Tata Memorial Hospital, Mumbai, Maharashtra, India

**CHARLES B. SIMONE II, MD**
Department of Radiation Oncology, Hospital of the University of Pennsylvania, University of Pennsylvania, Philadelphia, Pennsylvania

**IDA SONNI, MD**
Division of Nuclear Medicine and Molecular Imaging, Department of Radiology, Stanford University, Stanford, California

**RATHAN M. SUBRAMANIAM, MD, PhD, MPH**
Russell H. Morgan Department of Radiology and Radiological Sciences; Department of Oncology, Sidney Kimmel Comprehensive Cancer Centre; Armstrong Institute for Patient Safety and Quality, Johns Hopkins School of Medicine; Department of Health Policy and Management, Johns Hopkins Bloomberg School of Public Health, Johns Hopkins University, Baltimore, Maryland

**SUMEET SURESH MALAPURE, MD**
Assistant Professor, Department of Nuclear Medicine, Kasturba Medical College, Manipal University, Manipal, Karnataka, India

**ELENA TABACCHI, MD**
Nuclear Medicine, AOU di Bologna Policlinico S. Orsola-Malpighi, Bologna, Italy

**HEIDI R. WASSEF, MD**
Assistant Professor of Clinical Radiology, Department of Radiation Therapy, LAC-USC Medical Center, Keck School of Medicine of USC, Los Angeles, California

**ANUSHA YANAMADALA, MD**
Russell H. Morgan Department of Radiology and Radiological Sciences, Johns Hopkins School of Medicine, Baltimore, Maryland

# Contents

**Preface** xv

Sandip Basu and Abass Alavi

**PET-Based Personalized Management in Clinical Oncology: An Unavoidable Path for the Foreseeable Future** 203

Sandip Basu and Abass Alavi

It is imperative that the thrust of clinical practice in the ensuing years would be to develop personalized management model for various disorders. PET-computed tomography (PET-CT) based molecular functional imaging has been increasingly utilized for assessment of tumor and other nonmalignant disorders and has the ability to explore disease phenotype on an individual basis and address critical clinical decision making questions related to practice of personalized medicine. Hence, it is essential to make a concerted systematic effort to explore and define the appropriate place of PET-CT in personalized clinical practice in each of malignancies, which would strengthen the concept further. The potential advantages of PET based disease management can be classified into broad categories: (1) Traditional: which includes assessment of disease extent such as initial disease staging and restaging, treatment response evaluation particularly early in the course and thus PET-CT response adaptive decision for continuing the same regimen or switching to salvage schedules; there has been continuous addition of newer application of PET based disease restaging in oncological parlance (eg, Richter transformation); (2) Recent and emerging developments: this includes exploring tumor biology with FDG and non-FDG PET tracers. The potential of multitracer PET imaging (particularly new and novel tracers, eg, 68Ga-DOTA-TOC/NOC/TATE in NET, 68Ga-PSMA and 18F-fluorocholine in prostate carcinoma, 18F-fluoroestradiol in breast carcinoma) has provided a scientific basis to stratify and select appropriate targeted therapies (both radionuclide and nonradionuclide treatment), a major boost for individualized disease management in clinical oncology. Integrating the molecular level information obtained from PET with structural imaging further individualizing treatment plan in radiation oncology, precision of interventions and biopsies of a particular lesion and forecasting disease prognosis.

**Personalized Management Approaches in Lymphoma: Utility of Fluorodeoxyglucose-PET Imaging** 209

Emily C. Ayers, Sara Fardin, Saeid Gholami, Abass Alavi, and Anthony R. Mato

PET/computed tomography (CT) imaging has gained a prominent role in the diagnosis and staging of malignancies. In lymphoma the role of PET/CT imaging continues to evolve as the understanding of its use in prognostication and response assessment improves. Currently, many groups are studying the potential function of PET/CT imaging in helping to direct management decisions for treating clinicians. This article summarizes the most up-to-date literature surrounding the topic of PET/CT-adaptive treatment of different lymphoma subjects. Although more studies are necessary to solidify the role of PET/CT, it is clear that this imaging modality holds much promise for the development of response-adaptive treatment algorithms in the future.

and gynecologic malignancies, focusing on the most promising targets for therapies and for molecular imaging using PET.

**Personalized Clinical Decision Making in Gastrointestinal Malignancies: The Role of PET** **273**

Søren Hess, Ole Steen Bjerring, Per Pfeiffer, and Poul Flemming Høilund-Carlsen

Gastrointestinal malignancies comprise a heterogeneous group of diseases that include both common and rare diseases with very different presentations and prognoses. The mainstay of treatment is surgery in combination with preoperative and adjuvant chemotherapy depending on clinical presentation and initial stages. This article outlines the potential use of fluorodeoxyglucose-PET/CT in clinical decision making with special regard to preoperative evaluation and response assessment in gastric cancer (including the gastroesophageal junction), pancreatic cancer (excluding neuroendocrine tumors), colorectal cancer, and gastrointestinal stromal tumors.

**The Possible Role of PET Imaging Toward Individualized Management of Bone and Soft Tissue Malignancies** **285**

Elena Tabacchi, Stefano Fanti, and Cristina Nanni

This article presents fluorodeoxyglucose PET/computed tomography for the evaluation of soft tissue sarcomas. Its clinical impact is discussed analyzing all the clinical information provided when applied in different phases of the disease. A special paragraph is dedicated to the use of functional imaging for driving the biopsy.

**PET/Computed Tomography in Breast Cancer: Can It Aid in Developing a Personalized Treatment Design?** **297**

Sumeet Suresh Malapure, Kalpa Jyoti Das, and Rakesh Kumar

PET with fluorodeoxyglucose (FDG-PET)/computed tomography (CT) imaging has significantly improved the management of breast cancer. FDG, however, is not tumor-specific and various image interpretation pitfalls may occur due to false-positive and false-negative causes of FDG uptake. PET/CT imaging with more specific radiopharmaceuticals may provide useful information about the pathophysiology in such cases. In the present article, we reviewed the use of whole-body FDG-PET/CT and $^{18}$F-16α-17β-Fluoroestradiol PET/CT imaging to determine if these can be used to develop personalized treatment design for the better management of breast cancer.

**PET Imaging of Skeletal Metastases and Its Role in Personalizing Further Management** **305**

Abhishek Mahajan, Gurdip Kaur Azad, and Gary J. Cook

In oncology, the skeleton is one of the most frequently encountered sites for metastatic disease and thus early detection not only has an impact on an individual patient's management but also on the overall outcome. Multiparametric and multimodal hybrid PET/computed tomography and PET/MR imaging have revolutionized imaging for bone metastases, but irrespective of tumor biology or morphology of the bone lesion it remains unclear which imaging modality is the most clinically relevant to guide individualized cancer care. In this review, we

# PET CLINICS

**FORTHCOMING ISSUES**

***October 2016***
**PET/MRI: Clinical Applications**
Drew A. Torigian, Andreas Kjær, Habib Zaidi, and Abass Alavi, *Editors*

***January 2017***
**Molecular Imaging and Precision Medicine, Part I**
Rathan M. Subramaniam, *Editor*

***April 2017***
**Prostate Cancer Imaging and Therapy**
Cristina Nanni and Richard P. Baum, *Editors*

**RECENT ISSUES**

***April 2016***
**PET/MRI: Advances in Instrumentation and Quantitative Procedures**
Habib Zaidi, *Editor*

***January 2016***
**Special Techniques and Technical Advances in PET/CT Imaging**
Rakesh Kumar, *Editor*

***October 2015***
**PET-Based Interventions**
Rakesh Kumar, *Editor*

**PROGRAM OBJECTIVE**

The goal of *PET Clinics* is to keep practicing radiologists and radiology residents up to date with current clinical practice in positron emission tomography by providing timely articles reviewing the state of the art in patient care.

**TARGET AUDIENCE**

Practicing radiologists, radiology residents, and other health care professionals who provide patient care utilizing radiologic findings.

**LEARNING OBJECTIVES**

Upon completion of this activity, participants will be able to:

1. Review the evolving role of PET personalized clinical decision making.
2. Discuss the use of PET imaging in individualized treatment in radiation oncology, malignancies, and percutaneous needle biopsy.
3. Recognize the use of PET-based imaging in infectious and inflammatory disorders.

**ACCREDITATION**

The Elsevier Office of Continuing Medical Education (EOCME) is accredited by the Accreditation Council for Continuing Medical Education (ACCME) to provide continuing medical education for physicians.

The EOCME designates this enduring material for a maximum of 15 *AMA PRA Category 1 Credit*(s)™. Physicians should claim only the credit commensurate with the extent of their participation in the activity.

All other health care professionals requesting continuing education credit for this enduring material will be issued a certificate of participation.

**DISCLOSURE OF CONFLICTS OF INTEREST**

The EOCME assesses conflict of interest with its instructors, faculty, planners, and other individuals who are in a position to control the content of CME activities. All relevant conflicts of interest that are identified are thoroughly vetted by EOCME for fair balance, scientific objectivity, and patient care recommendations. EOCME is committed to providing its learners with CME activities that promote improvements or quality in healthcare and not a specific proprietary business or a commercial interest.

**The planning committee, staff, authors and editors listed below have identified no financial relationships or relationships to products or devices they or their spouse/life partner have with commercial interest related to the content of this CME activity:**

Abass Alavi, MD, MD (Hon), PhD (Hon), DSc (Hon); Emily C. Ayers, MD; Gurdip Kaur Azad, MBBS, MRCP, FRCR; Sandip Basu, MBBS (Hons), DRM, DNB, MNAMS; Ole Steen Bjerring, MD; Gang Cheng, MD, PhD; Patrick Colletti, MD; Gary J. Cook, MBBS, MSc, MD, FRCR, FRCP; Kalpa Jyoti Das, MD; Ghassan El-Haddad, MD; Stefano Fanti, MD; Sara Fardin, MD; Anjali Fortna; Saeid Gholami, MD; Poul Flemming Høilund-Carlsen, MD, DMSc; Nevine Hanna, MD; Søren Hess, MD; Sina Houshmand, MD; Andrei Iagaru, MD; Anusha Kalbasi, MD; Rakesh Kumar, MD, PhD; Abhishek Mahajan, MBBS, MD, MRes; Anthony R. Mato, MD; Cristina Nanni, MD; Vikas Ostwal, MBBS, MD, DM; Per Pfeiffer, MD, PhD; Rohit Ranade, MBBS, DRM; Ali Salavati, MD, MPH; Erin Scheckenbach; Shailesh V. Shrikhande, MBBS, MS; Charles B. Simone II, MD; Ida Sonni, MD; Rathan M. Subramaniam, MD, PhD, MPH; Sumeet Suresh Malapure, MD; Elena Tabacchi, MD; John Vassallo; Rajakumar Venkatesan; Heidi R. Wassef, MD; Anusha Yanamadala, MD.

**The planning committee, staff, authors and editors listed below have identified financial relationships or relationships to products or devices they or their spouse/life partner have with commercial interest related to the content of this CME activity:**

**Esther Mena, MD** has research support from the National Institutes of Health.

**UNAPPROVED/OFF-LABEL USE DISCLOSURE**

The EOCME requires CME faculty to disclose to the participants:

1. When products or procedures being discussed are off-label, unlabelled, experimental, and/or investigational (not US Food and Drug Administration [FDA] approved); and
2. Any limitations on the information presented, such as data that are preliminary or that represent ongoing research, interim analyses, and/or unsupported opinions. Faculty may discuss information about pharmaceutical agents that is outside of FDA-approved labelling. This information is intended solely for CME and is not intended to promote off-label use of these medications. If you have any questions, contact the medical affairs department of the manufacturer for the most recent prescribing information.

**TO ENROLL**

To enroll in the *PET Clinics* Continuing Medical Education program, call customer service at 1-800-654-2452 or sign up online at http://www.theclinics.com/home/cme. The CME program is available to subscribers for an additional annual fee of USD $235.

**METHOD OF PARTICIPATION**

In order to claim credit, participants must complete the following:

1. Complete enrolment as indicated above.
2. Read the activity.
3. Complete the CME Test and Evaluation. Participants must achieve a score of 70% on the test. All CME Tests and Evaluations must be completed online.

**CME INQUIRIES/SPECIAL NEEDS**

For all CME inquiries or special needs, please contact elsevierCME@elsevier.com.

# Preface

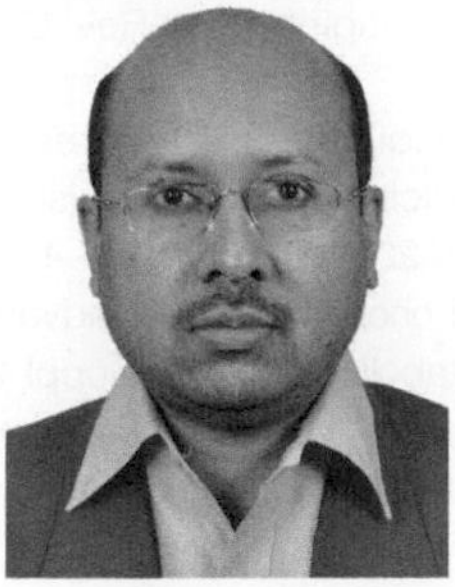
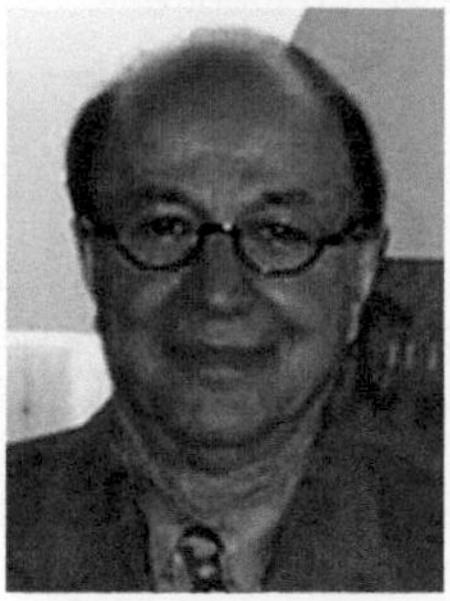

Sandip Basu, MBBS (Hons), DRM, DNB, MNAMS

Abass Alavi, MD, MD (Hon), PhD (Hon), DSc (Hon)

*Editors*

Increasingly, the concept of "Personalized Medicine" is being emphasized as the future trend in clinical practice, particularly in the field of Oncology. While the "triple-omics" has been at the forefront of this endeavor, the editors of this issue believe molecular imaging with PET will play the pivotal role in realization of personalized approach and management of a wide variety of cancers. It is therefore very timely to examine and forecast evolving and potential applications of this powerful modality and explore the various decision-making domains, where PET could play a critical role in such settings.[1–5] While over the years some efforts have been made to describe this rapidly evolving trend in medicine, as far as we could determine, there is no systematic and comprehensive review of this subject in the literature that may serve as a guide to the practicing clinicians. Therefore, in this issue of *PET Clinics*, we have made an attempt to introduce the ongoing research and clinical initiatives for developing PET-based personalized management models in various malignancies. The issue includes 13 reviews, which are drafted by a group of highly qualified colleagues who are authorities in their respective disciplines. The first introductory article in this issue reviews the current state of this field and future prospects for this very promising concept with special reference to the contents and points made by the contributing authors in the subsequent communications.

The topics covered in the present issue include the major neoplastic disorders, such as lymphoma, head and neck tumors, lung carcinomas, and gastrointestinal malignancies, with a separate discourse on gastroenteropancreatic neuroendocrine tumors. We should emphasize that PET imaging has played and continues to play an important role in the clinical decision-making process in these cancers. However, we felt that systematic exploration of the role of PET in these malignancies was lacking in the literature and there was a clear need to describe the evolving role of PET as a tool for personalized disease management. The role of molecular imaging for individualized management of certain disease conditions, such as gynecologic malignancies, breast carcinomas, bone and soft tissue tumors, skeletal metastases, and inflammatory disorders, is somewhat futuristic at this junction. Therefore, in the respective reviews related to these disorders, the ongoing trends have been explored, and the authors have forecasted the potential trends. Finally, the last two scientific communications in this issue, PET/CT-guided metabolic biopsies and PET-CT-based radiation therapy planning, respectively, have emphasized the critical role of molecular imaging in individualizing the intended treatments.

The editors believe and hope this issue will generate a great deal of interest and enthusiasm about the evolving applications of PET, and this could enhance and revolutionize the concept of Personalized Medicine in the future.

PET Clin 11 (2016) xv–xvi
http://dx.doi.org/10.1016/j.cpet.2016.04.001
1556-8598/16/$ – see front matter © 2016 Published by Elsevier Inc.

Sandip Basu, MBBS (Hons), DRM, DNB, MNAMS
Radiation Medicine Centre
Bhabha Atomic Research Centre
Tata Memorial Hospital Annexe
Jerbai Wadia Road, Parel, Mumbai
Maharashtra, India, 400 012

Abass Alavi, MD, MD (Hon), PhD (Hon), DSc (Hon)
Division of Nuclear Medicine
Perelman School of Medicine
Hospital of the University of Pennsylvania
Philadelphia, PA 19104, USA

E-mail addresses:
drsanb@yahoo.com (S. Basu)
abass.alavi@uphs.upenn.edu (A. Alavi)

## REFERENCES

1. Basu S. Personalized versus evidence-based medicine with PET-based imaging. Nat Rev Clin Oncol 2010;7:665–8.
2. Kruse V, Belle SV, Cocquyt V. Imaging requirements for personalized medicine: the oncologists point of view. Curr Pharm Des 2014;20(14):2234–49.
3. Kalia M. Personalized oncology: recent advances and future challenges. Metabolism 2013;62(Suppl 1):S11–4.
4. Basu S. The scope and potentials of functional radionuclide imaging towards advancing personalized medicine in oncology: emphasis on PET-CT. Discov Med 2012;13(68):65–73.
5. Hess S, Basu S, Blomberg BA, et al. The FDG-PET revolution of medical imaging--four decades and beyond. Current Molecular Imaging 2015;4(1):2–19.

# PET-Based Personalized Management in Clinical Oncology

## An Unavoidable Path for the Foreseeable Future

Sandip Basu, DRM, DNB, MNAMS[a,*], Abass Alavi, MD[b]

**KEYWORDS**

• PET-CT • Personalized medicine • Precision medicine • Oncology • Lymphoma • Head-neck cancer

**KEY POINTS**

- There are specific advantages of functional PET/computed tomographic (CT) assessment of the tumor in augmenting the concept of personalized medicine with an emphasis on cancer management.
- The impact of PET/CT adaptive treatment is clear and obvious in oncology, and it has the potential to be extended to the nonmalignant diseases as well.
- The future direction is to develop a disease-specific personalized model based on the evidence generated in each clinical decision-making step, which would form the objective basis and aid in making the clinical practice more scientific.

### INTRODUCTION: PERSONALIZED OR PRECISION MEDICINE: ADVANTAGES OF INTEGRATING PET/COMPUTED TOMOGRAPHIC IMAGING IN CLINICAL MANAGEMENT PROTOCOL

Personalized and Precision Medicine has been the major thrust of present day clinical management of both oncologic and nononcologic disorders. Many of the current and traditional utilities of PET/computed tomographic (CT) imaging in routine clinical oncology have been examples of personalization of disease management itself. These examples include (i) appropriate initial disease staging and thus selecting the optimal treatment approach, and (ii) early and end-of-treatment response assessment and thus continuing or switching to salvage regimens.[1–3] The stage of migration with PET with fludeoxyglucose (FDG-PET) in various malignancies, the so-called Will Rogers phenomenon, and the consequences of selection of appropriate therapy for disease outcome have been increasingly emphasized in literature over the past decade.[2] Over recent years, multiple newer and novel PET applications have emerged that have the potential to explore tumor and disease biology at an individual level. This has been the major strength of PET-based functional imaging for playing a pivotal role in personalized clinical decision-making and further

The authors have nothing to disclose.

[a] Radiation Medicine Centre, Bhabha Atomic Research Centre, Tata Memorial Hospital Annexe, Jerbai Wadia Road, Parel, Mumbai 400 012, India; [b] Division of Nuclear Medicine, Perelman School of Medicine, Hospital of the University of Pennsylvania, Philadelphia, PA, USA
* Corresponding author.
*E-mail address:* drsanb@yahoo.com

PET Clin 11 (2016) 203–207
http://dx.doi.org/10.1016/j.cpet.2016.03.002

clinical practice.[4] A systematic endeavor by the PET imaging community hence is required to define the place and role in each of the malignancies and the other nonmalignant disease conditions. This systematic endeavor should go hand-in-hand with the evolution of a personalized clinical decision-making model for various disorders, and in the authors' view, it is hoped would augment and strengthen its development. In the present article, the authors have primarily focused on the latter and briefly touched on the traditional utilities of PET in personalizing disease management that would form the basis of subsequent disease-specific reviews included in the thematic issue on PET-based personalized medicine.

## TRADITIONAL CLINICAL UTILITIES OF PET/COMPUTED TOMOGRAPHY IN PERSONALIZING DISEASE MANAGEMENT

Appropriate disease staging of malignancies at initial diagnosis has been a major thrust of the evolution of PET/CT in various malignancies. This disease staging has brought a paradigm shift in patient management strategy. The most prominent examples of this have been lymphoma, head-neck malignancies, and lung cancer. Abundant literature exists today emphasizing the role of PET/CT in the diagnosis and staging of lymphoma. Early appropriate treatment response assessment following systemic chemotherapy administration has been one of the major advantages: both escalation and deintensification of therapy based on PET/CT imaging of 1 to 3 cycles of chemotherapy have been a major thrust in the management of lymphoma; examples include following in Hodgkin lymphoma, escalation to BEACOPP (B, Bleomycin; E, Etoposide; A, Adriamycin; C, Cyclophosphamide; O, Oncovin; P, Procarbazine; P, Prednisolone) for PET/CT-positive patients after 2 cycles of first-line ABVD, foregoing radiation after ABVD (A, Adriamycin; B, Bleomycin; V, Vinblastine; D, Dacarbazine) based on PET/CT negativity, institution of radiotherapy after 6 cycles of escalated BEACOPP (eBEACOPP) based on PET/CT treatment response results, PET/CT results to determine need for bleomycin in ABVD after 2 cycles, thereby switching to a less pulmonary-toxic regimen. In non-Hodgkin diffuse B-cell large cell lymphoma subtype, the role of interim FDG-PET/CT has been explored for dose escalation to R-ICE or B-ALL protocol (PETAL [PET guided therapy of aggressive non-Hodgkin lymphomas] trial) or for deciding the need for consolidative radiotherapy. All these, when validated, can lead to better planning for a further course of treatment in lymphoma on an individual patient basis. Similar usefulness has also been obtained in assessing early response in gastrointestinal stromal tumors (to imatinib mesylate), neoadjuvant therapy in lung, esophagus, and breast cancer, in addition to better whole body disease assessment at baseline compared with the anatomical modalities alone.[5–10]

For staging head and neck malignancies, PET/CT demonstrates higher sensitivity than CT and MR imaging for ipsilateral and contralateral lymph nodes and distant metastases as well as diagnosing second primary malignancies. Furthermore, radiation therapy planning in a patient is enhanced by the introduction of FDG-PET/CT through better and more accurate tumor delineation and gross tumor volume. Accurate assessments of treatment response and better after-treatment surveillance are other discrete advantages of FDG-PET/CT that helps in disease management on an individual basis in this group of patients.

Epidermal growth factor receptor (EGFR) and Kristen rat sarcoma are the 2 most commonly studied and mutated proto-oncogenes in adenocarcinoma lung, and FDG-PET/CT has been used for early treatment assessment to identify individuals who benefit from treatment with EGFR-tyrosine kinase inhibitors, such as gefitinib and erlotinib. The article, Mena E, Yanamadala A, Cheng G, et al: The Current and Evolving Role of PET in Personalized Management of Lung Cancer, in this issue reviews the present literature in this domain whereby PET-documented early responses to these agents were associated with improved progression-free survival. They have also dealt with the potential of fluorothymidine-PET as an early predictor for response to therapy and survival with EGFR-targeted therapies.

The article, Mahajan A, Azad GK, Cook GJ: PET Imaging of Skeletal Metastases and Its Role in Personalizing Further Management, in this issue discusses the potential of PET/MR imaging to have higher diagnostic accuracy for detection of early bone marrow infiltration and for assessing bone tumors with low $^{18}$F-FDG uptake. The initial literature suggests improved treatment monitoring ability of this modality (with $^{18}$F-Choline-PET/MR imaging) for hormonal deprivation therapy as well as radiation therapy in prostate cancer.

## NEWER APPLICATIONS OF PET-BASED DISEASE RESTAGING WITH IMPLICATIONS FOR MANAGEMENT INDIVIDUALIZATION

Transformation of indolent lymphoma to aggressive subtype is associated with poor outcome and needs to be detected and intervened at the earliest opportunity. FDG-PET/CT has demonstrated high sensitivity and specificity in this area: detection of Richter syndrome (transformation of chronic lymphocytic leukemia into large B-cell lymphoma) by PET/CT has been described with literature evidence. (Please see Ayers EC, Fardin S, Gholami S, et al: Personalized Management Approaches in Lymphoma: Utility of Fluorodeoxyglucose-PET Imaging, in this issue.) Another example of PET/CT-based improved diagnosis (please see Wassef HR, Hanna N, Colletti P: PET/CT in Head-neck Malignancies: The Implications for Personalized Clinical Practice, in this issue) has been to detect the putative site of primary in carcinoma of unknown primary, which can guide endoscopic biopsy in the most metabolically active site. This has been dealt with by the addition of FDG-PET/CT-detected tumor between 30% and 37% following the failure of conventional imaging procedures, and 22% when panendoscopy was included in the protocol; all these aided individualized management with a change in patient management at around 35%.[10]

## EMERGING APPLICATIONS OF PET/COMPUTED TOMOGRAPHY IN PERSONALIZING DISEASE MANAGEMENT

### *Quantification of Metabolic Activity, Metabolic Tumor Volume, and Total Lesion Glycolysis as Disease Prognosticator*

There has been substantial interest in assessing disease biology and thereby prognosticating disease through PET metabolic activity. In the article concerning head and neck malignancies, the authors reviewed the various studies that have found correlation of outcome with maximum standard uptake value (SUVmax), mean SUV, metabolic tumor volume, gross tumor volume (by PET), and total lesion glycolysis with survival outcome, although a definitive model is yet to evolve that would incorporate FDG-PET/CT as a prognostic biomarker that could be adopted on an individualized basis. (Please see Wassef HR, Hanna N, Colletti P: PET/CT in Head-neck Malignancies: The Implications for Personalized Clinical Practice, in this issue.) In the parlance of breast carcinoma, higher SUVmax on FDG-PET has been typically described in triple-negative and HER2-positive tumors.[11]

### *PET-Based Risk Adaptive Management in Lymphoma and in Neoadjuvant Treatment Setting*

As mentioned before, FDG-PET-based assessment of response or residual disease, in addition to directing the subsequent therapies, also can serve as a prognostic indicator in certain lymphoma subtypes and other malignancies. Similarly, prognostic value of PET/CT-depicted disease burden before stem cell transplantation has been reported by various investigators in NHL.

### *Dual Tracer PET Imaging Approach in Individualizing Therapy*

The utility of dual tracer imaging, correlating the findings with tumor proliferation index (Ki-67/Mib1) has become an important approach for the individualized management in patients of neuroendocrine tumor. The authors have discussed in detail (please see Hess S, Alavi A, Basu S: PET-Based Personalized Management of Infectious and Inflammatory Disorders, in this issue) how the relative tracer uptake by dual tracer imaging approach (with somatostatin receptor targeted $^{68}$Ga-DOTA-TOC/NOC/TATE and GLUT receptor and glycolytic metabolism-specific FDG-PET) can be used to subsegment these patients, and personalized treatment could be used in patients of GEP-NET.[12]

### *As a Guide to Multitargets in Molecular-based Therapy*

In addition to the above, multitracer PET imaging can subserve as a valuable biomarker to select the most appropriate therapeutic agent in patients with cancer. The authors have initially examined the feasibility in bone-confined metastatic disease in medullary carcinoma of the thyroid and neuroendocrine tumor to decide on therapeutic options with $^{177}$Lu-DOTATATE versus $^{177}$Lu-EDTMP.[13] Similar issues could be encountered in metastatic prostate carcinoma as well as where one needs to weigh between bone-directed radionuclides (eg, $^{177}$Lu/$^{153}$Sm-EDTMP, $^{223}$Ra) and receptor-targeted agents (eg, $^{177}$Lu-PSMA). This aspect of PET imaging has also been highlighted in this issue. (Please see Mahajan A, Azad GK, Cook GJ: PET Imaging of Skeletal Metastases and Its Role in Personalizing Further Management.) There have been ongoing clinical trials in lung carcinoma whereby EGFR-targeted PET with experimental agents (eg, $^{11}$C-erlotinib, $^{11}$C-PD153035) or immuno-PET using radiolabeled monoclonal antibodies (eg, $^{89}$Zr-cetuximab and $^{89}$Zr-panitumumab) could help to identify patients who can benefit from the EGFR-targeted therapy. In the domain of urologic malignancies, PET imaging of therapeutic targets has immense potential for personalized management, and the explored areas include: (i) angiogenesis (with $^{89}$Zr-Bevacizumab for vascular endothelial growth factor receptor–targeted Bevacizumab therapy or $^{18}$F-SU11248 for sunitinib therapy), (ii) hormone receptors ($^{18}$F-FDHT for androgen receptor in prostate cancer, $^{18}$F-fluoroestradiol [FES] for estrogen receptor in endometrial and ovarian cancer), and (iii) cell surface antigens (eg, prostate-specific membrane antigen imaging $^{68}$Ga-PSMA in prostate cancer for $^{177}$Lu-PSMA therapy, $^{124}$I-cG250 PET/CT for cG250 targeted therapy in renal cell cancer). These areas are reviewed in a detailed manner in this issue. (Please see Sonni I, Iagaru A: PET Imaging Toward Individualized Management of Urological and Gynecologic Malignancies.) Similarly, the article (please see Suresh Malapure S, Das KJ, Kumar R: PET/Computer Tomography in Breast Cancer: Can It Aid in Developing a Personalized Treatment Design? in this issue) reviews the potential of noninvasive characterization of metastatic disease by receptor-based PET/CT with $^{18}$F-16α-17β-FES, and how it can be useful particularly in metastatic breast cancer in planning treatment strategies in a personalized manner. The article (please see Mahajan A, Azad GK, Cook GJ: PET Imaging of Skeletal Metastases and Its Role in Personalizing Further Management, in this issue) discusses the potential utility targeted PET imaging in skeletal metastases; for example, $^{89}$Zr-trastuzumab PET as a useful noninvasive method for characterizing HER2 expression in skeletal disease that could help in selecting this therapy with greater confidence.

### *Tumor Heterogeneity*

Exploring tumor heterogeneity is an important factor that has enormous implications for personalized cancer treatment. Intertumoral and even intratumoral heterogeneity of blood flow and angiogenesis, hypoxia, necrosis, cellular proliferation, gene mutation, and expression of specific receptors could be studied with FDG and non-FDG-PET tracers and can help in decision-making on an individual basis.[14] In the article Mena E, Yanamadala A, Cheng G, et al: The Current and Evolving Role of PET in Personalized Management of Lung Cancer, in this issue, the authors have highlighted this aspect of PET/CT imaging in the domain of lung cancer, with emphasis on hypoxia and angiogenesis imaging and its implications for radiotherapy and novel drugs targeting angiogenesis.

### *PET/Computed Tomography–guided Biopsy in Individualized Diagnosis and Appropriate Tumor Grading*

PET/CT functional imaging-driven biopsy has been of great advantage for individualized diagnosis and management. In the articles Tabacchi E, Fanti S, Nanni C: The Possible Role of PET Imaging Toward Individualized Management of Bone and Soft Tissue Malignancies and El-Haddad G: PET-Based Percutaneous Needle Biopsy, both in this issue, the authors have highlighted the utilities that could be of special help in large malignant lesions that could be heterogeneous and are able to guide biopsy to the area of highest uptake on $^{18}$F-FDG-PET/CT and reduces the probability of tumor grade underestimation. This important application is one clinical utility of FDG-PET/CT in depicting intratumoral heterogeneity that widely varies in each patient and tumor.

### *Detection of Synchronous and Metachronous Primaries and Other Sequelae of Toxic Therapies*

Many of the patients with cancer have a predilection for harboring second malignancies, whereby whole body FDG-PET/CT can be of specific advantage because of its exquisite sensitivity. The article (please see Wassef HR, Hanna N, Colletti P: PET/CT in Head-neck Malignancies: The Implications for Personalized Clinical Practice, in this issue) reviews this in the setting of head-neck malignancies whereby, as stated by the authors, PET-CT is an effective imaging modality in detecting most second cancers in either the lung, esophageal, or a second head and neck cancer.

## SUMMARY

The impact of PET/CT adaptive treatment is clear and obvious in oncology, and it has the potential to be extended to the nonmalignant diseases as well. The future direction is to develop a disease-specific personalized model based on the evidence generated in each clinical decision-making step, which would form the objective basis and would aid in making the clinical practice more scientific.

## REFERENCES


1. Basu S, Alavi A. Unparalleled contribution of 18F-FDG PET to medicine over 3 decades. J Nucl Med 2008;49(10):17N–21N, 37N.
2. Hess S, Basu S, Blomberg BA, et al. The FDG-PET revolution of medical imaging—four decades and beyond. Current Molecular Imaging 2015;4(1):2–19.
3. Basu S, Alavi A. Staging with PET and the "Will Rogers" effect: redefining prognosis and survival in patients with cancer. Eur J Nucl Med Mol Imaging 2008;35(1):1–4.
4. Basu S. Personalized versus evidence-based medicine with PET-based imaging. Nat Rev Clin Oncol 2010;7:665–8.

5. Basu S, Mohandas KM, Peshwe H, et al. FDG-PET and PET/CT in the clinical management of gastrointestinal stromal tumour (GIST). Nucl Med Commun 2008;29(12):1026–39.
6. Hazelton TR, Coppage L. Imaging for lung cancer restaging. Semin Roentgenol 2005;40(2):182–92.
7. Ozkan E. Positron emission tomography/computed tomography in locally advanced breast cancer. Exp Oncol 2013;35(4):253–7.
8. Izumi D, Yoshida N, Watanabe M, et al. Tumor/normal esophagus ratio in 18F-fluorodeoxyglucose positron emission tomography/computed tomography for response and prognosis stratification after neoadjuvant chemotherapy for esophageal squamous cell carcinoma. J Gastroenterol 2015. [Epub ahead of print].
9. Schmidt T, Lordick F, Herrmann K, et al. Value of functional imaging by PET in esophageal cancer. J Natl Compr Canc Netw 2015;13(2):239–47.
10. Pawaskar A, Basu S. Role of FDG PET-CT in carcinoma of unknown primary. PET Clin 2015;10(3):297–310.
11. Basu S, Chen W, Tchou J, et al. Comparison of triple-negative and estrogen receptor-positive/progesterone receptor-positive/HER2-negative breast carcinoma using quantitative fluorine-18 fluorodeoxyglucose/positron emission tomography imaging parameters: a potentially useful method for disease characterization. Cancer 2008;112(5):995–1000.
12. Basu S, Ranade R, Thapa P. Correlation and discordance of tumour proliferation index and molecular imaging characteristics and their implications for treatment decisions and outcome pertaining to peptide receptor radionuclide therapy in patients with advanced neuroendocrine tumour: developing a personalized model. Nucl Med Commun 2015;36(8):766–74.
13. Basu S, Ranade R, Thapa P. 177Lu-DOTATATE versus 177Lu-EDTMP versus cocktail/sequential therapy in bone-confined painful metastatic disease in medullary carcinoma of the thyroid and neuroendocrine tumour: can semiquantitative comparison of 68Ga-DOTATATE and 18F-fluoride PET-CT aid in personalized treatment decision making in selecting the best therapeutic option? Nucl Med Commun 2016;37(1):100–2.
14. Basu S, Kwee TC, Gatenby R, et al. Evolving role of molecular imaging with PET in detecting and characterizing heterogeneity of cancer tissue at the primary and metastatic sites, a plausible explanation for failed attempts to cure malignant disorders. Eur J Nucl Med Mol Imaging 2011;38(6):987–91.

# Personalized Management Approaches in Lymphoma

## Utility of Fluorodeoxyglucose-PET Imaging

Emily C. Ayers, MD[a], Sara Fardin, MD[b], Saeid Gholami, MD[b], Abass Alavi, MD[b], Anthony R. Mato, MD[c,*]

**KEYWORDS**

• Lymphoma • PET imaging • Response-adaptive treatment • PET-directed therapy

**KEY POINTS**

- Response-adaptive therapy for lymphoma using guidance by PET/CT imaging provides a way to minimize treatment toxicity and radiation exposure for patients with malignant lymphoma.
- Interim PET/CT imaging can be used to tailor radiation therapy in patients with Hodgkin lymphoma.
- Escalation of treatment in patients with positive interim PET/CT imaging leads to better outcomes than historically recorded.
- New computer software improves accuracy and sensitivity of PET imaging to calculate a corrected total disease activity level.

Although an abundance of literature over the past decade addresses the use and relevance of PET/computed tomography (CT) imaging in the diagnosis and staging of lymphoma, a more recent area of immense clinical importance has been to evaluate the role of this imaging modality in risk-adaptive treatment approaches. This article focuses on the most recent literature surrounding the topic of PET/CT-guided therapy including a summary of the evidence on the use of PET/CT imaging as a prognostic indicator in certain lymphoma subtypes, most up-to-date evidence on therapeutic adjustment based on PET/CT results, evidence supporting the use of PET/CT imaging to optimize the use radiation therapy (RT) in lymphoma management, and ongoing research on using PET/CT to escalate or deintensify lymphoma-directed treatment.

## HODGKIN LYMPHOMA

Hodgkin lymphoma (HL) occurs with an incidence of roughly 9000 cases per year in the United States. Over the course of the last few decades, standard of care in HL has improved dramatically such that cure is achieved in 75% to 90% of patients depending on stage and risk factors. Major efforts have been made over the last decade to minimize toxicity while maintaining the efficacy of treatment. Within this movement, fluorodeoxyglucose (FDG)-PET imaging has emerged as a promising tool.

Current guidelines recognize the use of PET/CT in the diagnosis and staging of HL.[1] The inclusion of combined PET/CT imaging in the primary evaluation of HL has led to higher diagnostic accuracy with consequentially more frequent upstaging compared with CT scan alone.[2,3] This increased

Disclosure Statement: The authors have nothing to disclose.

[a] Department of Medicine, Hospital of the University of Pennsylvania, 100 Centrex, 3400 Spruce Street, Philadelphia, PA 19104, USA; [b] Department of Radiology, Hospital of the University of Pennsylvania, 3400 Spruce Street, 4283, Philadelphia, PA 19104, USA; [c] Department of Hematology/Oncology, Perelman Center for Advanced Medicine, West Pavilion, 2nd Floor, 3400 Civic Center Boulevard, Philadelphia, PA 19104, USA
* Corresponding author.
*E-mail address:* anthony.mato@uphs.upenn.edu

PET Clin 11 (2016) 209–218
http://dx.doi.org/10.1016/j.cpet.2016.02.001
1556-8598/16/$ – see front matter 

sensitivity in initial staging has had a valuable impact on treatment selection for these patients.

PET/CT has also been well validated as a prognostic tool in HL. Literature supports the use of interim and posttherapy PET/CT to prognosticate progression-free survival (PFS) and overall survival (OS), with a very high negative predictive value upward of 94%.[4] A positive mid-treatment PET/CT is associated with decreased PFS and OS.[5] However, positive predictive value of interim PET/CT is markedly lower than the negative predictive value (53.8% vs 100%, respectively).[5]

Perhaps most exciting over the last decade, however, has been investigation into the role of PET/CT in driving management decisions for HL. Active exploration seeks to address whether chemotherapy should be de-escalated based on negative interim scans or intensified in response to positive interim scans. Additionally, there is much interest to identify a subset of patients who benefit most from adjuvant RT based on PET/CT imaging.

Given that HL is a disease of younger patients with long life expectancies, optimizing exposure to RT is of utmost importance. Lower total doses of RT and minimized fields may result in fewer toxicities, which include coronary angiopathy, secondary malignancies, thyroid abnormalities, and pulmonary toxicities.[6]

In 2013, Girinsky and colleagues[7] demonstrated that the addition of PET to CT imaging improved delineation of involved node RT with increased clinical target volumes but without increased volume of radiation delivered. Therefore, the addition of PET identified, with higher precision and sensitivity, targetable lymph nodes for RT without necessitating larger radiation volumes.

Others have addressed the possibility of eliminating the need for RT entirely. For example, Radford and colleagues[8] described the UK RAPID study, in which 602 patients with negative PET/CT (defined by the International Harmonization Project [IHP] criteria)[9] after three cycles of adriamycin, bleomycin, vinblastine, and dacarbazine (ABVD) were randomized to RT versus no RT. The 3-year PFS was 94.6% and 90.8% in the RT and no-RT groups, respectively. Although the study did not show noninferiority in terms of PFS, the authors concluded that patients with a negative PET/CT have an excellent prognosis with and without consolidative RT following chemotherapy.[8]

In contrast, Raemaekers and colleagues[10] demonstrated early treatment failure without RT in patients with negative PET/CT. This study enrolled 1137 patients with stage I/II HL and omitted involved-node RT in patients with a negative PET/CT after two cycles of ABVD. A preplanned interim futility analysis with the goal to stop recruitment in the case of inferiority in the investigational arm demonstrated futility in the favorable and unfavorable subgroups who did not receive RT ($P = .017$ and 0.026, respectively). In light of this analysis, the study was terminated, because the data predicted that the group was unlikely to observe efficacy between the standard and experimental arms.

Additionally, in the RATHL study, Engert and colleagues[11] investigated PET-directed RT following six cycles of escalated bleomycin, etoposide, adriamycin, cyclophosphamide, vincristine, procarbazine and prednisone (eBEACOPP) in advanced HL. In this study, only 11% of patients ultimately received RT for mass lesions measuring greater than or equal to 2.5 cm on PET/CT imaging. The group concluded that six cycles of BEACOPP followed by PET-directed RT interpreted according to the London criteria was more effective in terms of freedom from treatment failure with less toxicity than eight cycles of escalated BEACOPP.[12] Thus, there are promising data suggesting that PET-directed RT is effective and safe in HL but, because data are still somewhat conflicting, further investigation is warranted before the use of PET/CT to determine the need for consolidative RT is incorporated into standard practice.

Several groups have tested the hypothesis that escalation of therapy based on PET/CT imaging after one to three cycles of initial chemotherapy may salvage patients predicted to have a poor prognosis with standard-dose chemotherapy based on positive PET/CT results.

Gallamini and colleagues[13] in 2011 published results from 219 patients who received response-adapted treatment based on PET/CT performed after two cycles of ABVD. Patients who were PET/CT positive according to the London Criteria after two cycles of ABVD were escalated to BEACOPP.[13] The 2-year PFS was 91% for the entire cohort. PFS was 95% for PET-negative and 62% for PET-positive patients. These results were believed to be better than historic ABVD control subjects who would have continued this therapy in the setting of a positive interim PET/CT scan, leading the authors to conclude that escalation of therapy based on interim PET/CT imaging can lead to improved outcomes without exposing all patients to increased toxicity of more intense chemotherapeutic regimens, such as BEACOPP.

Several other clinical trials are currently ongoing to investigate the role of PET/CT in response-adapted therapy, which are discussed next. The RATHL study used PET/CT to investigate the role of prolonged bleomycin exposure in patients with HL undergoing combination chemotherapy with ABVD. Patients with negative PET/CT according to the London criteria after two cycles of ABVD are randomized to either four additional cycles of ABVD or AVD. Fewer cases of pulmonary toxicity were observed in the AVD arm. At 36 months, PFS was 85.4% (95% confidence interval [CI], 81.6–88.5) among the ABVD group and 84.4% (95% CI, 80.7–87.6) among the AVD group.[14]

In the Israeli H2 study group, 356 patients with advanced HL were assigned to initial treatment based on International Prognostic Score (IPS) score. Patients with an IPS of 0 to 1 received two initial cycles of ABVD and those patients with an IPS greater than or equal to 2 received two initial cycles of eBEACOPP.[15] PET/CT scan after the first two cycles was then used to direct therapy. Patients with negative interim PET/CT by the London criteria completed four additional cycles of ABVD, whereas patients with positive PET/CT were escalated to eBEACOPP with consolidative RT in the setting of bulky mediastinal disease. The 3-year PFS was 89% overall for patients with early stage disease (91% and 74% for PET/CT negative and positive, respectively). For patients with advanced HL, 3-year PFS was 85% (86% and 75% in PET/CT-negative and -positive patients, respectively). No difference was seen based on initial IPS score among patients controlled for PET/CT status. This study demonstrates that de-escalation of therapy is safe in advanced disease in the setting of a negative interim PET/CT following two cycles of chemotherapy.

In the French LYSA trial, the experimental arm allows for de-escalation of therapy from eBEACOPP to four cycles of ABVD in patients with a negative interim PET/CT, whereas those patients with positive interim PET/CT continue with eBEACOPP.[16] This study is ongoing (clinical trial NCT01358747).

In summary (**Table 1**), interim PET/CT carries important prognostic value in HL. What remains less clear, however, are the ways in which clinicians can use this prognostic tool to further direct therapy. There is conflicting evidence regarding the use of PET/CT to identify candidates for consolidative RT; although there seems to be a statistically significant difference in PFS favoring those who undergo RT, one must balance the risks of RT with the added PFS (but not OS) benefit. Further clarification may come when results are available of multiple trials that are currently investigating the role PET/CT can play in escalating or de-escalating HL therapy based on interim PET/CT status.

## DIFFUSE LARGE B-CELL LYMPHOMA

Diffuse large B-cell lymphoma (DLBCL) is the most common subtype of non-HL, accounting for 30% to 35% of cases. DLBCL has a median age of diagnosis in the seventh decade of life, with roughly half of patients presenting with advanced-stage disease. The current standard of care remains rituximab-cyclophosphamide, doxorubicin, vincristine, and prednisone (R-CHOP) as front-line therapy at time of diagnosis with 5-year survival rates ranging from 83% to 32% for patients with IPI scores of 0 to 3, respectively.[17]

In contrast to HL, the prognostic utility of interim PET/CT imaging is not supported in clinical practice at this time.[18] Before the inclusion of rituximab in DLBCL management, the literature supported a strong correlation between interim PET/CT and outcomes. In more recent years, however, the data suggest a high false-positive rate for interim PET/CT scans in DLBCL, rituximab-treated patients possibly because of an exaggerated inflammatory response following rituximab exposure.[19]

**Table 1**
**Hodgkin lymphoma**

| Trial | No of Patients | Study Summary |
|---|---|---|
| Radford et al,[8] 2015 (UK RAPID) | 602 | PET/CT negativity can be used to forego radiation after ABVD |
| Raemaekers et al,[10] 2014 | 1137 | PET/CT status cannot be used to obviate radiotherapy |
| Engert et al,[11] 2012 (HD15) | 2182 | PET/CT-directed RT after six cycles of eBEACOPP is effective and less toxic |
| Gallamini et al,[13] 2011 | 219 | Treatment escalation to BEACOPP for PET/CT-positive patients after two cycles of ABVD |
| RATHL | 1214 | PET/CT status to determine need for bleomycin in ABVD after two cycles |
| Israeli H2 | 356 | Interim PET/CT to dictate chemotherapeutic regimen after treatment based on IPS score after two cycles |
| French LYSA | Ongoing | De-escalation from eBEACOPP to ABVD after negative interim PET/CT |

Multiple studies demonstrate a strong association between interim PET/CT status and PFS. Itti and colleagues[20] argued that both standard uptake value (SUV) semiquantification and visual inspection of PET/CT scan after four cycles of induction chemotherapy can be used to prognosticate PFS. Similarly, two other studies show a high negative predictive value of visual and quantitative interpretation of interim PET/CT in predicting outcomes.[21,22]

However, others argue against the prognostic significance of interim PET/CT. In 2010, Moskowitz and colleagues[23] provided further insight into this argument. In this study, 98 patients at Memorial Sloan-Kettering received four cycles of R-CHOP after which time interim PET/CT was performed. Here, PET/CT positivity was defined as any FDG uptake greater than local background activity. Those patients with PET/CT positivity underwent confirmatory biopsy, which further directed care. Positive biopsies for DLBCL led to ifosfamide, carboplatin, and etoposide (ICE) chemotherapy followed by autologous stem cell transplant (SCT), whereas those patients who were PET-positive and biopsy-negative received ICE consolidation without SCT. At 44 months, survival was identical between PET-negative and PET-positive/biopsy negative groups, suggesting that interim PET/CT positivity in itself does not independently carry predictive power. Notably, of 38 patients who underwent biopsy for positive PET scan, 33 (86.8%) patients had negative biopsy, supporting the hypothesis of an unacceptably high false-positive rate.

Similarly, mixed evidence exists regarding the use of posttherapy PET/CT scan in DLBCL as a well-validated prognostic tool.[24] Multiple studies show poor positive predictive value of a positive posttherapy PET with both the mediastinal blood pool criteria[19] and the IHP criteria.[25] In 2013, Manohar and colleagues[26] compared various criteria of PET/CT interpretation to determine the most accurate way to prognosticate in patients without HL. In this paper, the authors demonstrate that the Gallamini (a semiquantitative approach using an $SUV_{max}$ cutoff of 3.5) criteria and the Deauville criteria have higher accuracies (88% and 88.4%, respectively) in detecting residual disease than the IHP criteria (71%; *P* value = .0001). These results are of immense importance as a reminder of the differences in which PET/CTs are evaluated and the limitations and advantages of each modality in clinical practice and interpreting clinical trial results. **Table 2** compares methods commonly used in PET/CT interpretation.

There are multiple trials presently investigating the potential role for PET/CT imaging in tailoring DLBCL therapy. In 2008, Sehn and colleagues[27] explored the need for involved field RT following induction chemotherapy based on interim PET/CT imaging for patients with nonbulky stage I and stage II disease. In this study, participants received three cycles of R-CHOP followed by PET/CT scan. Patients with positive PET/CT received involved field RT, whereas those who were PET-negative received additional cycles of R-CHOP. This study demonstrated that patients with negative interim PET/CT scans can avoid involved field RT with a PFS of 93% and only one relapse among the 49 included patients.

In 2014, Sehn[28] demonstrated excellent PFS and OS by tailoring therapy based on interim PET/CT. In this study, PET/CT was performed following four cycles of R-CHOP in 150 patients. Patients with negative PET/CT according to the IHP criteria were assigned to complete two additional cycles of R-CHOP therapy. Patients with positive interim PET/CT received four cycles of R-ICE. Posttherapy PET/CT was used to determine necessity for RT. In this study, total cohort PFS and OS were 79% and 87%, respectively. The study results demonstrated that patients with negative PET/CT may not require RT consolidation. Additionally, patients with a positive interim PET/CT may benefit from escalation of therapy to R-ICE as compared with historical data of receiving R-CHOP. Of note, 19% of the PET-positive cohort did not complete R-ICE secondary to intolerable toxicities.

The PETAL trial evaluated 851 patients in an intent-to-treat analysis to determine the utility in treatment escalation for patients with unfavorable PET/CT scans.[29] Here, a favorable interim PET/CT was defined by that in which the maximum SUV was reduced by greater than 66%. Enrolled subjects received two cycles of R-CHOP with subsequent PET/CT scan. Patients with favorable PET/CT received an additional four cycles of R-CHOP, whereas those with unfavorable PET/CT imaging were randomized to either six additional cycles of R-CHOP or a more aggressive protocol that included the following: hyperfractionated cyclophosphamide and ifosfamide, methotrexate, cytarabine, rituximab, doxorubicin, vincristine, vindesine, etopiside, and dexamethasone. The authors found no statistically significant difference in time to treatment failure or OS between patients with favorable and unfavorable PET/CT, therefore failing to demonstrate the alternate intensified regimen improved outcomes. Furthermore, patients who received intensified treatment suffered more severe leukopenia with comparable deaths with the R-CHOP cohort.

Finally, the "OPTIMAL greater than 60 trial for Improvement of Therapy in Elderly Patients with

**Table 2**
**PET imaging criteria**

| IHP Criteria | London Criteria | Gallamini Criteria | Deauville Score |
|---|---|---|---|
| • PET reviewed (attenuation corrected recommended) by visual assessment after completion of therapy<br>• Results are interpreted as positive or negative<br>• Lesions ≥2 cm: use mediastinal blood pool activity as reference background<br>• Lesions ≤2 cm: positive if its activity is more than that of the surrounding background<br>• Liver, spleen, lung, and bone marrow assessment by specific criteria | • PET scans with score 1–3 are considered negative<br>• PET scans with score 4–5 are considered positive<br>• Uses the Deauville 5-point score (see right) | • Pretreatment PET imaging required<br>• Disease evaluated site by site for involved lymph node and organs<br>• Negative result: no pathologic FDG uptake at any site (including those with previously increased uptake)<br>• Positive result: presence of focal FDG concentration outside physiologic uptake areas (increased relative to background)<br>• Patients with PET showing minimal residual uptake are considered PET-negative (SUV 2.0–3.5) | • Five-point scale of uptake<br>• Score 1: No uptake<br>• Score 2: Uptake ≤ mediastinum<br>• Score 3: Uptake ≥ mediastinum and < liver<br>• Score 4: moderately increased from the liver, at any site<br>• Score 5: Markedly increased uptake at any site, including new areas of disease |

CD20 + DLBCL" uses postinduction PET/CT status to select patients for RT in elderly patients with an aggressive B-cell lymphoma. Additionally, the study will compare standard immunochemotherapy (R-CHOP) with both R-CHLIP in which liposomal vincristine replaces conventional vincristine and R-CHOP with optimized rituximab dosing. This study is ongoing (clinical trial NCT0147852).

In summary (**Table 3**), in DLBCL the literature is inconclusive regarding the role of PET-directed personalized therapies. Data, although mixed, are suggestive that, as in HL, negative interim PET/CT scan may potentially be used to obviate RT; however, because of its false-positive rate we cannot recommend interim PET/CT imaging outside of the context of clinical research. The same is true for use of interim imaging to modify chemoimmunotherapy and at this time remains a research question only.

## OTHER NON-HODGKIN LYMPHOMA SUBTYPES

In contrast to the data available for HL and DLBCL, literature addressing the use of PET/CT-guided personalized therapy in other malignant lymphoma subtypes is less robust.

### *Follicular Lymphoma and Mantle Cell Lymphoma*

PET/CT imaging has recently been implemented in the use of initial staging and assessment of treatment response as part of the official guidelines in the management of follicular lymphoma (FL).[18]

**Table 3**
**Diffuse large B-cell lymphoma**

| Trial | No. of Patients | Study Summary |
|---|---|---|
| Sehn,[28] 2014 | 150 | Treatment escalation to R-ICE following positive interim PET/CT is more effective with increased toxicity |
| PETAL | 851 | Escalation to B-ALL protocol for positive interim PET/CT does not improve treatment efficacy |
| OPTIMAL >60 | — | Role of postinduction PET/CT in directing radiotherapy |

This imaging modality has allowed clinicians to identify more comprehensively the sites of nodal and extranodal disease involvement.[30] As with other lymphoma subtypes, there is much interest into the use of PET/CT imaging as a prognostication tool.

Dupuis and colleagues[31] published a prospective study of 121 patients with FL in which posttreatment PET/CT scan results were able to predict PFS. In this study, negative posttreatment PET/CT predicted superior PFS at 87% versus 51% in those patients with positive PET/CT scans, designated as a score greater than or equal to four on the five-point Deauville score.[32] Additionally, the PRIMA study demonstrated that interim PET/CT is strongly predictive of outcome in patients with FL.[33] In this study, 122 patients with high-tumor burden FL received PET/CT scans after induction R-CHOP or R-CVP. Analysis indicated that positive PET/CT, as determined locally, was associated with an inferior PFS of 32.9% compared with 70.7% in PET-negative patients at 42 months ($P<.001$).

Although it seems this improvement in staging and response assessment will likely impact the clinician's management decisions, the exact effect of PET/CT results on therapeutic choices has yet to be defined in the literature. There is limited evidence regarding the use of PET/CT scans to direct personalized treatment in these patients.

With regards to mantle cell lymphoma (MCL), there is mixed evidence and limited retrospective data regarding the use of PET/CT imaging as a prognostic tool. In 2012, our group published a study of 53 patients with MCL receiving R-Hyper-CVAD who had available PET/CT imaging results both mid-treatment and posttreatment.[34] We concluded that, whereas interim PET/CT has limited prognostic value, posttreatment PET/CT was associated with a significant inferior PFS with an associated trend toward inferior OS (hazard ratio, 5.2; 95% CI, 2.0–13.6; $P = .001$). Kedmi and colleagues[35] examined 58 patients with MCL receiving R-CHOP and determined that neither interim nor posttreatment PET/CT imaging had prognostic utility.

Recently in 2015, Bachanova and colleagues[36] studied the prognostic value of PET/CT status performed at a median of 1 month before SCT in a heterogeneous population of patients with non-HL undergoing SCT. This study enrolled 336 patients undergoing hematopoietic SCT with FL, large cell lymphoma, MCL, and natural killer cell lymphoma and investigated the association of PET/CT positivity, as determined by the reporting transplantation centers, and survival. At 3 years, PFS was 43% versus 47% ($P = .47$) and OS was 58% versus 60% ($P = .73$) for patients with PET-positive versus PET-negative, respectively. Positive PET/CT scan did forecast higher risk of relapse (40% vs 26%; $P = 0.001$), but did not demonstrate a statistically significant increased risk of mortality (relative risk, 1.29; $P = .08$).

### *Chronic Lymphocytic Lymphoma*

Recently, there has been promising progress in the use of FDG-PET imaging in the management of chronic lymphocytic lymphoma (CLL). Although PET/CT imaging has not been included on a routine basis in the management of CLL, the latest data suggest that PET/CT may be integral in the detection and treatment of transformed CLL into large B-cell lymphoma or Hodgkin lymphoma (Richter transformation).

Bruzzi and colleagues[37] were the first to demonstrate the high sensitivity and specificity of FDG-PET for Richter syndrome transformation. With 37 patients with CLL undergoing PET/CT scans, an SUVmax of greater than 5 demonstrated a 91% sensitivity for detection of disease transformation. In those patients with false-positive scans, one-third was ultimately diagnosed with alternative malignancy.

In 2014, Falchi and colleagues[38] examined 332 patients with CLL who had PET/CT imaging and available lymph node histology. In this paper, the group identified that SUVmax greater than 5 again held a high sensitivity of 91% in the detection of Richter transformation. Furthermore, the group discovered that an SUVmax greater than 10 was highly predictive of inferior OS (56.7 months vs 6.9 months). These findings will likely prove essential in the detection and management of patients with histologically aggressive CLL and CLL with Richter transformation. Especially in patients for whom biopsy is not attainable, PET/CT imaging can be used to guide therapy decisions when aggressive disease is suspected.

In the era of kinase inhibitor therapy, it remains unknown if PET/CT will effectively distinguish progression of CLL as compared with large B-cell transformation. Studies in this area are warranted.

## CONCLUDING REMARKS RELATED TO THE EVOLVING ROLE OF NOVEL QUANTITATIVE TECHNIQUES IN PERSONALIZED LYMPHOMA MANAGEMENT

PET in general and FDG-PET/CT in particular have revolutionized management of patients with lymphoma and have brought about individualized treatment of this malignancy. Although qualitative visual assessment with PET has played a major role in detecting disease activity in this population, quantitative data generated by this powerful imaging modality have provided, and continue to provide, a means for accurate monitoring of disease activity in patients with various lymphomas. However, there are some concerns about the accuracy of the quantitative values that are generated by the current analysis schemes for measuring the true concentration of FDG and other tracers in the lymph nodes and other involved structures. It is well established that lesions smaller than 3 to 4 cm in size cannot be assessed for their accurate metabolic activity. This is caused by a phenomenon called partial volume effect, which prevents accurate measurement of disease activity in small lesions.[39] This effect becomes even more significant when motions caused by respiratory and cardiac cycles affect the location of the lesion and the involved organ. Therefore, over the past decade, it has become apparent that partial volume correction must be adopted on a routine basis for most lesions that are visualized by PET in patients with lymphoma.[40]

Furthermore, the typical analysis of disease activity by PET only includes SUVs measured in two to three lesions that are then followed over time in the same locations. This clearly is a suboptimal approach for assessing the overall disease activity

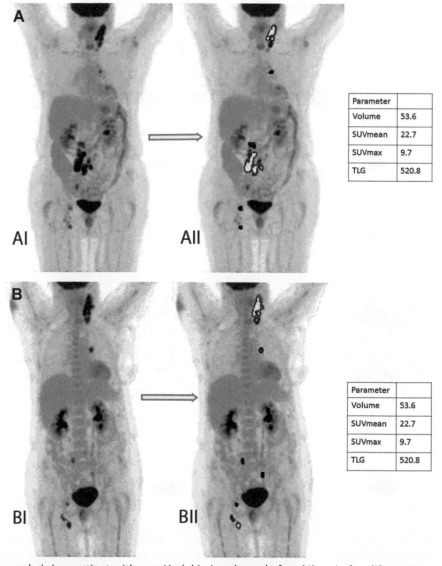

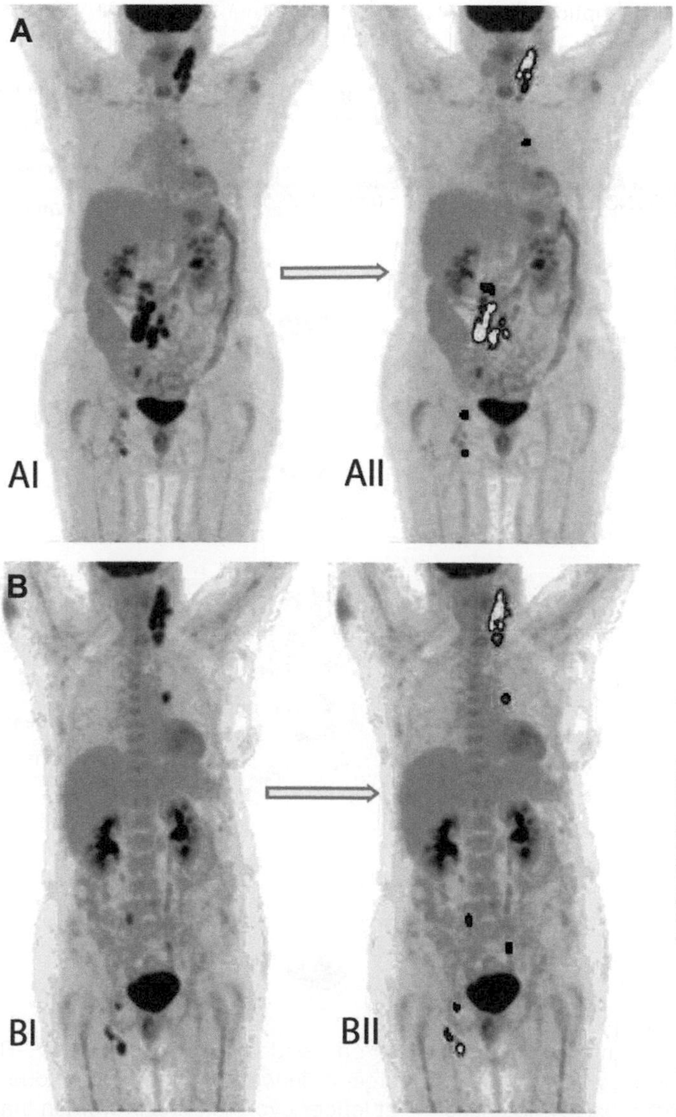


| Parameter | |
|---|---|
| Volume | 53.6 |
| SUVmean | 22.7 |
| SUVmax | 9.7 |
| TLG | 520.8 |

| Parameter | |
|---|---|
| Volume | 53.6 |
| SUVmean | 22.7 |
| SUVmax | 9.7 |
| TLG | 520.8 |

**Fig. 1.** Image analysis in a patient with non-Hodgkin lymphoma before (*A*) and after (*B*) treatment with radioimmunotherapy. (*A*) Patient with extensive involvement of neck, abdomen, and hip areas at baseline (AI). Lesions have been delineated by quantitative analysis software (Rover) on the right side (AII). (*B*) Involvement of abdominal area has significantly decreased (BI and BII) after radioimmunotherapy, which is reflected by quantitative segmentation and volumetric numbers in the tables. TLG, total lesional glycolysis (MTV*SUVmean); volume, metabolic tumor volume.

in this population, and therefore, there is a dire need to refine the current methodologies for this purpose and adopt a means that allows measurement of global disease burden.

Recent advances in computer-based software have overcome previously mentioned deficiencies, and therefore provide values with substantially improved accuracy and relevant information about the overall disease activity in this cancer.[41] These new tools correct for partial volume effect and provide correct metabolic activity for each lesion. Furthermore, this approach can measure the

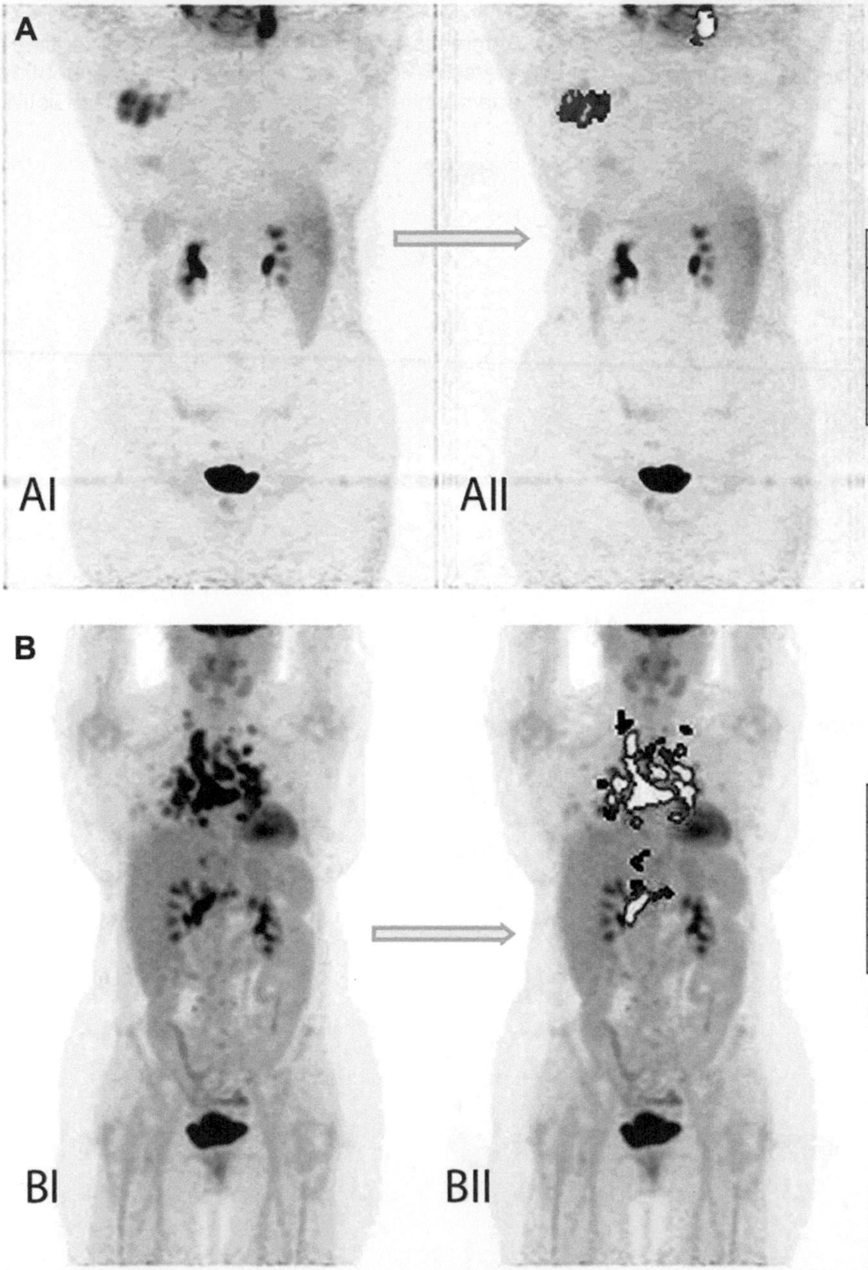

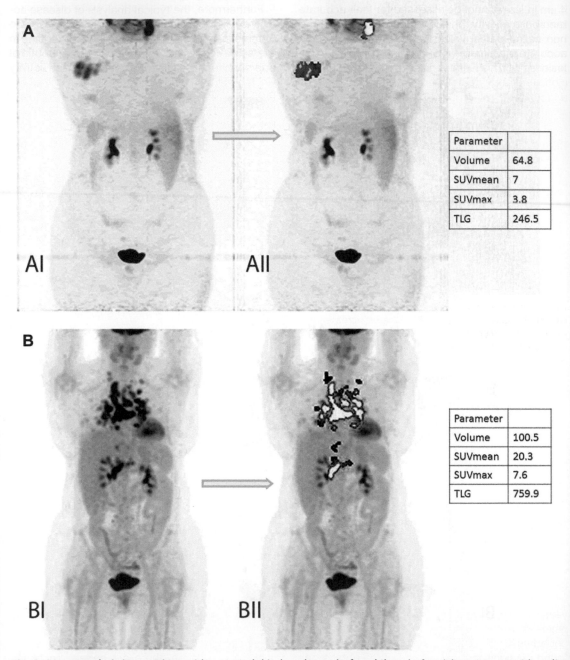

| Parameter | |
|---|---|
| Volume | 64.8 |
| SUVmean | 7 |
| SUVmax | 3.8 |
| TLG | 246.5 |

| Parameter | |
|---|---|
| Volume | 100.5 |
| SUVmean | 20.3 |
| SUVmax | 7.6 |
| TLG | 759.9 |

**Fig. 2.** Image analysis in a patient with non-Hodgkin lymphoma before (*A*) and after (*B*) treatment with radioimmunotherapy. (*A*) Patient with some involvement of neck and axillary area at baseline (AI). Lesions have been delineated by quantitative analysis software (Rover) on the right side (AII). (*B*) Involvement of neck and axillary areas disappeared after therapy but new extensive lesions are present in the thoracic and abdominal areas (BI and BII), which seem to be more extensive than baseline as per quantitative segmentation and volumetric numbers in the tables. TLG, total lesional glycolysis (MTV*SUVmean); volume, metabolic tumor volume.

metabolic volume of lesions based on PET images alone either in the lymph nodes or other organs. These measurements have been shown to be accurate and are almost identical to those on CT images. By generating a corrected metabolic activity value of each lesion along with its exact volume, readers are able to calculate total disease activity in each lesion. By summing the values from each lesion, one can calculate the whole body disease burden. The above figures are representative of such measurements in two patients with lymphomas who have undergone radiolabeled monoclonal antibody treatment of their disease (**Figs. 1** and **2**).

## REFERENCES


1. Eichenauer DA, Engert A, Andre M, et al. Hodgkin's lymphoma: ESMO clinical practice guidelines for diagnosis, treatment and follow-up. Ann Oncol 2014;25(Suppl 3):iii70–5.
2. El-Galaly TC, Hutchings M, Mylam KJ, et al. Impact of 18F-fluorodeoxyglucose positron emission tomography/computed tomography staging in newly diagnosed classical Hodgkin lymphoma: fewer cases with stage I disease and more with skeletal involvement. Leuk Lymphoma 2014;55:2349–55.
3. Hutchings M, Loft A, Hansen M, et al. Position emission tomography with or without computed tomography in the primary staging of Hodgkin's lymphoma. Haematologica 2006;91:482–9.
4. Barrington SF, Mikhaeel NG, Kostakoglu L, et al. Role of imaging in the staging and response assessment of lymphoma: consensus of the International Conference on Malignant Lymphomas Imaging Working Group. J Clin Oncol 2014;32:3048–58.
5. Miltenyi Z, Barna S, Garai I, et al. Prognostic value of interim and restaging PET/CT in Hodgkin lymphoma. Results of the CHEAP (chemotherapy effectiveness assessment by PET/CT) study - long term observation. Neoplasma 2015;62:627–34.
6. Gotti M, Fiaccadori V, Bono E, et al. Therapy related late adverse events in Hodgkin's lymphoma. Lymphoma 2013;2013. http://dx.doi.org/10.1155/2013/952698.
7. Girinsky T, Auperin A, Ribrag V, et al. Role of FDG-PET in the implementation of involved-node radiation therapy for Hodgkin lymphoma patients. Int J Radiat Oncol Biol Phys 2014;89:1047–52.
8. Radford J, Illidge T, Counsell N, et al. Results of a trial of PET-directed therapy for early-stage Hodgkin's lymphoma. N Engl J Med 2015;372:1598–607.
9. Juweid ME, Stroobants S, Hoekstra OS, et al. Use of positron emission tomography for response assessment of lymphoma: consensus of the Imaging Subcommittee of International Harmonization Project in Lymphoma. J Clin Oncol 2007;25:571–8.
10. Raemaekers JM, Andre MP, Federico M, et al. Omitting radiotherapy in early positron emission tomography-negative stage I/II Hodgkin lymphoma is associated with an increased risk of early relapse: clinical results of the preplanned interim analysis of the randomized EORTC/LYSA/FIL H10 trial. J Clin Oncol 2014;32:1188–94.
11. Engert A, Haverkamp H, Kobe C, et al. Reduced-intensity chemotherapy and PET-guided radiotherapy in patients with advanced stage Hodgkin's lymphoma (HD15 trial): a randomised, open-label, phase 3 non-inferiority trial. Lancet 2012;379:1791–9.
12. Meignan M, Gallamini A, Haioun C. Report on the first international workshop on interim-PET-scan in lymphoma. Leuk Lymphoma 2009;50:1257–60.
13. Gallamini A, Patti C, Viviani S, et al. Early chemotherapy intensification with BEACOPP in advanced-stage Hodgkin lymphoma patients with an interim-PET positive after two ABVD courses. Br J Haematol 2011;152:551–60.
14. Johnson P. Response rates and toxicity reduction by response-adapted therapy in advanced Hodgkin lymphoma (HL): initial results from the international RATHL study. 2013 NCRI Cancer Conference, Poster: B42. Liverpool, United Kingdom, November 3–6, 2013.
15. Dann EJ. Tailored therapy in Hodgkin lymphoma, based on predefined risk factors and early interim PET/CT: Israeli H2 study. 56th ASH Annual Meeting and Exposition (Abstract no. 4409). San Francisco, CA, December 6–9, 2014.
16. Casanovas R. AHL 2011: a LYSA randomized phase III study of a treatment driven by early pet response compared to a standard treatment in patients with Ann arbor stage III–IV or high-risk IIB Hodgkin lymphoma. J Clin Oncol 2013;31(Suppl; Abstract TPS8615).
17. Smith SD, Press OW. Diffuse large B-cell lymphoma and related diseases. In: Kaushansky K, Lichtman LA, Prchal JT, et al, editors. Williams Hematology. 9th edition. New York: McGraw-Hill; 2015. Available at: http://accessmedicine.mhmedical.com/content.aspx?bookid=1581&Sectionid=108074647. Accessed March 16, 2016.
18. Cheson BD, Fisher RI, Barrington SF, et al. Recommendations for initial evaluation, staging, and response assessment of Hodgkin and non-Hodgkin lymphoma: the Lugano classification. J Clin Oncol 2014;32:3059–68.
19. Han HS, Escalon MP, Hsiao B, et al. High incidence of false-positive PET scans in patients with aggressive non-Hodgkin's lymphoma treated with rituximab-containing regimens. Ann Oncol 2009;20:309–18.
20. Itti E, Meignan M, Berriolo-Riedinger A, et al. An international confirmatory study of the prognostic value of early PET/CT in diffuse large B-cell lymphoma: comparison between Deauville criteria and DeltaSUVmax. Eur J Nucl Med Mol Imaging 2013;40:1312–20.

21. Yang DH, Ahn JS, Byun BH, et al. Interim PET/CT-based prognostic model for the treatment of diffuse large B cell lymphoma in the post-rituximab era. Ann Hematol 2013;92:471–9.
22. Zinzani PL, Gandolfi L, Broccoli A, et al. Midtreatment 18F-fluorodeoxyglucose positron-emission tomography in aggressive non-Hodgkin lymphoma. Cancer 2011;117:1010–8.
23. Moskowitz CH, Schoder H, Teruya-Feldstein J, et al. Risk-adapted dose-dense immunochemotherapy determined by interim FDG-PET in advanced-stage diffuse large B-cell lymphoma. J Clin Oncol 2010; 28:1896–903.
24. Cheson BD. The International Harmonization Project for response criteria in lymphoma clinical trials. Hematol Oncol Clin North Am 2007;21:841–54.
25. Cashen AF, Dehdashti F, Luo J, et al. 18F-FDG PET/CT for early response assessment in diffuse large B-cell lymphoma: poor predictive value of International Harmonization Project interpretation. J Nucl Med 2011;52:386–92.
26. Manohar K, Mittal BR, Raja S, et al. Comparison of various criteria in interpreting end of therapy F-18 labeled fluorodeoxyglucose positron emission tomography/computed tomography in patients with aggressive non-Hodgkin lymphoma. Leuk Lymphoma 2013;54:714–9.
27. Sehn L, Savage K, Hoskin P, et al. Limited-stage DLBCL patients with a negative PET scan following three cycles of R-CHOP have an excellent outcome following abbreviated immuno-chemotherapy alone. Ann Oncol 2008;19(Suppl 4; Abstract 052).
28. Sehn L. Phase 2 trial of interim PET scan-tailored therapy in patients with advanced stage diffuse large B-cell lymphoma in British Columbia. 56th ASH Annual Meeting and Exposition (Abstract no. 392). San Francisco, CA, December 6–9, 2014.
29. Duhrsen U, Huttmann A, Jockel KH, et al. Positron emission tomography guided therapy of aggressive non-Hodgkin lymphomas: the PETAL trial. Leuk Lymphoma 2009;50:1757–60.
30. Luminari S, Biasoli I, Arcaini L, et al. The use of FDG-PET in the initial staging of 142 patients with follicular lymphoma: a retrospective study from the FOLL05 randomized trial of the Fondazione Italiana Linfomi. Ann Oncol 2013;24:2108–12.
31. Dupuis J, Berriolo-Riedinger A, Julian A, et al. Impact of [(18)F]fluorodeoxyglucose positron emission tomography response evaluation in patients with high-tumor burden follicular lymphoma treated with immunochemotherapy: a prospective study from the Groupe d'Etudes des Lymphomes de l'Adulte and GOELAMS. J Clin Oncol 2012;30: 4317–22.
32. Biggi A. Analysis of the Deauville criteria for the assessment of interim PET in advanced stage Hodgkin lymphoma patients enrolled in the IVS study: II. Reliability of score and concordance among reviewers. J Nucl Med 2012;53:154.
33. Trotman J, Fournier M, Lamy T, et al. Positron emission tomography-computed tomography (PET-CT) after induction therapy is highly predictive of patient outcome in follicular lymphoma: analysis of PET-CT in a subset of PRIMA trial participants. J Clin Oncol 2011;29:3194–200.
34. Mato AR, Svoboda J, Feldman T, et al. Post-treatment (not interim) positron emission tomography-computed tomography scan status is highly predictive of outcome in mantle cell lymphoma patients treated with R-HyperCVAD. Cancer 2012;118:3565–70.
35. Kedmi M, Avivi I, Ribakovsky E, et al. Is there a role for therapy response assessment with 2-[fluorine-18] fluoro-2-deoxy-D-glucose-positron emission tomography/computed tomography in mantle cell lymphoma? Leuk Lymphoma 2014;55:2484–9.
36. Bachanova V, Burns LJ, Ahn KW, et al. Impact of pretransplantation (18)F-fluorodeoxy glucose-positron emission tomography status on outcomes after allogeneic hematopoietic cell transplantation for Non-Hodgkin lymphoma. Biol Blood Marrow Transplant 2015;21:1605–11.
37. Bruzzi JF, Macapinlac H, Tsimberidou AM, et al. Detection of Richter's transformation of chronic lymphocytic leukemia by PET/CT. J Nucl Med 2006;47: 1267–73.
38. Falchi L, Keating MJ, Marom EM, et al. Correlation between FDG/PET, histology, characteristics, and survival in 332 patients with chronic lymphoid leukemia. Blood 2014;123:2783–90.
39. Hickeson M, Yun M, Matthies A, et al. Use of a corrected standardized uptake value based on the lesion size on CT permits accurate characterization of lung nodules on FDG-PET. Eur J Nucl Med Mol Imaging 2002;29:1639–47.
40. Berkowitz A, Basu S, Srinivas S, et al. Determination of whole-body metabolic burden as a quantitative measure of disease activity in lymphoma: a novel approach with fluorodeoxyglucose-PET. Nucl Med Commun 2008;29:521–6.
41. Houshmand S, Salavati A, Hess S, et al. An update on novel quantitative techniques in the context of evolving whole-body PET imaging. PET Clin 2015; 10:45–58.

# PET/CT in Head-neck Malignancies

## The Implications for Personalized Clinical Practice

Heidi R. Wassef, MD[a,*], Nevine Hanna, MD[b], Patrick Colletti, MD[a]

**KEYWORDS**

- Fluorodeoxyglucose F 18 • FDG • Positron emission tomography/computer tomography • PET/CT • Head and neck • Squamous cell carcinoma • HNSCC

**KEY POINTS**

- PET/CT has been shown to help localize head and neck cancers and provide more accurate staging, post-treatment assessment, and restaging than standard imaging.
- PET/CT detects synchronous and metachronous cancers and sequelae of therapy and provides prognostic information for each patient.
- Information provided by PET/CT allows for more individualized therapeutic and surveillance plans for patients with head and neck squamous cell carcinoma (HNSCC).

## INTRODUCTION

Approximately 60,000 Americans develop head and neck cancer annually and it is the cause of death for 12,000 Americans per year. It accounts for 3% of all cancers in the United States.[1] Most head and neck cancers are squamous cell carcinomas (HNSCC) arising from the mucosal lining of the upper aerodigestive tract. The most common sites of HNSCCs are the larynx (including the supraglottis, glottis, and subglottis), oral cavity (tongue, floor of mouth, hard palate, buccal mucosa, and alveolar ridges), and oropharynx (base of tongue, tonsils, and soft palate). Less common sites include the nasopharynx, nasal cavity, paranasal sinuses, hypopharynx, thyroid, and salivary glands.

The incidence of HNSCC increases with age. Most patients are between 50 and 70 years and it is more common in men than women. The incidence in women has been increasing because of their increased tobacco use and in younger patients due to increased exposure to human papilloma virus (HPV). Even though treatment is the same for both types of HNSCC, HPV-related head and neck cancer has a better prognosis than non–HPV-related cancer.[2] Patients are treated with radiation therapy (RT) with or without chemotherapy and surgical resection and lymph node dissection. Contrast-enhanced CT and MRI have been used in conjunction with physical examination and endoscopy for diagnosis and management of HNSCC. PET/CT has assumed a greater role in the management of these patients because it helps localize unknown primaries and provides more accurate staging, post-treatment assessment, and restaging than standard imaging.

The authors have nothing to disclose.

[a] Department of Radiation Therapy, LAC-USC Medical Center, Keck Medical School of USC, 1983 Marengo Street, D&T Building, 4th Floor 4D334, Los Angeles, CA 90033, USA; [b] Department of Radiation Oncology, Huntsman Cancer Hospital, 1950 Circle of Hope, Room 1570, Salt Lake City, UT 84112, USA
* Corresponding author.
*E-mail address:* wassef@med.usc.edu

PET Clin 11 (2016) 219–232
http://dx.doi.org/10.1016/j.cpet.2016.02.002

PET/CT also provides prognostic data and detects synchronous and metachronous cancers and sequelae of therapy.

## FLUORODEOXYGLUCOSE F 18 PET/CT

PET allows semiquantitative and quantitative assessment of biochemical processes in the body. Because most cancers are characterized by increased glucose utilization, PET using the glucose analog 18F-fluorodeoxyglucose (18F-FDG) PET/CT has a major role in staging, radiotherapy planning, assessing response to therapy and detection of recurrence of HNSCC. The increased FDG uptake in HNSCC is due to overexpression of GLUT-1 glucose transporters and increased hexokinase activity. The distribution of FDG is determined by the localization of annihilation photons emitted by fluorine-18. Coregistered CT data provide not only attenuation correction of the PET data but also excellent spatial resolution, helping to provide better localization and characterization of hypermetabolic lesions. FDG-PET is thought to detect cancers when they reach approximately $10^9$ cells, which correlates to a size of 4 mm to 10 mm. After therapy, tumor metabolism decreases faster than the decrease in size.[3] Thus PET/CT provides earlier and more sensitive evaluation of response to therapy.

## PET/CT PROTOCOL

In addition to the standard 4-hour to 6-hour fast, patients are instructed to avoid talking from 30 minutes prior to FDG injection and throughout the uptake phase to the time of imaging, to avoid FDG uptake in the vocal cord muscles. Patients should not drink during the uptake phase.[4] Scheduling these patients in midmorning minimizes uptake in the genioglossus muscle and anterior floor of the mouth. The genioglossus muscle holds the tongue at the base of the mouth and prevents it from obstructing the airway when the patient is supine for a long time, such as during sleep. Patients should not be supine during the uptake phase. A bite device, which provides for a stable open mouth position, improves tumor localization.[5] The open mouth position is recommended because it separates the palate, tongue, and the alveolar ridge, especially the retromolar trigone. The silicon device also allows the mouth to be imaged in the same position during PET and CT.[4] PET/CT images are to be acquired with the same immobilization device used during RT. Other techniques have been reviewed recently by Kumar and colleagues.[6] **Table 1** summarizes the advantages of the puffed cheek, open mouth, and phonation methods and the modified Valsalva maneuver.

Most centers acquire whole-body (WB) and dedicated head and neck PET/CTs at 60 minutes whereas others have reported acquiring WB PET/CT at 90 minutes and the dedicated head and neck portion at 150 minutes following FDG injection.[9] Intravenous contrast is given unless contraindicated. The addition of dedicated head and neck PET/CT with thinner collimation, longer bed time, greater matrix size, and smaller pixel size allows for the detection of metastatic disease in small lymph nodes (<15 mm).[9] A matrix of 400 compared with 200 was found to demonstrate more lymph nodes and have higher sensitivity for the detection of lesions.[10] Time of flight was found to have no effect on the detectability of small lymph nodes but image quality improved and the apparent maximum standardized uptake value (SUVmax) increased. Although the difference did not reach statistical significance, dedicated head and neck PET/CT was 7.4% more sensitive than WB PET/CT in the detection of cervical nodes, all of which were between 5 mm and 10 mm, but

**Table 1**
**Studies evaluating special techniques in PET/CT in the evaluation of head and neck cancer**

| Technique | Location of Cancer | Advantage for Head and Neck Cancer |
|---|---|---|
| Puffed cheek[7] | Oral cavity | Delineate extent and location<br>Decrease dental amalgam artifact |
| Open mouth[8] | Oral cavity<br>Oropharynx | Prevent dental amalgam artifact from obscuring cancer |
| Modified Valsalva maneuver[8] | Hypopharynx<br>Laryngeal vestibule | Increase tumor visibility<br>Delineate tumor extension<br>May open fossa of Rosenmüller |
| Phonation (patient says "e")[8] | Supraglottic<br>Infraglottic | Improve evaluation of true vocal cord thickness<br>Better visualization of ventricle, which helps differentiate supraglottic vs glottic location |

specificity was lower due to FDG uptake in inflammatory nodes containing granulocytes and macrophages.[11]

Patients with HNSCC have risk factors for lung and esophageal cancers; thus, the thorax should be imaged. Patients at high risk for distant metastases (DMs) may benefit from imaging of the abdomen and pelvis. Precise criteria for high risk of metastatic disease have not been well established.[12] In a retrospective study by Garavello and colleagues[13] of 1972 patients, 181 developed DMs. The risk of developing DMs was found influenced by site of primary cancer, local and/or regional extension, histologic grade, achievement of locoregional control, and, to a lesser extent, age. Hypopharyngeal primary had the highest risk and the oral cavity had the lowest risk of DMs. Age less than 45 years was associated with a higher risk of DM. Most centers image from skull base to midthighs in addition to the dedicated head and neck PET/CT with contrast to evaluate for possible DMs.

## QUANTIFICATION OF METABOLIC ACTIVITY AND TUMOR VOLUME

An advantage of PET/CT is the ability to quantify biologic functions. There are several methods and parameters used to quantify metabolic activity of tumors. Standardized uptake value (SUV) based on lean body mass or surface area is more accurate than SUV based on weight. Peak standardized uptake (SUVpeak) is the SUV mean (SUVmean) over a 1-cm sphere centered on the location of SUVmax (the maximum single-voxel uptake in a user-defined 3-D sphere). SUVmax is sensitive to noise and artifacts whereas SUVpeak is more reliable.[14] Metabolic tumor volume (MTV) aims to measure the volume of tumor using hypermetabolism to delineate the tumor margins. The threshold technique uses a cutoff value, for example, 40% of SUVmax to delineate the tumor. The gradient method using software, such as MIM Software (Cleveland, Ohio), analyzes the change in activity to determine the edges of the tumor. Total lesion glycolosis (TLG) is calculated as SUVmean $\times$ MTV and thus combines the volume of tumor and metabolic activity into one parameter.

## MOLECULAR AND GENETIC CHARACTERIZATION OF HEAD AND NECK SQUAMOUS CELL CARCINOMA

Gene expression studies can differentiate between subtypes of HNSCC. Initially, this allowed for differentiation of HPV-positive and HPV-negative tumors. With continued advancement in DNA analysis and mutation detection, HNSCCs are already being subdivided based on distinct genetic mutations. The Cancer Genome Atlas has studied various genomic alterations in 279 HNSCCs.[15] The molecular variations are reflected in different clinical courses. Knowledge of the different mutations may allow for personalized prognosis, treatment, and monitoring schedules in the different cancer subtypes. The various mutations may also provide targets for therapy and information regarding drug resistance and susceptibility.[16]

## PET/CT IN HEAD AND NECK SQUAMOUS CELL CARCINOMA AND PERSONALIZED MANAGEMENT

In addition to biology and genetics, FDG-PET is also advancing personalized medicine for patients with HNSCC. The role of PET in localizing the primary site in patients with cervical lymph nodes and unknown primary cancer, providing more accurate staging, and increasing the sensitivity of detection of second primaries will be discussed. PET is also a predictive biomarker helping to predict local control and disease-free survival (DFS) and overall survival (OS) rates in patients with HNSCC.

## UNKNOWN PRIMARY

Among head and neck cancers, 2% to 9% present with cervical lymph nodes with unknown primary; 90% of these are squamous cell carcinomas (SCC) prior to PET/CT and the remainder are adenocarcinoma, melanoma, and other rare histologies.[17] PET/CT aids in the localization of the primary tumor. A meta-analysis by Rusthoven and colleagues[18] from 1994 to 2003 found that PET/CT detected the primary tumor in 24.5% of cases with unknown HNSCC after standard work-up. Standard work-up varies greatly in different institutions and can include panendoscopy with random mucosal biopsies from sites that are likely to be the primary site. The detection rate for PET/CT in the 10 studies that included panendoscopy was 22%. The detection rate of PET/CT is higher when PET/CT was performed prior to panendoscopy. The detection rate of the primary by PET/CT performed before panendoscopy was 44.2% (23/52) in a study, including all histologies.[19,20] PET/CT can guide endoscopic biopsy to the most metabolically active site and help avoid necrotic tissue.

The most common false-positive sites are oropharynx and hypopharynx.[18,20,21] Extensive physiologic metabolic activity makes evaluation of the head and neck challenging. On the other hand, CT artifacts from dental amalgam may be less problematic on PET[22] (**Fig. 1**). One approach proposed by Koppula and Rajendran[23] is to perform a PET/CT if clinical examination, in-office endoscopy, and MR imaging do not reveal the primary tumor. If a suspect site is identified on PET, panendoscopy with frozen-section evaluation of this site can be performed first and, only if necessary, biopsies from other common sites of squamous cell carcinoma can be obtained. By helping identify the primary site of tumor, FDG-PET/CT helps direct the biopsy and the therapeutic plan.

## STAGING

### *Primary Tumor*

PET determines tumor volume more accurately than CT. In a study of 41 patients, PET determined primary tumor volume was smaller than that determined by CT, resulting in improved dosimetry and lower radiation dose to adjacent at-risk organs, including salivary glands and lens.[24] Gross tumor volume (GTV) determined by PET was found to be significantly different from that obtained by CT in another study of 185 patients with locoregionally advanced HNSCC. In 86% of patients, PET/CT-based GTV was smaller and thus decreased the required area of radiation, and in 14%, CT-based GTV was erroneously smaller due to multifocal disease or lymph node metastases detected only on PET/CT. An average of 6.5 years of follow-up in this study showed that OS and disease-specific survival (DSS) correlated with the GTV based on PET.[25] Anderson and colleagues[26] evaluated GTV determined by CT, PET/CT, and MR imaging in a study of 14 patients with HNC. They found that GTV derived by PET/CT was smallest and was associated with the least interobserver variability (**Fig. 2**). The limitations of both PET/CT and MR imaging are superficial

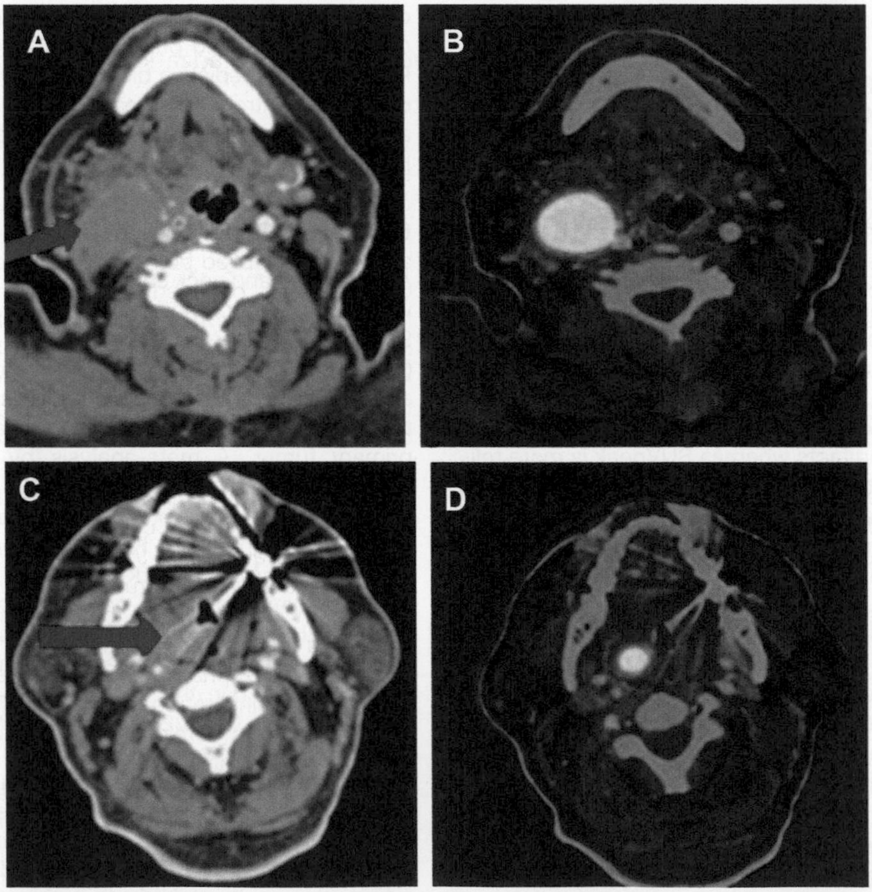


**Fig. 1.** A 62-year-old man with right neck mass. Primary tumor remained unknown after flexible laryngoscopy. (*A*) Contrast-enhanced CT and (*B*) fused FDG-PET/CT PET demonstrate hypermetabolic right cervical adenopathy (*arrow* in *A*). (*C*) Contrast-enhanced CT demonstrates beam hardening artifact from dental fillings with no definite abnormality at this level (*arrow*) but (*D*) PET/CT localized the primary tumor to the right tonsil/pharyngeal wall. Patient underwent transoral robotic surgery and right modified radical neck dissection followed by adjuvant chemoradiation.

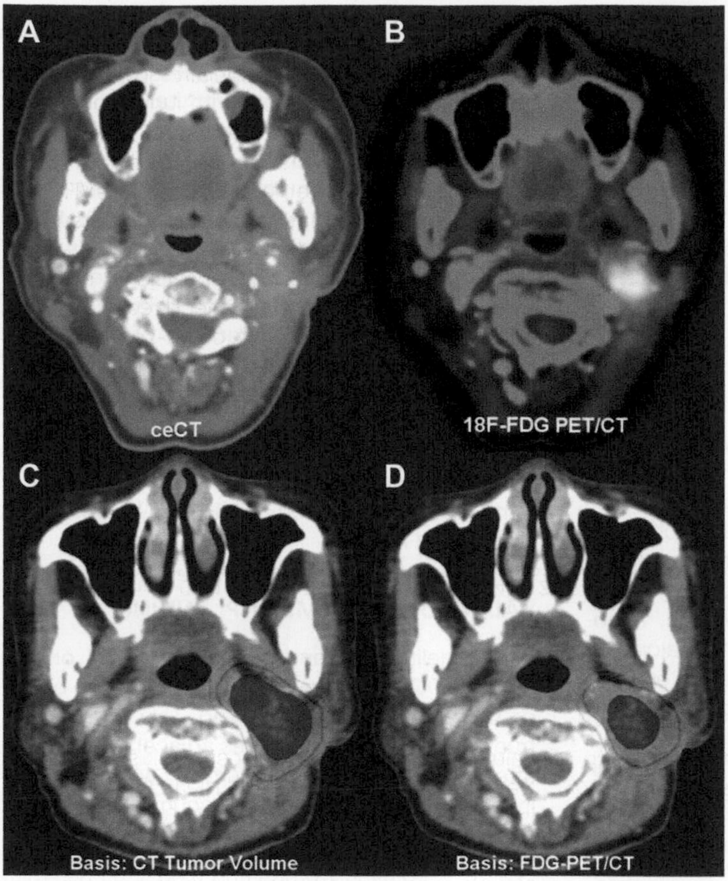


**Fig. 2.** A 62-year-old man with recurrent nasopharyngeal squamous cell cancer. Soft tissue in the left carotid space is seen (*A*) on contrast-enhanced CT (ceCT). PET/CT (*B*) allows differentiation of recurrent tumor from post-treatment fibrosis, allowing accurate radiation planning. The smaller radiation field based on PET (*D*) compared with the area based on ceCT (*C*) helps avoid radiation of at-risk structures in the neck and the associated sequelae. Red, GTV; purple, CTV; and blue, PTV.

lesions and micrometastases. Tumors with thickness less than or equal to 3 mm, such as those in the oral cavity, may present as false negative on PET/CT.[4] Overall, PET/CT is superior to other imaging modalities because it provides more accurate, reproducible, and smaller tumor volumes for better therapeutic planning.

## *Lymph Nodes*

FDG-PET/CT is more sensitive and accurate than CT and MR imaging in the detection of metastatic lymph nodes. PET does not rely on lymph node size or morphology and can identify pathologic lymph nodes in unexpected locations (**Fig. 3**). In a study of 2719 resected nodes, more than 40% of cervical lymph node metastases were found to be smaller than 1 cm[27]; FDG-PET/MR has not been found to significantly improve accuracy for cervical lymph node metastases compared with PET or MR imaging.[28]

The sensitivity of PET/CT is higher than CT and MR imaging for both ipsilateral and contralateral

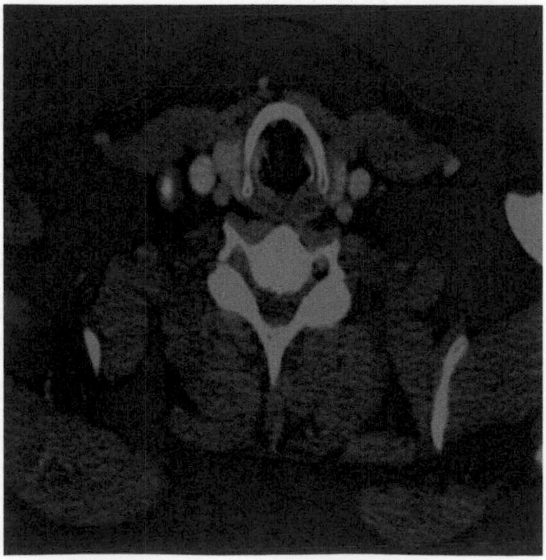

**Fig. 3.** A 42-year-old man with squamous cell carcinoma of the right tonsil (not shown). PET/CT reveals a subcentimeter metastasis, which is nonpathologic by size criteria.

lymph nodes. The sensitivity of detection of contralateral lymph nodes is lower than for ipsilateral lymph nodes using all 3 modalities because of their smaller size and lower incidence. The sensitivity of PET/CT is 94% and of CT and MR imaging 86% for the detection of ipsilateral lymph nodes whereas the sensitivity is only 58% and 35%, respectively, for contralateral lymph nodes. There was no added benefit from FDG-PET/MR or MR imaging compared to FDG-PET/CT in 25 patients with HNSCC in local staging and detection of recurrence.[29,30]

### *Sentinel lymphoscintigraphy*

A meta-analysis of 26 studies from 1970 to 2011 included 766 patients who underwent sentinel lymph node biopsy prior to neck dissection. They found that the sensitivity and negative predictive value (NPV) of pre-operative sentinal lymphoscintigraphy was 95% and 96% for all head and neck tumors; 94% and 96% for oral cavity tumors; and 100% and 100% for oropharyngeal, hypopharyngeal, and laryngeal cancers. A majority of these patients (693/766) were stage T1 or T2.[31] Increased utilization of lymphoscintigraphy in this group of patients will further individualize therapy, reserving neck dissection for those patients who have lymph node involvement confirmed by lymphoscintigraphy.

### *Distant Metastases*

The development of DM makes the possibility of cure very low and markedly decreases survival. DMs commonly become clinically apparent during the 2 years after diagnosis.[13] The incidence of DM was 9.2% and 9.5% in 2 studies evaluating 1972 and 1880 patients with HNSCC, respectively.[13,32] The percentage of patients with lung, bone, liver, and multiple sites of metastases was 55.8%, 9.9%, 3.9%, and 30.4% respectively.[13] Chan and colleagues[33] compared PET/CT and whole body MR imaging in 103 oropharyngeal and hypopharyngeal squamous cell carcinomas. PET/CT had higher sensitivity for the detection of DMs, primarily due to the superiority of CT over MR imaging for the detection of pulmonary nodules. A meta-analysis by Xu and colleagues[34] found that the sensitivity and specificity of PET/CT to detect both DMs and second primary cancers were 89% and 95%. The high sensitivity of PET/CT in the detection of metastatic disease makes it the ideal imaging study for HNSCC staging and restaging (**Fig. 4**).

## RADIATION TREATMENT PLANNING

Tumor delineation and thus GTV based on the FDG-PET/CT is more accurate than that based on CT, as previously discussed. This is especially true when the tumor infiltrates adjacent structures; after initial treatment or surgery when residual inactive tissue and residual/recurrent tumor are difficult to separate on CT; and in areas of artifacts on CT, such as the oral cavity with dental fillings.[22] FDG-PET commonly provides smaller GTV, clinical target volume (CTV), and planning target volume (PTV) compared with CT for HNSCC. RT adds a margin for microscopic/subclinical disease

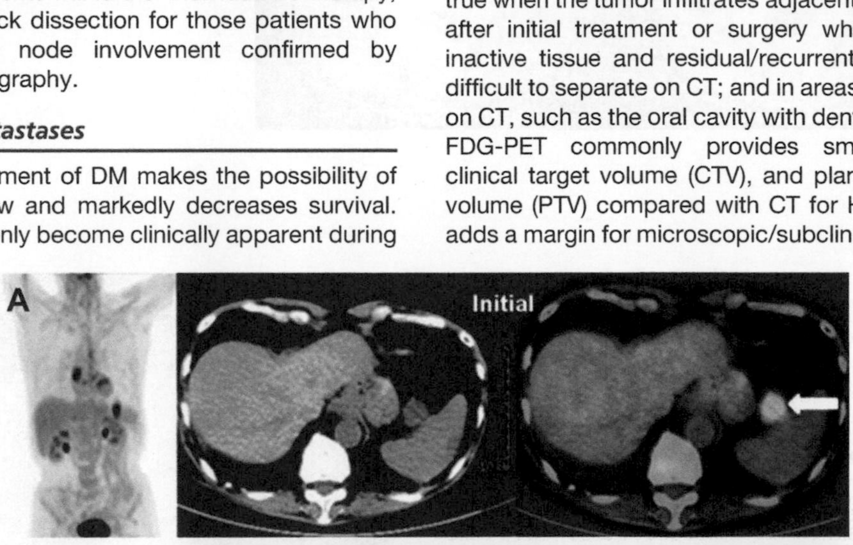

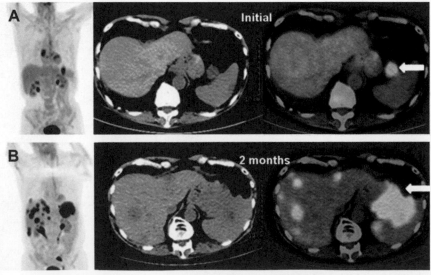


**Fig. 4.** (*A*) Post-treatment maximum intensity projection (MIP), CT, and PET/CT in a patient with resolution of base of tongue squamous cell carcinoma (not shown) shows a new left upper quadrant mass (*arrow, right*). (*B*) Interval development of liver metastases and marked increase in the left upper quadrant mass, are seen on MIP (*left*), CT (*middle*) and PET/CT (*arrow, left*) 2 months later.

spread not seen on imaging to the GTV to obtain the CTV. The PTV is obtained by adding a security margin of 4 mm to 5 mm around the CTV, which accounts for many factors of geometric uncertainty, such as machine error, patient movement, and weight loss. Smaller radiation volumes also correspond to lower doses to organs at risk, potentially resulting in lower incidence of side effects. There was no recurrence in the area outside CTV determined by PET and within that determined by CT in 41 patients with a median follow-up of 3 years.[24] This is good evidence that the tumor volume determined by PET is accurate in addition to being smaller than the tumor volume determined by CT.

In addition, PET/CT identifies metastases and synchronous primaries that may not otherwise be detected, prompting changes in the radiation field. Finally, because many tumors have heterogeneous metabolic activity, PET/CT allows initial dose painting for intensity-modulated RT and adaptive dose painting during therapy. Early studies in head and neck cancer seem promising. Adaptive dose painting resulted in an increase in minimum and decrease in maximum doses in target volumes and in decreases in dose per volume in organs at risk, such as parotid glands and speech and swallowing structures.[35] Higher radiation dose to the larynx is associated with poor speech outcome and higher radiation dose to the supraglottic larynx, and adjacent lateral pharyngeal walls is associated with weight loss, restricted diet, and poor quality-of-life outcomes.[36] To further increase the usefulness of PET/CT, limitations of spatial resolution, edge delineation, partial volume effects, motion, and misregistration need to be studied further and minimized.[37] In summary, PET/CT has a significant impact on the personalization of RT volume, dose, and distribution.

## ASSESSMENT OF RESPONSE TO THERAPY

Accurate assessment of treatment response is critical. Some patients may avoid unnecessary surgery with its associated morbidity and others may be promptly assigned further treatment, thus improving their chance at achieving a cure. Prior to the development of PET/CT, clinical examination, CT, and MR imaging were used to assess response to treatment. CT and MR imaging may be limited due to their reliance on size criteria for lymph nodes and potentially extensive post-treatment fibrosis and scar formation, which confound the detection of residual disease. In addition, metabolic change occurs earlier than morphologic change. FDG-PET/CT can detect residual tumor in small lymph nodes and is superior to CT alone in differentiating residual disease from post-therapy changes (see **Fig 2**). In addition to evaluating the response to therapy, several studies have found newly detected DMs on the post-therapy PET/CT in 8% to 10% of patients.[38,39]

In a study of 170 patients, FDG-PET was more accurate in post-treatment surveillance of head and neck squamous cell carcinoma compared with ceCT.[40,41] The addition of contrast enhancement to the PET/CT may offer minimal clinical advantage.[40] Gupta and colleagues[42] found higher diagnostic accuracy when the follow-up PET/CT was more than 12 weeks after completion of therapy. Prestwich and colleagues[38] then evaluated PET/CT at 16 weeks post-therapy. This retrospective study of 44 patients treated with chemotherapy and radiotherapy demonstrated overall sensitivity, specificity, positive predictive value (PPV), and NPV of 100%, 84%, 54%, and 100%, respectively. Zundel and colleagues[39] found that PET/CT at 4 to 6 months had sensitivity and specificity of 100% and 64.6%, respectively. Using a Likert scale, such as the Deauville criteria, reduced the number of equivocal post-treatment lymph nodes compared with using SUVmax; 79% of equivocal cases by visual inspection were correctly categorized as responders or nonresponders using the Deauville criteria. The area under the curve was 0.82 for the Deauville criteria and 0.67 for SUVmax.[43] The Deauville criteria are listed in **Table 2**.

**Table 2**
**Deauville criteria**

| Deauville Score | Fluorodeoxyglucose F 18 Uptake | Interpretation |
|---|---|---|
| 1 | None | No tumor |
| 2 | Less than or equal to blood pool | Probably no tumor |
| 3 | Greater than blood pool but less than liver | Probably post-treatment inflammation |
| 4 | Moderately greater than liver | Probably tumor |
| 5 | Markedly greater than liver | Tumor |

With kind permission from Springer Science+Business Media: Sjövall J, Bitzén U, Kjellén E, et al. Qualitative interpretation of PET scans using a Likert scale to assess neck node response to radiotherapy in head and neck. Eur J Nucl Med Mol Imaging 2015;43:609–16.

The high NPV of PET/CT observed in several studies allows for the avoidance of surgery in those patients.[38,44] Although the PPV for PET/CT has been reported as high as 78%, it is typically low due to the presence of post-therapy inflammation.[42] The PPV for the primary site alone (43%) was lower than for the lymph nodes in the neck (63%).[38] This is a significant limitation of PET/CT. Post-treatment inflammation may be difficult to differentiate from residual tumor. Optimum timing between therapy and PET/CT may improve the PPV. The ideal time for follow-up PET/CT is uncertain but should be at least 6 weeks post-RT based on previous studies.

## SURVEILLANCE

In recent years, functional imaging with PET has taken a greater role in surveillance. The pooled sensitivity and specificity of scans performed 4 to 12 months after treatment were found to be 0.95 (95% CI, 0.91–0.97) and 0.78 (95% CI, 0.70–0.84), respectively.[45] MR imaging sensitivity to detect recurrence was 67% and PET/MR imaging was 92%, according to Nakamoto and colleagues.[46] PET/CT is well suited for surveillance in patients with HNSCC (**Fig. 5**).

## PROGNOSIS

FDG-PET/CT is a prognostic biomarker for many tumors including HNSCC. The prognostic information PET/CT provides for each HNSCC tumor subtype has the potential to guide earlier changes to the treatment plan.[47] SUVmax of 4.15 or higher was found related to extracapsular spread and cervical lymph node metastases in a retrospective review of 54 patients.[48] A limited shrinkage of positive lymph nodes during treatment is associated with poor outcome in terms of locoregional relapse. In a study of 81 patients with locoregionally advanced laryngeal and hypopharyngeal cancer, pretherapy MTV was an independent prognostic factor. Patients with MTV greater than 18 mL had a poor survival outcome.[49] Adaptive threshold-based pretreatment MTV was found predictive of therapy response in a study of 62 patients with locally advanced head and neck cancer and no DMs and showed statistically significant predictive value for local recurrence-free survival, DFS, and OS, whereas $SUV_{max}$ did not show any significance.[50] A Radiation Therapy Oncology Group study of 940 patients confirmed that MTV was a strong predictor of progression-free survival.[51]

A meta-analysis of 13 studies, which included 1180 patients with HNSCC, concluded that MTV and TLG are prognostic predictors of outcome. The hazard ratio with MTV was 3.06 for progression or recurrence and 3.14 with TLG.[52] PET/CT-based GTV predicted DSS. When $GTV_{PET}$ prior to therapy was greater than 40 $cm^3$, 10 $cm^3$ to 40 $cm^3$, and less than 10 $cm^3$, the DSS rates were 8.4 ± 0.96 months, 28.8 ± 4.9 months, and

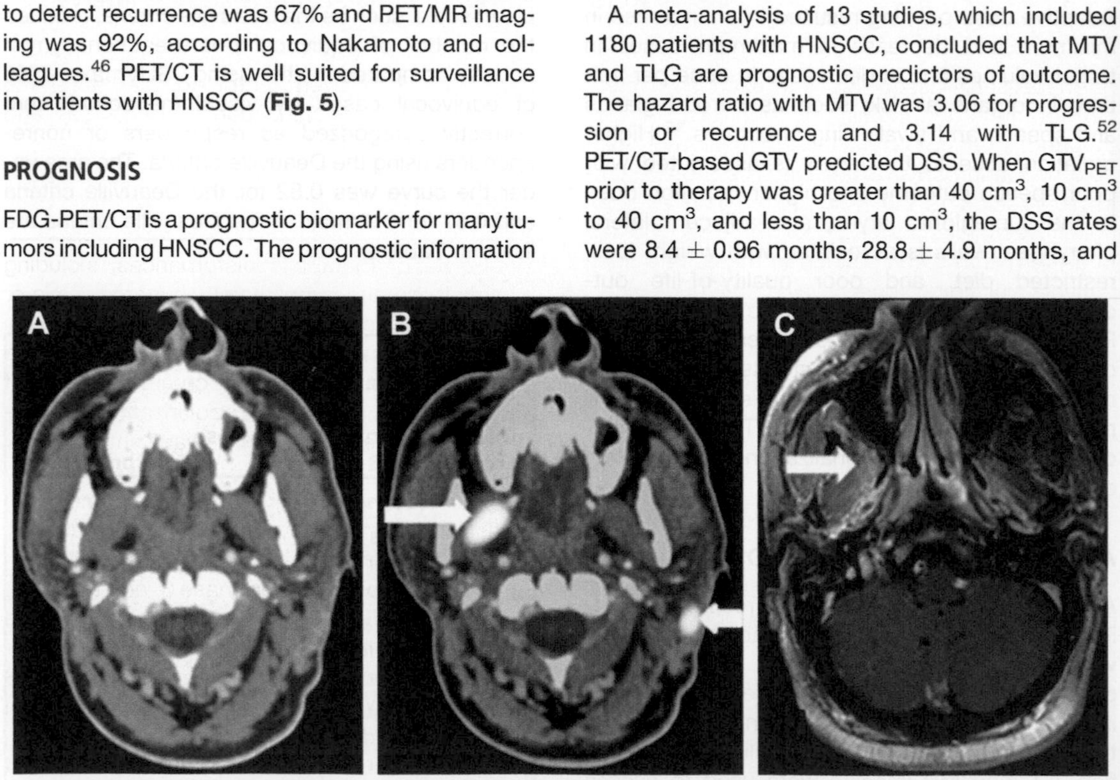


**Fig. 5.** Patient with history of laryngeal squamous cell carcinoma who is status post–oropharyngectomy and laryngectomy with local recurrence in the neopharynx (not shown). (*A*) Contrast-enhanced CT at the level of right medial pterygoid is unremarkable. (*B*) Fused PET/CT demonstrates hypermetabolism within the right medial pterygoid (SUVmax 20) and a subcentimeter lymph node (SUVmax 13) (*arrows*). (*C*) Contrast-enhanced T1-weighted MR at the same level demonstrates subtle increased enhancement within the anterior R medial pterygoid muscle (*arrow*), seen only in retrospect after PET/CT examination. Nodal and right medial pterygoid metastases could be missed without FDG. Patient treated with chemotherapy instead of surgical resection because of recurrence within the neopharynx. (*Courtesy of* Pareen Mehta, MD, Los Angeles, CA.)

82.1 ± 6.1 months, respectively.[25] In a prospective study of 51 patients with advanced pharyngeal cancer, the SUVmax reduction ratio of primary tumor after definitive chemoradiotherapy with cumulative radiation dose of 41.4 to 46.8 Gy was prognostic of the OS and DFS. When the reduction ratio was less than 0.64, 2-year OS and DFS rates were only 47% and 41%, respectively, compared with 2-year OS and DFS rates of 66% and 64%, respectively, when the reduction ratio was greater than or equal to 0.64%.[53] PET/CT can identify patients at high risk for treatment failure, thus allowing oncologists to plan a more aggressive treatment plan from the start with more frequent surveillance.[54]

## DETECTION OF SYNCHRONOUS AND METACHRONOUS PRIMARIES

Most synchronous cancers are lung, esophageal, or a second head and neck cancer (**Fig. 6**). Alcohol and tobacco use is a risk factor shared by these cancers.[54] Douglas and colleagues[55] reported that 14% of head and neck cancer patients develop lung cancer, 31% of which are synchronous. PET/CT detected second primaries in 4.4% (8/182) of patients with locoregionally advanced HNSCC in another study.[25] PET/CT was found more sensitive than WB MR imaging in the detection of secondary primaries in patients with oropharyngeal and hypopharyngeal squamous cell carcinoma (**Fig. 7**).[33] In a study of 589 patients, Strobel and colleagues[56] found not only a 10% prevalence of second primaries but also that the therapeutic management was changed in 80% of patients.

## DETECTION OF SEQUELAE OF THERAPY

HNSCC patients often undergo radiation, chemotherapy, and surgery. Oncologists, surgeons, and radiotherapists take all available precautions to prevent complications of treatment. The amount

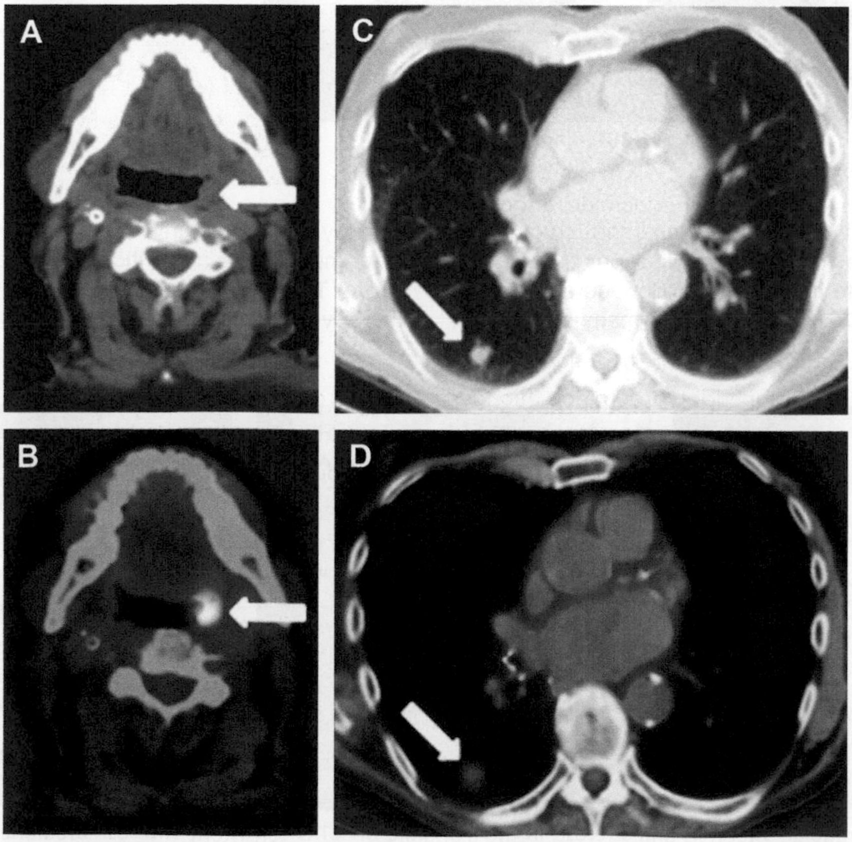


**Fig. 6.** (*A*) CT and (*B*) PET/CT show squamous cell cancer of the left tonsil in an 84-year-old man. An incidentally detected lung nodule seen on (*C*) CT and (*D*) PET/CT of the same day was subsequently biopsied. Synchronous adenocarcinoma of the right lower lobe was detected on the PET/CT for initial staging of the tonsillar carcinoma. (*Courtesy of* Pareen Mehta, MD, Los Angeles, CA.)

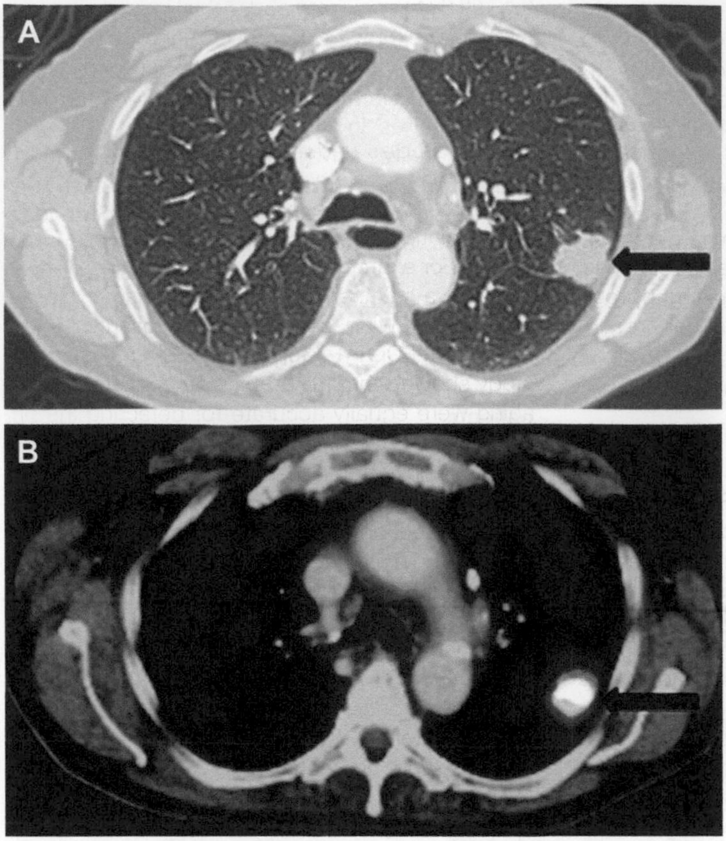

**Fig. 7.** A 72-year-old man with hyopharyngeal and laryngeal squamous cell cancer with hypermetabolic lung mass seen on (*A*) CT and (*B*) fused PET/CT. Surveillance PET/CT detected interval development of a metachronous biopsy-proved primary squamous cell lung cancer. (*Courtesy of* Pareen Mehta, MD, Los Angeles, CA.)

and proximity of critical organs and structures in the neck may result in complications that may be serious or life threatening. Follow-up and surveillance PET/CT is able to detect many sequelae of therapy (**Fig. 8**). Early detection and treatment of complications are critical in improving quality of life. **Table 3** lists some of the complications of therapy that occur in the neck.

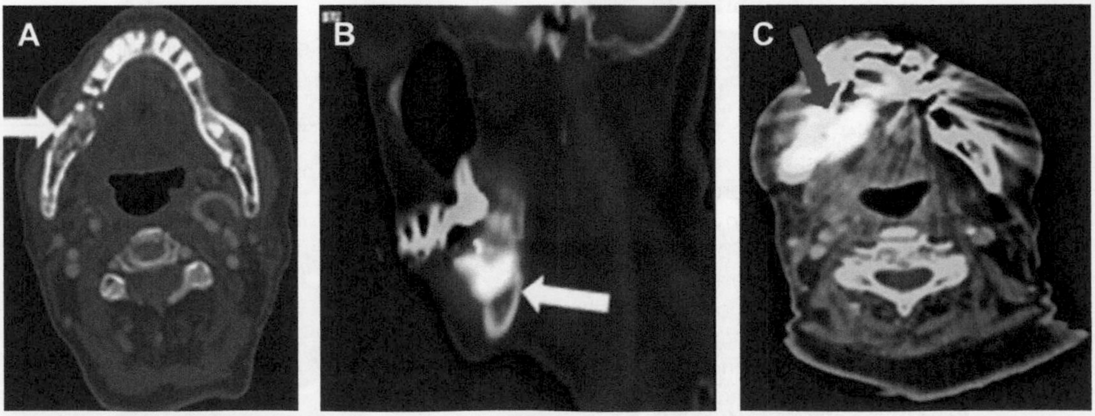

**Fig. 8.** (*A*) Irregular osteolysis and sclerosis in the mandible on CT is consistent with osteoradionecrosis 2 years after radiotherapy. (*B*) Hypermetabolism is seen in the area of osteoradionecrosis on PET/CT. Biopsy-proven tongue carcinoma was discovered on surveillance PET/CT (*C*) three years after radiation. Surveillance PET/CTs may detect second primaries in this patient population with high incidence of secondary head and neck, lung, and esophageal cancers.

**Table 3**
**Sequelae of therapy for head and neck carcinoma**

| | Acute | Chronic |
|---|---|---|
| Radiation | Fatigue<br>Nausea/vomiting<br>Xerostomia<br>Parotitis<br>Dysphagia<br>Mucositis<br>Infection<br>Dysgeusia<br>Dermatitis<br>Esophagitis<br>Aspiration pneumonia | Xerostomia<br>Parotitis<br>Poor dentition/periodontitis<br>Dermatitis, subcutaneous fibrosis<br>Osteoradionecrosis<br>Dysgeusia<br>Trismus<br>Laryngeal alterations, hoarseness<br>Neuropathic pain<br>Cervical dystonia<br>Secondary cancers<br>Hearing loss<br>Thyroid insufficiency<br>Myelo-radiculo-plexo-neuro-myopathy<br>Baroreflex dysfunction |
| Surgery | • Functional disturbances with<br>◦ Speaking<br>◦ Mastication<br>◦ Swallowing<br>• Vascular compromise<br>• Dermatitis | • Functional disturbances with<br>◦ Speaking<br>◦ Mastication<br>◦ Swallowing<br>• Vascular compromise<br>• Nerve damage<br>• Muscular atrophy<br>• Subcutaneous fibrosis<br>• Cosmetic alterations |
| Chemotherapy | Oral mucositis<br>Dysgeusia<br>Hearing loss<br>Neuropathy<br>Infections<br>Mucositis<br>Nausea/vomiting<br>Renal dysfunction<br>Liver dysfunction<br>Diarrhea<br>Fatigue<br>Immune dysfunction | Leumia<br>Secondary cancers |

## *Summary*

FDG-PET/CT can localize the primary tumor in 22% to 44% of patients with unknown primary after standard work-up. PET/CT has a higher sensitivity and specificity for staging HNSCC compared with contrast-enhanced CT or MR imaging. After therapy, changes in tumor metabolism occur before morphologic changes. This allows PET/CT to provide earlier and more accurate evaluation of response to treatment and restaging. PET data provide important prognostic information for more individualized surveillance and therapy planning. It is hoped that PET will be able to differentiate tumors that would not respond to RT, so that surgical resection can be performed early and patients spared RT, from tumors that would respond to radiation therapy with or without chemotherapy and can be spared neck dissection. PET has high sensitivity in identifying recurrent, synchronous, and metachronous tumor on surveillance imaging. In addition, PET is able to reveal post-treatment adverse effects earlier so they can be treated promptly. Accurate personalized treatment and surveillance are possible because of the extensive information that PET/CT provides.

## *The Future of PET-based Individualized Management of Head and Neck Squamous Cell Carcinoma*

Other PET radiopharmaceuticals and techniques have the potential to provide further insights into the molecular, clinical, and therapeutic variations of HNSCC and guide localization and biopsy, contributing to even further personalized management. Buchbender and colleagues[57] proposed the use of virtual 3-D FDG-PET/CT panendoscopy, showing that it is technically feasible, can evaluate the subglottic region in intubated patients, and can guide biopsy and surgery. A study of 17 patients found that pretherapy FDG SUVmax showed no difference between the patients who had residual/recurrent disease and those who were disease free post-therapy, whereas (62)Cu-ATSM SUVmax, a tumor hypoxia marker, has demonstrated a statistically significant difference ($P$<.05) in DFS. All patients who were disease free had a (62)-Cu-ATSM SUVmax less than 5.0, and 6 of 10 patients with recurrent/residual disease had SUVmax greater than 5.0.[58] This PET radiopharmaceutical would allow for early treatment modification if extensive hypoxia exists which is associated with resistance to radiotherapy and chemotherapy. Dynamic PET/CT also seems promising. Anderson's group evaluated 84 patients with triphasic FDG-PET/CT at 60, 90 and 120 minutes 3 months after RT. Their findings suggest that inflammatory tissue have a decrease in the slope of SUVmax after 90 minutes. Residual or recurrent tumor has similar or increased slope of SUVmax after 90 minutes.[59] The role of PET/CT in personalized clinical management in patients diagnosed with HNSC will continue to grow.

## REFERENCES


1. Siegel RL, Miller KD, Jemal A. Cancer statistics. CA Cancer J Clin 2015;2015(65):5–29.
2. Vermorken JB, Psyrri A, Mesia R, et al. Impact of tumor HPV status on outcome in patients with recurrent and/or metastatic squamous cell carcinoma of the head and neck receiving chemotherapy with or without cetuximab: retrospective analysis of the phase III EXTREME trial. Ann Oncol 2014;25(4):801–7.
3. Wahl RL, Jacine H, Kasamon Y, et al. From RECIST to PERCIST: evolving Considerations for PET response criteria in solid tumors. J Nucl Med 2009; 1:122S–50S.
4. Pentenero M, Cistaro A, Brusa M, et al. Accuracy of $^{18}$F-FDG-PET/CT for staging of oral squamous cell carcinoma. Head Neck 2008;30(11):1488–96.
5. Abouzied MM, Crawford ES, Nabi AN. $^{18}$F-FDG imaging: pitfalls and artifacts. J Nucl Med Technol 2005;33:145–55.
6. Kumar R, Mukherjee A, Mittal BR. Special techniques in PET/computed tomography imaging for evaluation of head and neck Cancer. PET Clin 2016;11:13–20.
7. Chang CY, Yang BH, Lin KH, et al. Feasibility and incremental benefit of puffed-cheek 18F -FDG PET/CT on oral cancer patients. Clin Nucl Med 2013;38(10): e374–8.
8. Henrot P, Blum A, Toussaint B, et al. Dynamic maneuvers in local staging of head and neck malignancies with current imaging techniques: principles and clinical applications. Radiographics 2003;23(5): 1201–13.
9. Rodrigues RS, Bozza FA, Christian PE, et al. Comparison of whole-body PET/CT, Dedicated high-resolution head and neck PET/CT, and contrast-enhanced CT in preoperative staging of clinically M0 Squamous Cell carcinoma of the head and neck. J Nucl Med 2009;50(8):1205–13.
10. Li CY, Klohr S, Sadick H, et al. Technique on the diagnostic performance of $^{18}$F-FDG PET/CT for assessment of lymph node metastases in head and neck squamous cell carcinoma. J Nucl Med Technol 2014;42:181–7.
11. Yamamoto Y, Wong TZ, Turkington TG, et al. Head and neck cancer: dedicated FDG PET/CT protocol for detection—phantom and initial clinical studies. Radiology 2007;244:263–72.
12. Wong TZ, Fras M. PET/CT protocols and practical issues for the evaluation of patients with head and neck cancer. PET Clin 2007;2:413–21.
13. Garavello W, Ciardo A, Spreafico R, et al. Risk factors for distant metastases in head and neck squamous cell carcinoma. Arch Otolaryngol Head Neck Surg 2006;132:762–6.
14. Houshmand S, Salvati A, Hess S, et al. An update on novel quantitative techniques in the context of evolving whole-body PET imaging. PET Clin 2015; 10(1):45–58.
15. Cancer Genome Atlas Network. Comprehensive genomic characterization of head and neck squamous cell carcinomas. Nature 2015;517: 576–82.
16. Gross AM, Cohen EE. Towards a personalized treatment of head and neck cancer. Am Soc Clin Oncol Educ Book 2015;35:28–32.
17. Jereczek-Fossa BA, Jassem J, Orecchia R. Cervical lymph node metastases of squamous cell carcinoma from an unknown primary. Cancer Treat Rev 2004;30: 153–64.
18. Rusthoven KE, Koshy M, Paulino AC. The role of fluorodeoxyglucose positron emission tomography in cervical lymph node metastases from an unknown primary tumor. Cancer 2004;101:2641–9.
19. Waltonen JD, Ozer E, Hall NC, et al. Metastatic carcinoma of the neck of unknown primary origin: evolution and efficacy of the modern workup. Arch Otolaryngol Head Neck Surg 2009;135:1024–9.
20. Johansen J, Petersen H, Godballe C, et al. FDG-PET/CT for detection of the unknown primary head and neck tumor. Q J Nucl Med Mol Imaging 2011;55:500–8.
21. Dong MJ, Zhao K, Lin XT, et al. Role of fluorodeoxyglucose-PET versus fluorodeoxyglucose-PET/computed tomography in detection of unknown

primary tumor: a meta-analysis of the literature. Nucl Med Commun 2008;29:791–802.
22. Lauridsen JK, Rohde M, Thomassen A. Positron emission tomography/computed tomography in malignancies of the thyroid and in head and neck squamous cell carcinoma. a review of the literature. PET Clin 2015;10:75–88.
23. Koppula B, Rajendran JG. PET-CT in head and neck cancer. Appl Radiol 2010;4:20–7.
24. Leclerc M, Lartigau E, Lacornerie T, et al. Primary tumor delineation based on $^{18}$F FDG PET for locally advanced head and neck cancer treated by chemo-radiotherapy. Radiother Oncol 2015;116: 87–93.
25. Hideghéty K, Cserháti A, Besenyi Z, et al. Role of 18FDG-PET/CT in the management and gross tumor volume definition for radiotherapy of head and neck cancer; single institution experiences based on long-term follow-up. Magy Onkol 2015;59:103–10.
26. Anderson CM, Sun W, Buatti JM, et al. Interobserver and intermodality variability in GTV delineation on simulation CT, FDG-PET, and MR images of head and neck cancer. Jacobs J Radiat Oncol 2014; 1(1):006.
27. Van den Brekel MW, Stel H, Castelijns JA, et al. Cervical lymph node metastasis: assessment of radiologic criteria. Radiology 1990;177:379–84.
28. Platzek I, Beuthien-Basumann B, Schneider M, et al. FDG PET/MR for lymph node staging in head and neck cancer. Eur J Radiol 2014;83:1163–8.
29. Kastrinidis N, Kuhn FP, Hany TF, et al. 18F-FDG-PET/CT for the assessment of the contralateral neck in patients with head and neck squamous cell carcinoma. Laryngoscope 2013;123:1210–5.
30. Kim SY, Kim JS, Doo H, et al. Combined [18F] fluorodeoxyglucose positron emission tomography and computed tomography for detecting contralateral neck metastases in patients with head and neck squamous cell carcinoma. Oral Oncol 2011;47: 376–80.
31. Thompson CF, St John MA, Lawson G, et al. Diagnostic value of sentinel lymph node biopsy in head and neck cancer: a meta-analysis. Eur Arch Otorhinolaryngol 2013;270:2115–22.
32. Leon X, Quer M, Orus C, et al. Distant metastases in head and neck cancer patients who achieved locoregional control. Head Neck 2000;22:680–6.
33. Chan SC, Wang HM, Yen TC, et al. $^{18}$F-FDG PET/CT and 3.0-T whole-body MRI for the detection of distant metastases and second primary tumours in patients with untreated oropharyngeal/hypopharyngeal carcinoma: a comparative study. Eur J Nucl Med Mol Imaging 2011;38:1607–19.
34. Xu GZ, Guan DJ, He ZY. (18) FDG-PET/CT for detecting distant metastases and second primary cancers in patients with head and neck cancer. A meta-analysis. Oral Oncol 2011;47:560–5.
35. Olteanu LA, Berwouts D, Madani I, et al. Comparative dosimetry of three-phase adaptive and non-adaptive dose-painting IMRT for head-and-neck cancer. Radiother Oncol 2014;111:348–53.
36. Dornfeld K, Simmons JR, Karnell L, et al. Radiation doses to structures within and adjacent to the larynx are correlated with long-term diet- and speech-related quality of life. Int J Radiat Oncol Biol Phys 2007;68:750–7.
37. Wahl RJ, Herman JM, Ford E. The promise and pitfalls of positron emission tomography and single-photon emission computed tomography molecular imaging–guided radiation therapy. Semin Radiat Oncol 2011;21:88–100.
38. Prestwich RJD, Subesinghe M, Gilbert A, et al. Delayed response assessment with FDG-PET-CT following (chemo)radiotherapy for locally advanced head and neck squamous cell carcinoma. Clin Radiol 2012;67:966–97.
39. Zundel MT, Michel MA, Schultz CJ, et al. Comparison of physical examination and fluorodeoxyglucose positron emission tomography/computed tomography 4-6 months after radiotherapy to assess residual head-and-neck cancer. Int J Radiat Oncol Biol Phys 2011;81:825–83.
40. Suenaga Y, Kitajima K, Ishihara T, et al. FDG-PET/contrast-enhanced CT as a post-treatment tool in head and neck squamous cell carcinoma: comparison with FDG-PET/non-contrast-enhanced CT and contrast-enhanced CT. Eur Radiol 2015;26: 1018–30.
41. Andrade RS, Heron DE, Degirmenci B, et al. Post-treatment assessment of response using FDG-PET/CT for patients treated with definitive radiation therapy for head and neck cancers. Int J Radiat Oncol Biol Phys 2009;65:1315–22.
42. Gupta T, Master Z, Kannan S, et al. Diagnostic performance of post-treatment FDG PET or FDG PET/CT imaging in head and neck cancer: a systematic review and meta-analysis. Eur J Nucl Med Mol Imaging 2011;38:2083–95.
43. Sjövall J, Bitzén U, Kjellén E, et al. Qualitative interpretation of PET scans using a Likert scale to assess neck node response to radiotherapy in head and neck cancer. Eur J Nucl Med Mol Imaging 2015;43: 609–16. Available at: http://ejnmmigateway.net/ArticlePage.aspx?doi=10.1007/s00259-015-3194-3. Accessed November 15, 2015.
44. Porceddu SV, Pryor DI, Burmeister E, et al. Results of a prospective study of positron emission tomography-directed management of residual nodal abnormalities in node-positive head and neck cancer after definitive radiotherapy with or without systemic therapy. Head Neck 2011;33:1675–82.
45. Sheikhbahaei S, Taghipour M, Ahmad R, et al. Diagnostic Accuracy of Follow-up FDG PET or PET/CT in patients with head and neck cancer after definitive

treatment: a systematic review and meta-analysis. Am J Roentgenol 2015;205(3):629–39.
46. Nakamoto Y, Tamai K, Saga T, et al. Clinical value of image fusion from MR and PET in patients with head and neck cancer. Mol Imaging Biol 2009;1:46–53.
47. Belli ML, Fiorino C, Zerbetto F, et al. Early volume variation of positive lymph nodes assessed by in-room MVCT images predicts risk of loco-regional relapses in head and neck cancer patients treated with IMRT. Acta Oncol 2015;23:1–6.
48. Dequanter D, Shahla M, Aubert C, et al. Prognostic value of FDG PET/CT in head and neck squamous cell carcinomas. Onco Targets Ther 2015;8:2279–83.
49. Park GC, Kim JS, Roh JL, et al. Prognostic value of metabolic tumor volume measured by 18F-FDG PET/CT in advanced-stage squamous cell carcinoma of the larynx and hypopharynx. Ann Oncol 2013;24(1):208–14.
50. Akagunduz OO, Savas R, Yalman D, et al. Can adaptive threshold-based metabolic tumor volume (MTV) and lean body mass corrected standard uptake value (SUL) predict prognosis in head and neck cancer patients treated with definitive radiotherapy/chemoradiotherapy? Nucl Med Biol 2015; 42:899–904.
51. Schwartz DL, Harris J, Yao M, et al. Metabolic tumor volume as a prognostic imaging-based biomarker for head-and-neck cancer: pilot results from Radiation Therapy Oncology Group protocol 0522. Int J Radiat Oncol Biol Phys 2015;91:721–9.
52. Pak K, Cheon GJ, Nam HY, et al. Prognostic value of metabolic tumor volume and total lesion glycolysis in head and neck cancer: a systematic review and meta-analysis. J Nucl Med 2014;55:884–90.
53. Chen SW, Hsieh TC, Yen KY. Interim FDG PET/CT for predicting the outcome in patients with head and neck cancer. Laryngoscope 2014;124(12):2732–8.
54. Piccio M, Kirienko M, Mapelli P, et al. Predictive value of pre-therapy $^{18}$F-FDG PET/CT for the outcome of $^{18}$F-FDG PET-guided radiotherapy in patients with head and neck cancer. Eur J Nucl Med Mol Imaging 2014;41:21–31.
55. Douglas WG, Rigual NR, Loree TR, et al. Current concepts in the management of a second malignancy of the lung in patients with head and neck cancer. Curr Opin Otolaryngol Head Neck Surg 2003;11:85–8.
56. Strobel K, Haerle SK, Stoeckli SJ, et al. Head and neck squamous cell carcinoma (HNSCC)–detection of synchronous primaries with (18)F-FDG-PET/CT. Eur J Nucl Med Mol Imaging 2009;36(6):919–27.
57. Buchbender C, Treffert J, Lehnerdt G, et al. Virtual 3-D 18F-FDG PET/CT panendoscopy for assessment of the upper airways of head and neck cancer patients: a feasibility study. Eur J Nucl Med Mol Imaging 2012;39:1435–40.
58. Minagawa Y, Shizukuishi K, Koike I, et al. Assessment of tumor hypoxia by 62Cu-ATSM PET/CT as a predictor of response in head and neck cancer: a pilot study. Ann Nucl Med 2011;25:339–45.
59. Anderson CM, Chang T, Graham MM, et al. Change of maximum standardized uptake value slope in dynamic triphasic [18F]-fluorodeoxyglucose positron emission tomography/computed tomography distinguishes malignancy from postradiation inflammation in head-and-neck squamous cell carcinoma: a prospective trial. Int J Radiat Oncol Biol Phys 2015;91:472–9.

# PET-Based Molecular Imaging in Designing Personalized Management Strategy in Gastroenteropancreatic Neuroendocrine Tumors

Sandip Basu, DRM, DNB, MNAMS[a,*], Rohit Ranade, MBBS, DRM[a],
Vikas Ostwal, MBBS, MD, DM[b], Shailesh V. Shrikhande, MBBS, MS[c]

**KEYWORDS**

• Neuroendocrine tumor • Personalized management • Somatostatin receptor imaging
• FDG-PET/CT • Tumor biology • Tumor heterogeneity • Molecular imaging

**KEY POINTS**

- In recent years, PET-based molecular imaging has been increasingly used in neuroendocrine tumors (NETs) for tailoring of treatment strategies on an individual basis.
- For each particular patient, the relative tracer uptake by dual-tracer imaging approach is now frequently assessed along with the histopathologic tumor grades for selecting the optimal treatment approach for advanced/metastatic cases.
- The traditional advantages of PET/CT in terms of disease staging and treatment response monitoring are also applicable for personalization of management.
- From a surgical perspective, somatostatin receptor–based PET/CT is usually included in the preoperative staging, which strongly complements the conventional cross-sectional imaging for surgical decision making by providing improved and more complete information on the extent of the disease for an individual patient.

## INTRODUCTION: THERAPEUTIC STRATEGIES IN GASTROENTEROPANCREATIC NEUROENDOCRINE TUMORS

Traditionally, the management strategy of gastroenteropancreatic neuroendocrine tumors (GEP-NETs) involves multiple considerations, such as anatomic parameters (eg, site, size, invasiveness to surrounding structures), functionality in terms of hormone secretion, and status of metastasis. Surgery is the first consideration when curative surgery is feasible. With inoperable advanced/metastatic disease, multiple therapeutic options are

The authors have nothing to disclose.
[a] Radiation Medicine Centre, Bhabha Atomic Research Centre, Tata Memorial Hospital Annexe, Jerbai Wadia Road, Parel, Mumbai 400 012, India; [b] Department of Medical Oncology, Tata Memorial Hospital, Mumbai, India; [c] Gastrointestinal and Hepato-Pancreato-Biliary Service, Department of Surgical Oncology, Tata Memorial Hospital, Mumbai, India
* Corresponding author.
*E-mail address:* drsanb@yahoo.com

PET Clin 11 (2016) 233–241
http://dx.doi.org/10.1016/j.cpet.2016.02.004
1556-8598/16/$ – see front matter 

considered, including (1) somatostatin analogues, such as long-acting octreotide; (2) somatostatin receptor (SSTR) targeted peptide receptor radionuclide therapy (PRRT) with lutetium (Lu) 177/yttrium (Y) 90 DOTATATE/DOTATOC; (3) chemotherapy with conventional agents (cisplatinum-etoposide combination or more popularly in recent times capecitabine-temzolamide combination); and (4) targeted therapy with sunitinibor mTOR inhibitors, such as everolimus, locoregional ablative therapies, such as chemoembolization, or radiofrequency ablation or selective internal radiotherapy. Hence, tumor characteristics that aid in appropriate selection of therapy among these multiple options are a clinical need of present-day management.

## PERSONALIZED SELECTION OF THE APPROPRIATE THERAPEUTIC STRATEGY: THE TRADITIONAL DETERMINANTS AND THE EVOLVING PLACE OF DUAL-TRACER PET IMAGING

Traditionally, tumor grading has played a pivotal role, especially in deciding on appropriate systemic therapy in metastatic/advanced GEP-NETs. The widely heterogeneous GEP-NETs have been typically classified based on the Ki67 or Mib1 index: the well-differentiated NET comprises grade 1 (<2 mitoses/10 hpf and Ki67 <3%) and the intermediate grade/grade 2 (2–20 mitoses/10 hpf or Ki67 3%–20%), whereas poorly differentiated neuroendocrine cancers are high-grade or grade 3 tumors (>20 mitoses/10 hpf or Ki67 index >20%). Chemotherapy with cisplatin-etoposide has been typically effective in poorly differentiated subtypes of NETs, whereas this regimen in well-differentiated NETs demonstrates only 25% to 35% response rates that are usually less than 8 to 9 months.[1] In an early reported study, tumors negative on SSTR scintigraphy had a response to cisplatin-etoposide more than 70% compared with 10% in strongly positive somatostatin receptor scintigraphy (SRSS) carcinoid tumors with this chemotherapy regimen.[2] The preferred chemotherapy in low- to intermediate-grade tumors is a combination of capecitabine and temozolomide, which is preferred over cisplatin-etoposide. Somatostatin analogues for metastatic GEP-NETs, however, have been useful in low and intermediate well-differentiated NETs, which usually express abundant SSTRs. An indirect evidence of this was documented with long-acting octreotide in the PROMID study (Placebo-controlled prospective randomized study on the antiproliferative efficacy of Octreotide LAR in patients with metastatic neuroendocrine MIDgut tumors); average tumor stabilization was 14.3 months compared with 6 months for placebo.[3]

The strength of the in vivo dual-tracer whole-body PET imaging is its ability to perform a whole-body assessment, which has theoretical advantages over the limitations of histopathology obtained from a single site. This would, logically, enable better selection of the most appropriate therapy for an individual patient. The varying characteristics of management individualization are made through illustrations of appropriate cases with discussion of the evolving perspectives as appropriate.[4]

### *Case 1: Well-Differentiated (G1) Somatosatin Receptor–Positive and Fluorodeoxyglucose-Negative Pancreatic Neuroendocrine Tumors*

A 70-year-old man initially presented features of obstructive jaundice. Computed tomography (CT) scan of the upper abdomen showed an enhancing mass lesion in the region of head of the pancreas and multiple liver space occupying lesions (SOLs). He underwent biliary stenting for the obstructive jaundice. Biopsy from the mass showed well-differentiated pancreatic NET. The final diagnosis was of pancreatic NET with liver metastasis. Gallium (Ga) 68-DOTATATE PET/CT showed multiple SSTR-positive lesions in the liver, lesion in head of pancreas, and peripancreatic lymph nodes. 18F Fluorodeoxyglucose (FDG)-PET/CT scan was normal with no FDG-avid lesion (**Fig. 1**).

#### *Outcome*

The patient received five cycles of PRRT with 177Lu-DOTATATE (cumulative dose of 881 mCi) with the scan and biochemical findings demonstrating stable disease at 3.5 years following diagnosis.

#### *Learning point*

The classical molecular imaging characteristics of lower grade NETs are positivity on SSTR-targeted 68Ga-DOTATATE/NOC PET/CT and negativity on 18F FDG-PET/CT. PRRT with 177Lu-DOTATATE demonstrates good outcome even in advanced disease, such as in this patient who has progression-free survival of 42 months with stable disease.

### *Case 2: Poorly Differentiated (G3) Somatosatin Receptor–Negative and Fluorodeoxyglucose-Positive Neuroendocrine Cancer*

A 25-year-old female patient initially presented with vomiting and generalized weakness. CT scan of the abdomen showed a mass in the body and tail of the pancreas, and multiple liver lesions. CT-guided liver biopsy revealed it to be neuroendocrine carcinoma, with Mib1 index being 45%. 99mTc-HYNIC-TOC showed no SSTR-positive lesions. The right kidney was pushed to the front by the huge mass. 18F FDG-PET/CT showed intense 18F FDG-avid lesions in both

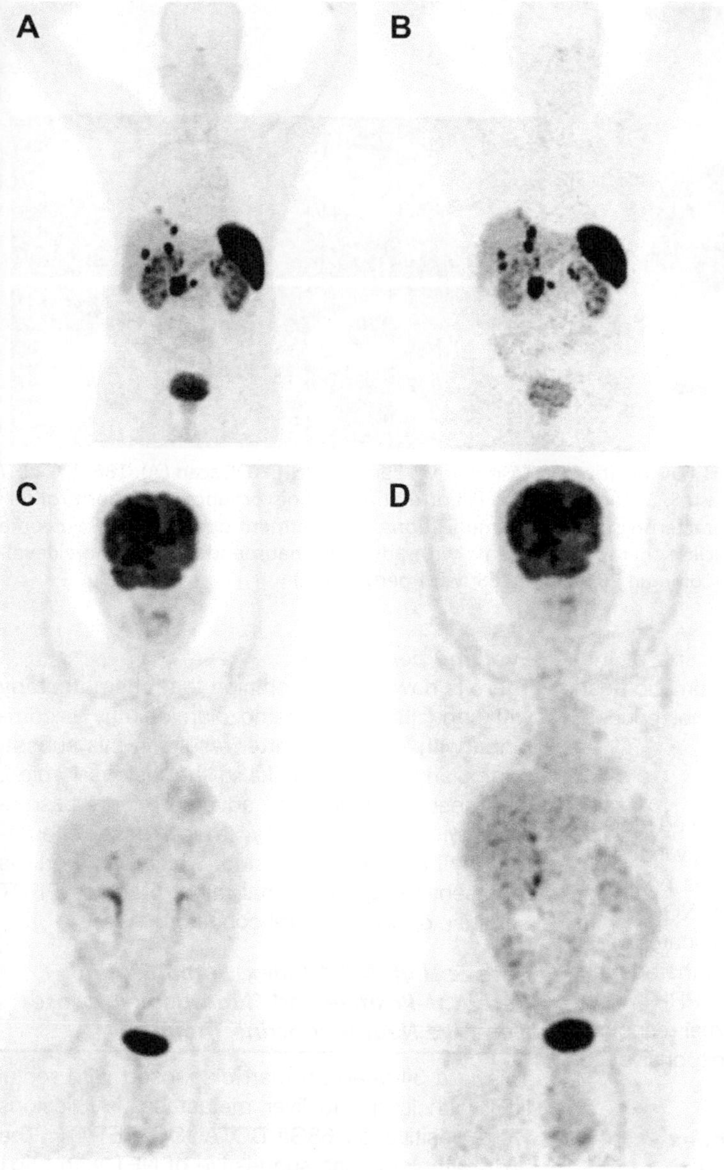


**Fig. 1.** Group I: Well-differentiated NET fluorodeoxyglucose (FDG)-negative. Baseline 68 gallium (Ga)-DOTA scan (*A*), post first cycle PRRT 68Ga-DOTA scan (*B*), baseline FDG-PET scan (*C*), and post fifth cycle PRRT FDG-PET scan (*D*).

lobes of the liver and in the body and tail of the pancreas (**Fig. 2**). The patient was considered for chemotherapy with carboplatin and etoposide.

### *Case 3: Well-Differentiated (G2) Intermediate Mib1 Index, Somatosatin Receptor–Positive and Fluorodeoxyglucose-Negative Neuroendocrine Tumors*

A 51-year-old man initially presented with features of abdominal distention and constipation. Colonoscopy revealed a rectal mass. Biopsy showed it as intermediate-grade NET with Mib 1 index 10% to 12%. CT scan showed a mass lesion in the rectum with retroperitoneal and mesenteric lymph nodes, pelvic and peritoneal deposits, with right tenth rib lesion. He had undergone three cycles of chemotherapy with cisplatin and etoposide without benefit before being referred for PRRT. 99m-Tc-HYNIC-TOC scan showed multiple SSTR-positive lesions in the liver, multiple skeletal lesions, and pelvic deposits. FDG-PET/CT was normal (**Fig. 3**). The patient was treated with three cycles of 177Lu-based PRRT with cumulative dose being 443 mCi (16.39 GBq).

#### *Outcome*

Follow-up 68Ga-DOTATATE PET/CT showed a good partial reduction in the number of SSTR-positive lesions (almost complete resolution in

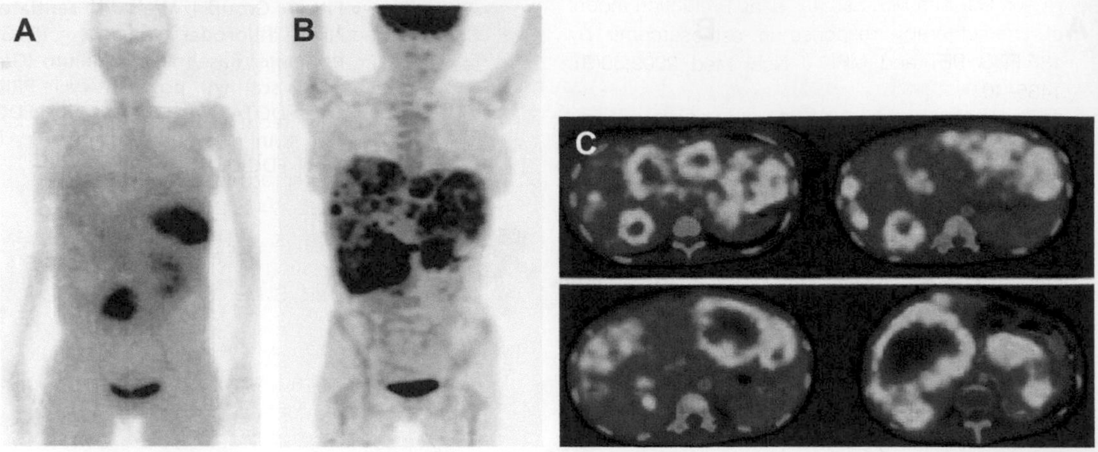


**Fig. 2.** Group II: Poorly differentiated NET FDG-positive/DOTA-negative. 99mTc-HYNIC-TOC scan (*A*), 18F FDG-PET/CT (*B*), and 18F FDG-PET/CT (*C*). (*From* Basu S, Ranade R, Thapa P. Correlation and discordance of tumor proliferation index and molecular imaging characteristics and their implications for treatment decisions and outcome pertaining to peptide receptor radionuclide therapy in patients with advanced neuroendocrine tumor: developing a personalized model. Nucl Med Commun 2015;36(8):768; with permission.)

the skeletal lesions with decrease in size of the liver lesions). The patient was asymptomatic post three cycles. Serum chromogranin A level reduced from 94 ng/mL to 55 ng/mL.

### Learning point

One of the major advantages of PET-based molecular imaging is assessing disease biology in the intermediate grade NETs. Along with the positivity on SSTR-targeted 68Ga-DOTATATE/NOC PET/CT, negativity on 18F FDG-PET/CT indicates preference toward PRRT as the preferred therapeutic approach. In the illustrated case, PRRT with 177Lu-DOTATATE showed good partial response after three cycles who was unresponsive to chemotherapy.

## Case 4: Intermediate/High Mib1 Index, Somatosatin Receptor–Positive and Fluorodeoxyglucose-Positive Neuroendocrine Tumors

This is a 51-year-old man with a known case of NET of uncinate process of pancreas with metastases to liver, all of which were positive on 68Ga-DOTANOC PET/CT. The histopathology was suggestive of grade 2 NET (with intermediate Ki67 of 10%). FDG-PET/CT demonstrated FDG-avid lesions in pancreas and liver. The patient complained of severe abdominal pain before the first cycle of PRRT and underwent PRRT with 733 mCi (27.12 GBq) in five sittings. He was asymptomatic at the last assessment, and 68Ga-DOTANOC and FDG-PET/CT showed stable disease. Serum CgA level dropped from 845 at baseline to 321.3 in January 2013 to June 2015 (**Fig. 4**).

### Evolving perspective

There is now evolving opinion that chemotherapy with capecitabine and temozolamide may be combined with PRRT for better results in this subset, particularly if FDG uptake in the lesions is high. One needs to weigh the adverse effects associated with chemotherapy (a low-dose chemotherapy has been suggested, which can work as radiosensitizing agent) that might preclude PRRT because of poor general condition.

## Case 5: High Mib1 Index, Somatosatin Receptor–Positive and Fluorodeoxyglucose-Negative Neuroendocrine Tumors

This is a 34-year-old man diagnosed with rectal NET with lung and liver metastases. All lesions were positive on 68Ga-DOTANOC PET/CT. The histopathology was suggestive of NET with Mib1 20%. However, FDG-PET/CT was normal with no FDG uptake in either of the lesions in the liver or lung. He presented with substantial pain in the right chest and upper abdomen and weakness, and underwent PRRT with 800 mCi (29.6 GBq) of 177Lu-DOTATATE in five sittings. At the time of last assessment at 55 months post first cycle of PRRT, he had complete resolution of all symptoms. FDG-PET/CT remained normal (**Fig. 5**).

### Learning point

In the subset of high Mib1 index including those having Mib1 between the gray zone of 20% to 30%, FDG nonavidity would indicate preference for PRRT if the lesions are positive on 68Ga-DOTA-NOC/TATE PET/CT. One can often experience adequate disease control with PRRT.

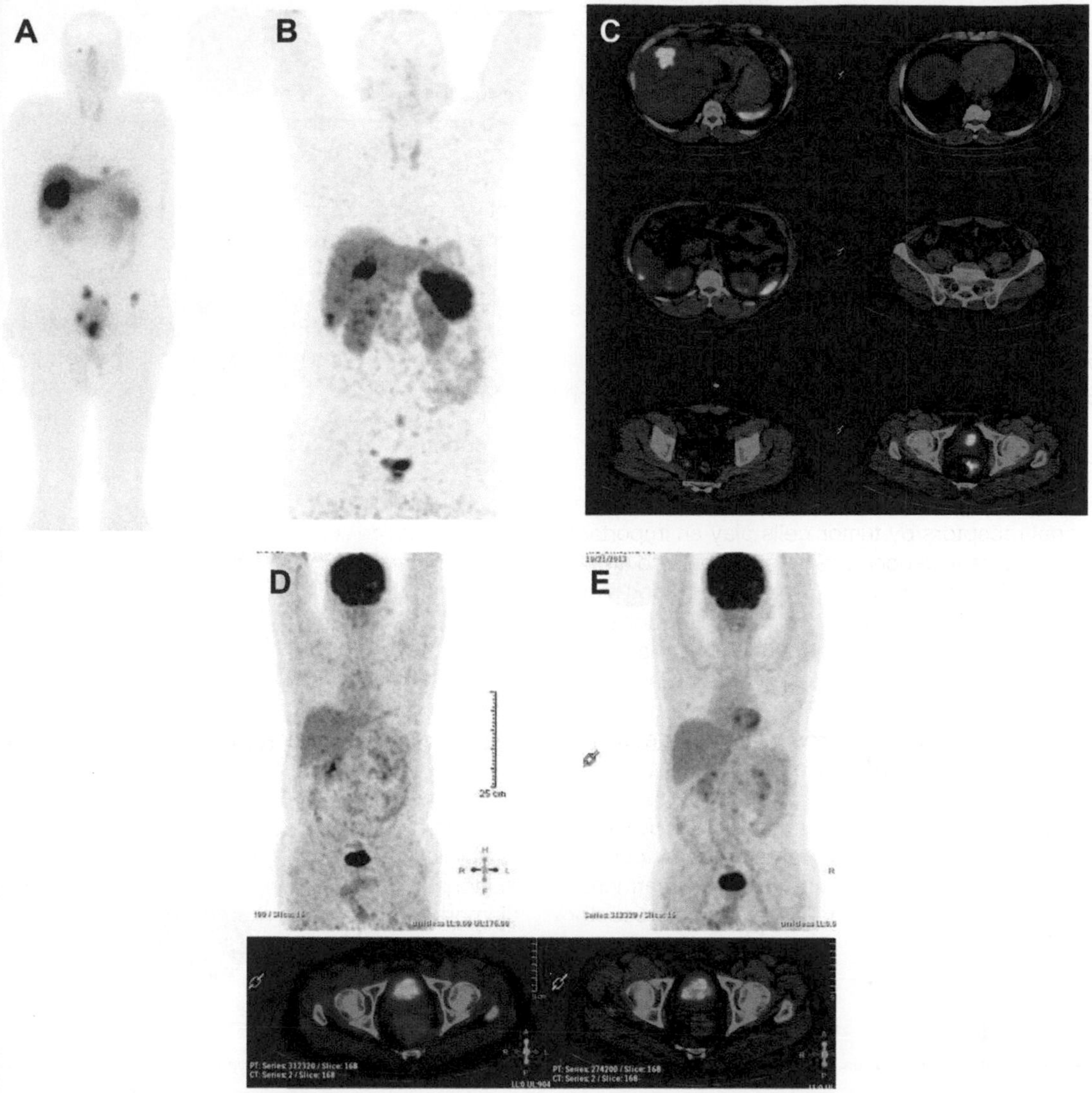


**Fig. 3.** Group III: Intermediate Mib1 grade FDG-negative. 177Lu-DOTATATE posttherapy scan (first cycle PRRT) (*A*), Ga-DOTATATE PET post three cycles of PRRT (*B*), post three cycles of PRRT Ga-DOTATATE (*C*), baseline FDG-PET/CT scan (*D*), and post three cycles PRRT FDG-PET/CT scan (*E*).

## PET IN DISEASE PROGNOSIS

In the clinical parlance of GEP-NET, an overexpression of SSTR2 has been equated with better prognosis, whereas overexpression of GLUT receptors and glycolytic metabolism are predictive of poor prognosis. The current PET-based molecular imaging explores this in vivo on a real-time basis and hence has the potential to explore tumor biology. A flip-flop between the 68Ga-DOTANOC and FDG-PET/CT is an usual observation, with low-grade tumors typically 68Ga-DOTANOC avid and the high grade poorly differentiated. Neuroendocrine carcinoma with lower survival is typically FDG avid. The tumors with intermediate Mib 1 index are variably positive on either of the tracer, which can be used for disease prognostication with histopathologic parameters.

## PET-BASED ASSESSMENT OF TREATMENT RESPONSE IN TREATMENT INDIVIDUALIZATION

Early treatment response monitoring has been a major advantage of PET, which could assess patients with NET on an individual basis. This is akin to several other malignancies where reduction in tracer uptake is suggestive of response to the administered therapy and thereby implies the effectivity of the particular regimen. Both 68Ga-DOTANOC and FDG-PET/CT can play an important role provided the baseline study

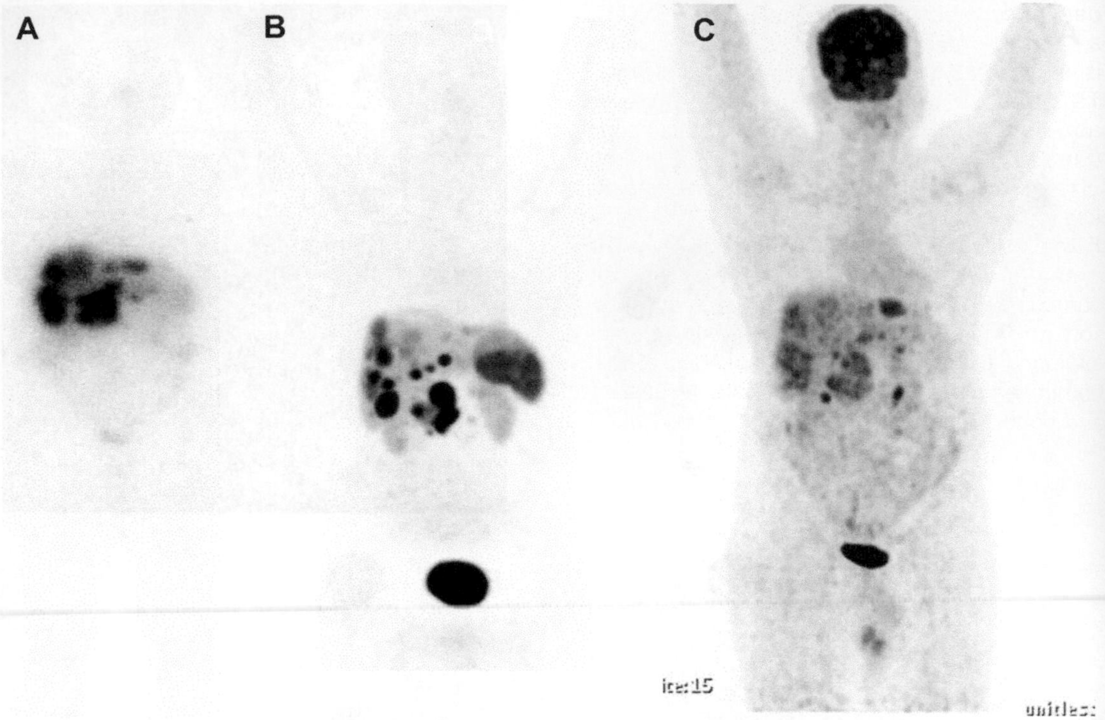


**Fig. 4.** Intermediate-grade FDG-positive. Posttherapy scan first PRRT (*A*), post fifth cycle PRRT Ga-DOTA scan (*B*), and baseline FDG-PET/CT (*C*).

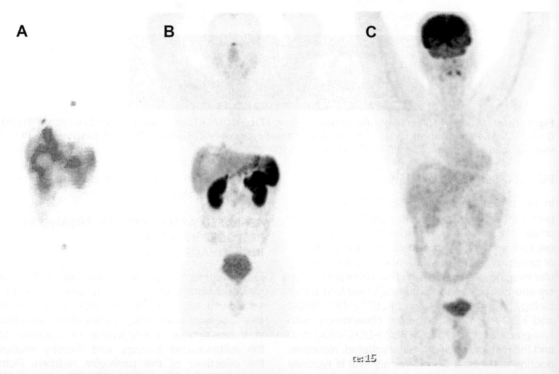


**Fig. 5.** High Mib1 FDG-negative. 177Lu-DOTATATE posttreatment (first PRRT) (*A*), post fifth cycle PRRT 68Ga-DOTATATE PET/CT (*B*), and baseline FDG-PET/CT (*C*).

demonstrate uptake of the particular tracer. Thus, a low-grade NET, which is typically FDG-negative, is monitored with SSTR-based 68Ga-DOTA-NOC/TATE PET/CT, whereas the FDG uptake can be an additional parameter for FDG-positive tumors (**Fig. 6**).

One particular interesting observation is that in low-grade NETs with low- to intermediate-grade FDG uptake, a reduction in uptake post-PRRT indicated treatment response and is associated with favorable outcome (see **Fig 6**).

### *Case 6*

A 55-year-old man with initial presentation of abdominal lump and CT abdomen finding of a solid cystic lesion in the peripancreatic region with multiple hypodense lesions in the liver had

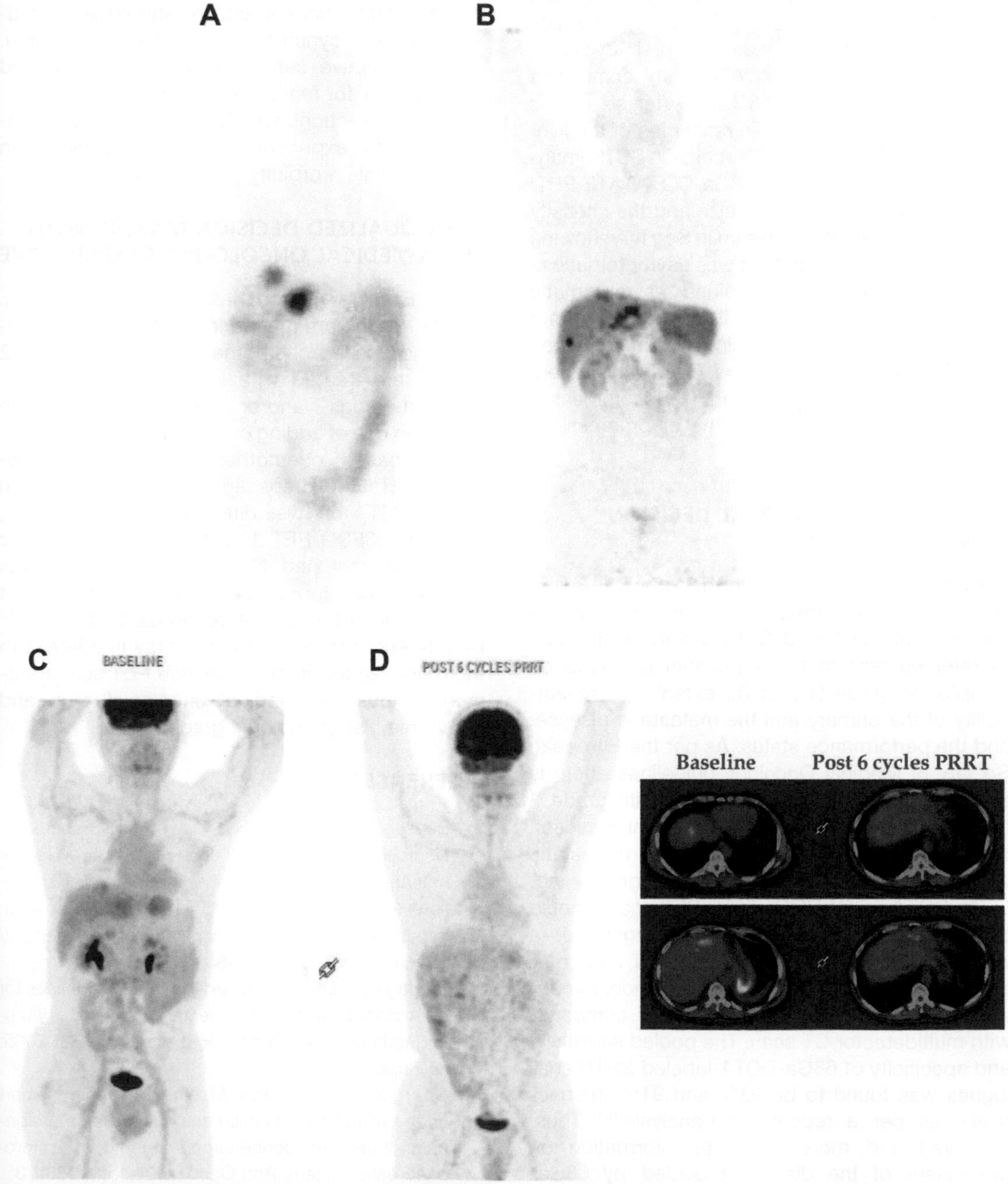


**Fig. 6.** Treatment response assessment in well-differentiated FDG-positive. First posttherapy 177Lu-DOATATE (*A*), post sixth cycle PRRT 68Ga-DOTATATE (*B*), baseline FDG-PET/CT (*C*), and post six cycles FDG-PET/CT (*D*).

undergone surgical excision of pancreatic mass (see **Fig. 6**). Histopathology of the peripancreatic mass revealed it as a well-differentiated NET. CT at 3 years postsurgery showed multiple enhancing lesions in liver with subsequent biopsy showing them as metastatic well-differentiated NET. The patient had undergone three cycles of chemotherapy with cisplatin and etoposide before being referred for PRRT. 99mTc-HYNIC TOC scan was done, which showed multiple SSTR-expressing lesions in the liver. Some of the lesions were FDG concentrating on 18F FDG-PET/CT scan. The patient was treated subsequently with six cycles of PRRT with 177Lu-DOTATATE with cumulative dose being 800 mCi (29.6GBq). After six cycles there is complete metabolic resolution of the liver lesions on 18F FDG-PET/CT scan. On SSTR imaging post six cycles PRRT, 68Ga-DOTATATE PET/CT showed decrease in the size and the intensity of all the lesions with the lesion in Seg IVA showing central necrosis. The patient was asymptomatic at presentation and has remained asymptomatic during six cycles of PRRT. The patient's tumor marker (serum chromogranin A) has remained almost stable during the period. Overall the patient showed partial response on PET/CT commensurate with his favorable outcome of progression-free survival at 38 months.

## INDIVIDUALIZED SURGICAL DECISION MAKING WITH PET

Surgery is the only approach that offers cure and is thus the preferred option for any patient who presents with a GEP-NET.[5] However, the decision to offer surgery to these patients is based on symptoms, grade (1/2 or 3), extent and resectability of the primary and the metastatic disease, and the performance status. As per the European Society of Medical Oncology guidelines, there is a general agreement that patients with grade 3 tumors should not be offered surgical resection because these tumors are already metastatic at the time of diagnosis. SSTR scintigraphy (eg, 68Ga-DOTA-TOC/-NOC/-TATE PET scan) should be included in the preoperative staging for a well-differentiated (grade 1 and 2) NET and complements the conventional cross-sectional imaging. It offers a higher sensitivity when compared with multidetector CT scan. The pooled sensitivity and specificity of 68Ga-DOTA-labeled SSTR analogues was found to be 93% and 91%, respectively, as per a recent meta-analysis.[6,7] Thus, improved and more complete information on the extent of the disease provided by 68Ga-DOTA-SSTR analogue PET/CT can help to make a decision in a multidisciplinary setting.

The guiding principles for deciding on surgical resection for a GEP-NET are as follows:

1. The primary (well-differentiated) should be resected even in the presence of liver metastases. The indolent nature of these tumors can allow the primary to lead to debility in the form of mesenteric fibrosis; bowel obstruction in case of a small intestinal primary; and obstructive jaundice, bowel obstruction, and gastrointestinal bleeding in case of a pancreatic primary.
2. Resectable liver metastases should be considered for a synchronous or staged resection. Cytoreductive surgery should be considered especially for functional tumors.
3. These resections should be performed in centers with experience so as to provide an acceptable morbidity and mortality.

## INDIVIDUALIZED DECISION MAKING WITH PET: A MEDICAL ONCOLOGIST'S PERSPECTIVE

GEP-NETs are treated based on differentiation. Grade 3 tumors respond well to platinum-etoposide-based chemotherapy.[8] Grade 1 and 2 tumors are treated with long-acting octreotide, targeted drugs, and/or PRRT.[9] There is an emerging role of adding capecitabine and temozolamide based chemotherapy in intermediate-grade NETs.[10] Octreoscan is more sensitive than 18FDG-PET for well-differentiated GEP-NETs, whereas 18FDG-PET has higher sensitivity for poorly differentiated NETs.[11] Histologic grades based on the biopsy from a single site may not correlate with the overall response to therapy.[12] Dedifferentiation of the tumors may interfere with the response to therapy.[12] Hence PET scan treatment guides the medical oncologist over and above the histopathologic grade.

## REFERENCES

1. Benson AB, Myerson RJ, Sasson AR. Pancreatic, Neuroendocrine GI, and adrenal cancers. Cancer management: a multidisciplinary approach. 13th edition. 2010. ISBN 978-0-615-41824-7. Available at: http://www.cancernetwork.com/cancer-management/pancreatic/article/10165/1802606.
2. Ramage JK, Davies AH, Ardill J, et al. Guidelines for the management of gastroenteropancreatic neuroendocrine (including carcinoid) tumours. Gut 2005;54(Suppl 4):iv1–16.
3. Oberg K, Kvols L, Caplin M, et al. Consensus report on the use of somatostatin analogs for the management of neuroendocrine tumors of the gastroenteropancreatic system. Ann Oncol 2004;15(6):966–73.
4. Basu S, Sirohi B, Shrikhande SV. Dual tracer imaging approach in assessing tumor biology and

heterogeneity in neuroendocrine tumors: its correlation with tumor proliferation index and possible multifaceted implications for personalized clinical management decisions, with focus on PRRT. Eur J Nucl Med Mol Imaging 2014;41(8):1492–6.

5. Öberg K, Knigge U, Kwekkeboom D, et al, ESMO Guidelines Working Group. Neuroendocrine gastro-entero-pancreatic tumors: ESMO clinical practice guidelines for diagnosis, treatment and follow-up. Ann Oncol 2012;23(Suppl 7):vii124–30.
6. Kumar R, Sharma P, Garg P, et al. Role of (68)Ga-DOTATOC PET-CT in the diagnosis and staging of pancreatic neuroendocrine tumours. Eur Radiol 2011;21(11):2408–16.
7. Treglia G, Castaldi P, Rindi G, et al. Diagnostic performance of gallium-68 somatostatin receptor PET and PET/CT in patients with thoracic and gastroenteropancreatic neuroendocrine tumours: a meta-analysis. Endocrine 2012;42(1):80–7.
8. Sorbye H, Strosberg J, Baudin E, et al. Gastroenteropancreatic high-gradeneuroendocrine carcinoma. Cancer 2014;120(18):2814–23.
9. Alexandraki KI, Kaltsas G. Gastroenteropancreatic neuroendocrine tumors: new insights in the diagnosis and therapy. Endocrine 2012;41(1):40–52.
10. Fine RL, Gulati AP, Krantz BA, et al. Capecitabine and temozolomide (CAPTEM) for metastatic, well-differentiated neuroendocrine cancers: The Pancreas Center at Columbia University experience. Cancer Chemother Pharmacol 2013;71(3):663–70.
11. Squires MH, VolkanAdsay N, Schuster DM, et al. Octreoscan versus FDG-PET for neuroendocrine tumor staging: a biological approach. Ann Surg Oncol 2015;22(7):2295–301.
12. Moertel CG, Kvols LK, O'Connell MJ, et al. Treatment of neuroendocrine carcinomas with combined etoposide and cisplatin: evidence of major therapeutic activity in the anaplastic variants of these neoplasms. Cancer 1991;68:227–32.

# The Current and Evolving Role of PET in Personalized Management of Lung Cancer

Esther Mena, MD[a], Anusha Yanamadala, MD[a],
Gang Cheng, MD, PhD[b],
Rathan M. Subramaniam, MD, PhD, MPH[a,c,d,e,*]

## KEYWORDS

• PET/CT imaging • Genomics • Personalized medicine • Management • Lung cancer

## KEY POINTS

- Recent applications of molecular targeting agents for genomically defined lung cancer patients have brought a new, exciting approach in the response assessment of lung cancer.
- Future research directions will involve incorporation of molecular characteristics and next generation probes into new strategies to improve early tumor to enrich the target population.
- Targeted therapies have revolutionized the field of lung cancer; next steps involve strategies for using PET imaging to identify and manage secondary resistances.
- Newer generation inhibitors and/or combination strategies to inhibit multiple pathways may ultimately overcome the issue of acquired resistance.
- New strategies against previously elusive targets will most likely be developed, and PET tracers will be used to diagnose and assess therapy.

## INTRODUCTION

Lung cancer remains the leading cause of cancer-related mortality worldwide, accounting for about 1.6 million deaths yearly.[1] Despite significant advances in both diagnostic and therapeutic approaches, patients' prognosis remain poor, and only about 16% of patients will survive for at least 5 years after diagnosis, in the United States.[1] Owing to differing heterogeneous malignancy patterns and treatment strategies, lung cancer has historically been divided into 2 main types: small cell lung cancer and non–small cell-lung cancer (NSCLC). The predominant histology NSCLC accounts for 85% to 90% of all lung cancers, of which 40% are adenocarcinoma, approximately 25% to 30% are squamous cell carcinoma and approximately 10% to 15% are large cell carcinoma.[2] Regardless of histologic subtype, lung cancer is one of the most genomically diverse

Dr R.M. Subramaniam is a consultant to GE Health Care. He received research grants for clinical trials from Bayer HealthCare. Dr E. Mena is supported by NIBI/NIH grant under the award T32EB006351. Dr A. Yanamadala and Dr G. Cheng have nothing to disclose.

[a] Russell H. Morgan Department of Radiology and Radiological Sciences, Johns Hopkins School of Medicine, 601 North Caroline Street, Baltimore, MD 21287, USA; [b] Department of Radiology, Hospital of the University of Pennsylvania, 3400 Spruce Street, Philadelphia, PA 19104, USA; [c] Department of Oncology, Sidney Kimmel Comprehensive Cancer Centre, Johns Hopkins School of Medicine, 401 North Broadway, Baltimore, MD 21231, USA; [d] Armstrong Institute for Patient Safety & Quality, Johns Hopkins School of Medicine, 750 East Pratt Street, Baltimore, MD 21202, USA; [e] Department of Health Policy and Management, Johns Hopkins Bloomberg School of Public Health, Johns Hopkins University, 624 North Broadway, Baltimore, MD 21205, USA
* Corresponding author. Russell H. Morgan Department of Radiology and Radiological Sciences, Johns Hopkins School of Medicine, 601 North Caroline Street, JHOC 3235, Baltimore, MD 21287.
*E-mail address:* rsubram4@jhmi.edu

PET Clin 11 (2016) 243–259
http://dx.doi.org/10.1016/j.cpet.2016.02.010

and deranged of all cancers, creating tremendous challenges for both prevention and treatment strategies.[3]

In the era of personalized medicine, recent advances in molecular biology have elucidated molecular mechanisms of lung cancer development and progression. Understanding molecular carcinogenesis, pharmacogenomics, and individual genetic differences may help in tailoring therapeutic approaches on an individual-by-individual basis. This is well-illustrated in patients harboring specific molecular alterations, such as epidermal growth factor receptor (EGFR) mutations, that have yielded improved response rates with targeting EGFR therapies when compared with conventional chemotherapies,[4] whereas the use of these treatment agents in the general NSCLC as a standard therapy had not shown survival benefits,[5,6] which might be explained by disease heterogeneity between patients with regards to histology and molecular features.[7]

Molecular imaging can be used for early disease detection, characterization, and real-time monitoring of therapeutic responses, as well as for improving drug development. Imaging might be the key component in the assessment of treatment response and to define disease progression during conventional chemotherapy, molecular targeting therapy, and combination of therapies. This review summarizes the recent genomic discoveries in lung cancer and their implications for imaging, highlighting emerging techniques in molecular imaging and functional imaging, including 18F-fluorodeoxyglucose (FDG) PET and novel PET tracers designed to characterize the mechanism-specific and pathway-specific for treatment selection, and follow-up response assessment to therapy.

## MOLECULAR GENETICS IN LUNG CANCER: VALUE OF PET IMAGING

The molecular origins of lung cancer lie in complex interactions between the environment and host genetic susceptibility. Understanding of the role of genetics in lung cancer etiology could play a role in personalizing specific targeted therapies and oncogenic mutations, which could revolutionize clinical and treatment approaches.[8]

Tumor molecular heterogeneity is a major reason that patients with NSCLC with a similar clinical stage and tumor histology can dramatically differ from outcomes and responses to therapy.[9] EGFR and Rat Sarcoma (RAS) are the 2 most commonly mutated protooncogenes in adenocarcinoma of the lung; EGFR mutations had been found to be more common in nonsmoking adenocarcinoma patients with well-differentiated tumors, whereas RAS mutations tend to occur in smokers with poorly differentiated adenocarcinoma tumors.[10] These gene expression profiles are associated with reduced in recurrence-free or overall survival (OS) in different subtypes of NSCLC.[9] Therefore, gene mutation testing seems to have an important role in determining patient's eligibility for personalized treatment[11] (**Fig. 1**).

### *Tumor Heterogeneity*

It is fair to say that clinical medicine has always been personalized; as a physician, one has to take into consideration patients' age, body weight/body surface area, renal and hepatic function, and other factors when determining a dose. This is especially important in oncology owing to serious side effects of a treatment and severe consequence of treatment failure. The practice of pathologic classification of tumor subtypes and selection of treatment strategy based on pathologic findings is another example of personalized approach in clinical oncology.[12]

However, the importance of personalized medicine in cancer therapy has been more widely accepted in recent years, as we increasingly recognize that tumors, even of the same subtype, are different in different patients. The most important factor underlying personalized cancer treatment is the presence of significant tumor heterogeneity, which may affect treatment strategy and outcome. Tumor heterogeneity is present not only in different subtypes of a malignancy, but also within the same pathologic subtypes, in different tumor tissues within the same person, and even within the same tumor mass. Multiple environmental factors and cellular and molecular characteristics contribute to tumor heterogeneity, such as regional blood flow and angiogenesis, hypoxia, necrosis, cellular proliferation and growth rate, gene mutation, and expression of specific receptors. Tumor heterogeneity within histopathologically the same subtype of malignancy is referred to as *intratumoral heterogeneity*, to differentiate from tumor heterogeneity among histopathologically different tumors or tumor subtypes, that is, intertumoral heterogeneity.[13] For instance, it is a common clinical finding that FDG uptake varies markedly within the same tumor mass. Tumor metabolism also varies considerably in primary and metastatic sites in patients with lung cancer.[14] Intratumoral heterogeneity is constantly observed in various tumors[15–18] and with newer PET tracers.[19,20] Although intertumoral heterogeneity is well-known, we have very limited knowledge about intratumoral heterogeneity

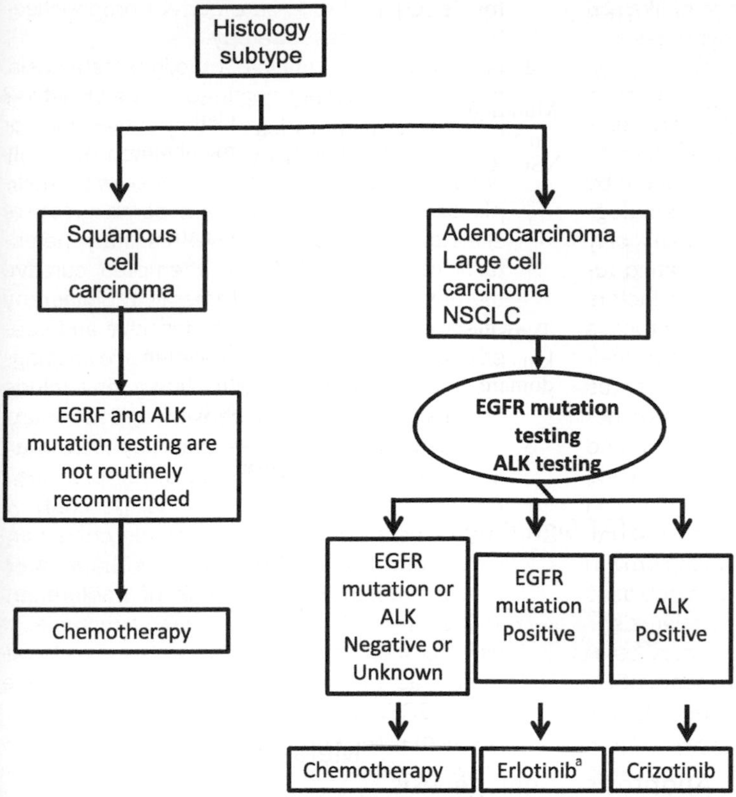


**Fig. 1.** Genomic-based approach for therapy decision in lung cancer. Tumors mutation testing plays an important role in identifying patients suitable for targeted abnormalities with effective agents and optimizing therapeutic approach in non–small cell lung cancer (NSCLC). [a] Erlotinib is recommended when *EGFR* mutation is discovered before first-line chemotherapy. If *EGFR* mutation is discovered during first-line chemotherapy, switching to maintenance erlotinib or adding erlotinib to current chemotherapy regimen is recommended; ALK, anaplastic lymphoma kinase; EGFR, epidermal growth factor receptor. (*Adapted from* Nishino M, Hatabu H, Johnson BE, et al. State of the art: response assessment in lung cancer in the era of genomic medicine. Radiology 2014;271(1):9.)

because it is more difficult to evaluate. Even a small subpopulation of tumor cells with different genetic or phenotypic characteristics may cause eventual treatment failure, because the outcome of a treatment is determined not by a cell subpopulation that is most susceptible to the therapy, but by a cell subpopulation that is least susceptible to the therapy. In fact, tumor heterogeneity is an important factor implicated in treatment failure, greater chance of metastasis, and OS.[21]

In recent years, we have seen the most spectacular advances in the field of tumor genomics, including mutational status and deregulated pathways in multiple malignancies, which has been shown as a very promising and powerful tool in delineating "personalized" characteristics of a malignancy, thus to improve treatment and prognosis in patients with cancer. At the same time, imaging studies have contributed significantly to our knowledge of tumor heterogeneity. In recent years, texture analysis in the medical imaging community has established strong correlation between image features and tumor heterogeneity, for either CT[22,23] or PET.[24–27] For instance, tumor heterogeneity in NSCLC, as assessed by CT texture analysis, offers a novel independent predictor of survival for NSCLC.[22] FDG PET may provide functional information of tumor heterogeneity. In addition to the maximum ($SUV_{max}$) and mean ($SUV_{mean}$) standardized uptake value, textural parameters in PET images also include other metabolic parameters such as metabolic tumor volume (MTV), total lesion glycolysis (TLG; MTV $\times$ $SUV_{mean}$). These volume-based parameters may provide more accurate assessment of the tumor burden and better prognostic value than $SUV_{max}$ for NSCLC.[24,27,28] In addition, the larger tumor size is associated with higher tumor heterogeneity.[27] However, it is difficult to correlate texture analysis with biological features of a malignancy, and current imaging studies are still not able to provide optimal characterization of tumor heterogeneity to guide effective therapeutic interventions.

## *Epidermal Growth Factor Receptor Mutation in Non–Small Cell Lung Cancer*

The EGFR is a transmembrane tyrosine kinase receptor involved in signaling cells pathways, which regulates tumorigenic processes, including cancer-cell proliferation, apoptosis, tumor-induced neoangiogenesis, and tumor invasion[29] (**Fig. 2**). EGFR amplification is associated with development of disease progression, and shortened survival in patients with NSCLC.[30] EGFR

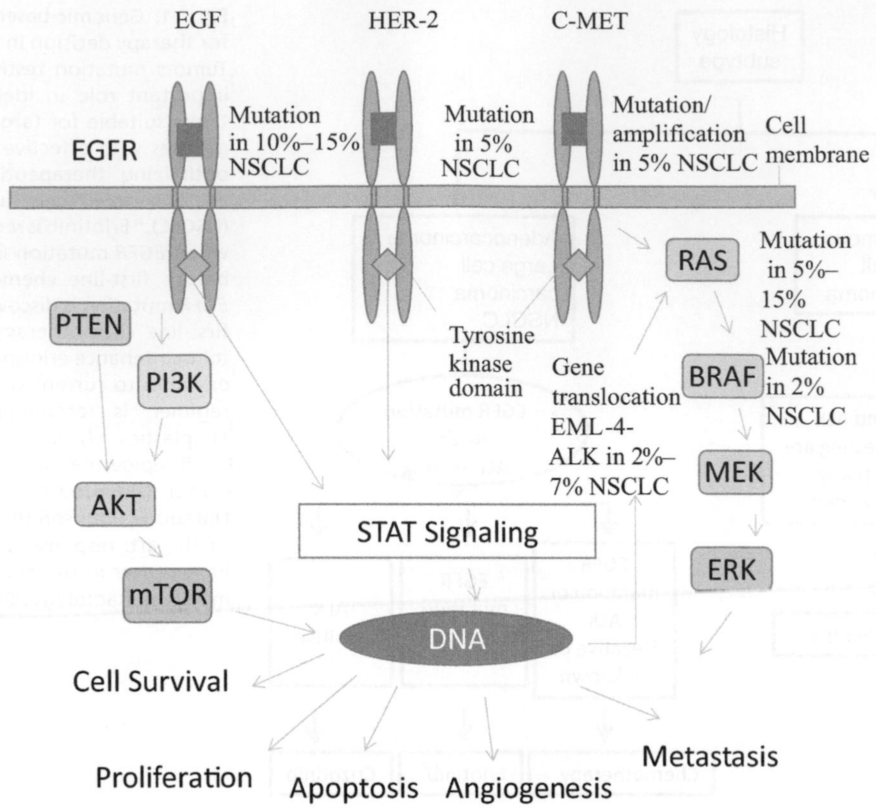


**Fig. 2.** Epidermal growth factor receptor (EGFR) pathway in non–small cell lung cancer (NSCLC). EGFR include Epidermal growth factor (EGF), human epidermal growth factor receptor (HER)-2, and mesenchymal–epithelial transition factor (C-MET). MAPK –Mitogen activated protein kinases/ERK-extracellular signal regulated kinases: Ras-Raf-MEK-ERK pathway. Mutations or overexpression of growth factors receptors such as EGFR, HER-2 and C-MET are most frequent in NSCLC tumors from nonsmokers patients. EML4/ALK fusion gene is associated to NSCLC from young and nonsmoking patients. KRAS mutations and signaling pathway depending to KRAS are most frequent in smoker patients. PI3K signaling pathway modifications are most frequently observed in squamous cell carcinomas.

mutations have found to be present in 10% of specimens from lung adenocarcinoma patients from the United States and, in about 30% to 50% of tumors from Asian patients,[31,32] and are more common in female gender, never-smokers, and well-differentiated adenocarcinoma histology.[10]

The presence of activating EGFR mutations has proven to be relevant for patient stratification for drug treatment. Recently, small-molecule tyrosine kinase inhibitors (TKIs) of the EGFR domain, have been developed and approved to treat patients with advanced stage EGFR-mutant NSCLC: erlotinib (Tarceva, Genentech, South San Francisco, CA) and gefitinib (Iressa, AstraZeneca, London, UK).[33,34] Several subtypes of EGFR mutations, such as exon 19 deletions or L858R point mutation in exon 21, seem to be associated with response to EFGR-thymidine kinase 1 therapy, and hence, are considered "sensitizing mutations," whereas exon 20 insertions seem to account for resistant and lack of response to EGFR inhibitors.[35] According to the recent American Society of Clinical Oncology recommendations, EGFR mutation should be tested for NSCLC patients to assess whether chemotherapy or an EGFR TKI is the appropriate first-line therapy.[32] NSCLC patients treated with gefitinib and erlotinib have demonstrated significant higher response rates (>70%) and improved progression-free survival (PFS) ranging from 9.7 to 13.1 months, when compared with conventional chemotherapy (carboplatin–paclitaxel).[4,36] Furthermore, EGFR messenger RNA expression has been found to be an important predictive factor of response to TKIs like gefitinib and patients with more number of copies of EGFR genes are more likely to have better OS rates after treatment with TKIs.[37–40]

The association between the presence of EGFR mutation in NSCLC and the remarkable response to therapy with TKI therapy led to the investigation of whether noninvasive functional PET imaging could play a role in predicting EGFR mutation. However, contradictory publications have been reported in this setting. Earlier studies reported a significant association between tumor FDG uptake and EFGR mutation status, with opposite direction of associations. Na and colleagues[39] stated that the $SUV_{max}$ was lower in the EGFR mutant group than in the wild-type group, whereas Huang and colleagues[40] reported that higher $SUV_{max}$ values in the EGFR mutant group. Subsequently, 2 larger cohorts studies by Lee and colleagues[41] and Mak and colleagues[42] with 206 and 100 NSCLC patients, respectively, stated that the $SUV_{max}$ was lower in the EGFR mutation group compared with the wild-type group. The $SUV_{max}$ was found to be an important and independent predictor of EGFR mutations in lung cancer in 71 patients with stage IV lung adenocarcinoma.[43] However, in the largest sample size series, the results suggested that FDG avidity in NSCLC had no significant clinical value in predicting EGFR mutation status. In addition, there was no significant difference in FDG uptake between the genotypes of EGFR mutation known to be associated with a poorer prognosis and those associated with a better prognosis.[41]

## *Kras Mutation: Value of PET Imaging*

KRAS mutations represent the most common molecular change in NSCLC, being identified in about 20% to 25% of lung adenocarcinoma tumor samples.[44] The presence of a RAS mutation has been shown to be associated with a poor prognosis for K-RAS mutant compared with wild-type mutations for specific studies in lung adenocarcinoma.[45,46] Clinical trials have shown that KRAS mutations seem to be correlated with primary resistance to TKI agents and NSCLC patients harboring KRAS gene mutations have decreased response to TKIs.[47,48] Hence, the topic of growing interest in concerning targeted therapy for NSCLC is to identify the EGFR and KRAS status for selecting patients who benefit from EGFR inhibitors.

At present, EGFR mutational status assessment is the preferred test for selecting patients for EGFR TKI therapy and, although recent studies do not support the routine use of determining KRAS mutation in assessing treatment response in lung cancer patients,[45] it has been suggested that testing for KRAS could have a role because presence of KRAS mutation excludes the presence of other molecular abnormalities such as ROS1 and anaplastic lymphoma kinase (ALK) rearrangements.[45] Furthermore, there are also intense efforts to develop new drugs that target mutant and new therapeutic agents for Kras mutant.[45,49]

It has been reported recently that either genotype of mutant KRAS-Gly12Cys or mutant KRAS-Gly12Val is associated with a worse prognosis compared with other mutant KRAS-type or wild-type groups. However, Lee and colleagues[41] did not find any significant differences of FDG avidity between groups. Caicedo and colleagues[50] found no difference in FDG uptake between the EGFR-positive and EGFR-negative groups in a cohort of 102 patients with stage III or IV NSCLC; in contrast, a significantly greater FDG uptake was found in KRAS-positive patients than in KRAS-negative patients.

In a retrospectively study of 93 stage IV NSCLC patients with known EGFR and KRAS mutant status, Brady and colleagues[51] reported that patients with mutations of the KRAS gene were not associated with decreased OS or PFS when offered treatment with standard chemotherapy. By contrast, in a larger metaanalysis including 17 studies and 1008 patients, 168 of them with KRAS mutation, Linardou and colleagues[47] reported significant association between the presence of KRAS mutation and the absence response to TKIs, with a sensitivity and specificity of 21% and 94%, respectively. KRAS mutations were highly specific negative predictors of treatment response to EGFR TKIs in advanced NSCLC.

PET imaging in this regard is useful and has been shown to be effective in determining the Kras and EGFR status. Caicedo and colleagues[50] assessed the association of FDG-PET parameters with KRAS and EGFR mutation status in 102 patients with stage III or IV NSCLC. Tumors with Kras mutation were found to have significantly greater uptake on FDG-PET than with EGFR or a wild-type mutation with no Kras mutation specimens. In a multivariate analysis, FDG-PET was shown to have a sensitivity and specificity of 78.6% and 62.2%, respectively, with area under the curve of 0.77 for identifying Kras mutant status in lung cancer patients; the $SUV_{mean}$ seemed to be a reliable predictor of Kras status in lung cancer patients. EGFR and KRAS gene status in paired NSCLC and metastatic tumors had been investigated by many studies, but remained controversial. Wang and Wang[48] performed a metaanalysis to determine the role of EGFR and KRAS mutations in primary and corresponding metastatic tumors of NSCLC. The discordant rates of EGFR and KRAS mutations in paired primary and metastatic NSCLC were found to be 14.5% and 16.7%, respectively. The frequency of occurrence of mutation was not shown to be different from the frequency of loss of mutation for EGFR (*P* = .093) and KRAS gene (*P* = .227). EGFR and KRAS mutations were found to be present at increased frequency in metastases and even before the occurrence of metastasis. Therefore, routine analysis of EGFR or KRAS gene status was not feasible in both primary and metastatic tumors.[52] Therefore, the utility of determining KRAS mutational status to predict clinical benefit to anti-EGFR therapies remains unclear in patients with NSCLC. The future implications of testing for KRAS mutational status can be to exclude the possibility of an EGFR mutation or to identify the group of patients with NSCLC in whom to implement a drug development strategy that targets the KRAS molecular pathway (**Fig. 3**).

### *Anaplastic lymphoma kinase and ROS-1 mutations*

Other new genomic abnormalities have been discovered and studied to develop targeting therapeutic agents in NSCLC. Chromosomal inversion results in fusion of the echinoderm microtubule-associated protein-like 4 (ELM4) gene with the ALK gene in about 2% to 7% of the NSCLC population. This was described initially in Japanese patients with adenocarcinoma of the lung,[53,54] and has been shown to be more prevalent in younger patients, women, never or light smokers, and with adenocarcinoma histology. Additionally, approximately 1% to 2% of patients with NSCLC present with tumors with genetic rearrangements involving the protooncogene receptor tyrosine kinase ROS1, which represent another specific disease subtype. On these patient groups, treatment with crizotinib (Xalkori, Pfizer, New York, NY), an adenosine triphosphate-competitive inhibitor of ALK receptor tyrosine kinase, has yielded promising efficacy results. In a large phase III clinical trial, including 347 patients with advanced-stage ALK-positive NSCLC, crizotinib resulted in higher response rates of up to 65% compared with the standard treatment with pemetrexed or docetaxel.[55] Likewise, in a clinical phase I trial Shaw and colleagues[56] reported response rates with crizotinib treatment of 72% in 50 patients with ROS1-positive NSCLC. To date, no published studies have visualized molecular ELM4–ALK or ROS1 targets using PET imaging. Radiolabeling inhibitors of NSCLC-associated fusion proteins, such as crizotinib, could enable PET-based quantification of the therapeutic targets that might improve treatment stratification, response rates, and outcomes.

## PET IMAGING IN ASSESSING RESPONSE TO THERAPY

Tumor response assessment has a foundation for advances in cancer therapy. Because of the increased use of effective molecular targeting therapy for specific genomic abnormalities in

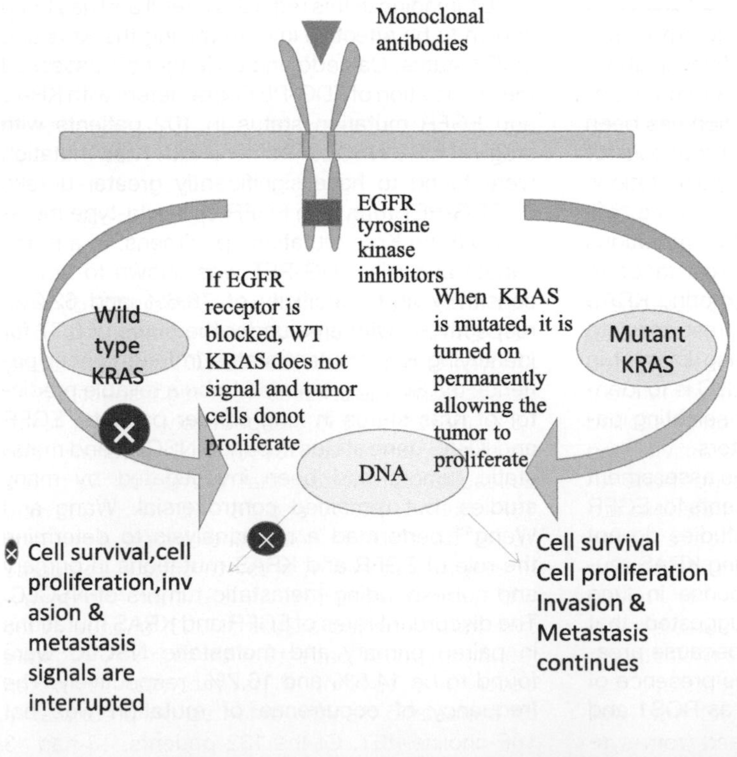


**Fig. 3.** Diagram of signaling pathways reviewing the underling effects of epidermal growth factor receptor (EGFR)-specific monoclonal antibodies (ie, cetuximab and panitumumab), and their role in antitumor response.

NSCLC patients, recent investigations have attempted to address the utility of FDG-PET in quantifying metabolic response of tumors to targeted therapy[57] (**Figs. 4–6**). This is summarized in **Table 1**. Several prospective studies had been conducted to assess the predictive value of FDG-PET in assessing PFS and OS in NSCLC patients treated with targeted therapies, such as TKI. Kahraman and colleagues[58] and de Langen and colleagues[59] prospectively assessed the value of PET in predicting PFS benefit from TKI in 30 and 40 NSCLC patients, respectively. A decrease in SUV of greater than 30% by 1 week and greater than 20% by 3 weeks after therapy was related with longer PFS ($P$ = .003 and $P$ = .01, respectively) and FDG-PET was able to identify patients who benefit from TKI treatment and allow earlier response evaluation than conventional methods. Dingemans and colleagues[60] prospectively studied 40 patients with stage IIIb or IV NSCLC, assessing treatment response to erlotinib and bevacizumab, supporting that a decrease of 20% in SUV at 3 weeks after treatment predicted longer PFS (9.7 vs 2.8 months; $P$ = .01). Investigators concluded that early response evaluation with FDG-PET imaging was the best predictive test for PFS. The presence of KRAS (n = 10) or EGFR mutations (n = 5) did not influence patients' outcome.

Kobe and colleagues[61] retrospectively reviewed 30 patients with stage IV NSCLC using FDG and $^{18}$F-fluorothymidine (FLT) PET at 1 and 6 weeks after starting erlotinib treatment. The investigators reported that patients with lower early and late residual FLT and FDG tumor uptake after 6 weeks of therapy were associated with prolonged PFS compared with patients with higher residual tumor FLT and FDG uptake (282 vs 118 days; $P$ = .022).[62] Bengtsson and colleagues[62] evaluated the predictive value of FDG-PET for OS in 125 lung cancer patients treated with erlotinib, reporting that presence of new lesions at 2 weeks after therapy was a significant predictive factor, and may potential surrogate biomarker for OS in NSCLC.[63,64]

In a multicenter prospective trial including 51 NSCLC patients treated with second- and third-line erlotinib, Mileshkin and colleagues[63] concluded that patients with early metabolic partial response, with a decrease in $SUV_{max}$ of 15% or greater had associated improved PFS (5.5 vs 25 months) and OS (11.6 vs 7.6 months) compared with nonresponders. Another study with 22 patients with NSCLC treated with erlotinib showed that patients without metabolic response in the early follow-up PET had shorter PFS (47 vs 119 days; $P$<.001) and shorter OS (87 vs 828 days; $P$ = .01) than patients with metabolic response, with a decrease of greater than 30% in SUV. Therefore, FDG PET/CT performed early in the treatment assessment of TKI could help to identify patients who can benefit from this targeted therapy. In a phase II study with 38 patients with stage IIIB and IV NSCLC treated with erlotinib, O'Brien and colleagues[65] prospectively assessed whether FDG-PET/CT could identify the nonresponding patients and minimize the time of exposure to erlotinib. FDG-PET/CT was able to identify the nonresponders as early as 6 weeks after starting treatment and treatment could have been stopped early on the basis of the FDG PET/CT scan results, which could avoid unnecessary exposure to ineffective treatment.[65] Aukema and colleagues[66] also evaluated the role of integrated FDG-PET/CT for the early identification of response to erlotinib, comparing the metabolic response, that is, a decrease of 25% or greater in SUV, with the pathologic response, obtained by histopathologic examination. FDG-PET/CT could predict response to TKI as early as 1 week after initiating the treatment.

There are wide variations of the measured FDG-PET parameters and the metabolic tumor response criteria between existing publications. In addition, most studies accrued patients based on clinical factors, instead of selecting patients based on the specific genomic abnormalities known to be sensitive to EGFR TKIs. Even the studies performed on *EGFR* mutation testing had a small fraction of patients with *EGFR* mutation (see **Table 1**). Because *EGFR* mutation testing is recommended for NSCLC patients, who are being considered for first-line EGFR TKI therapy, investigation of the role of FDG PET in response assessment should be carried out in specific genomically defined patients,[32] enriching the target population.

## BEYOND $^{18}$F-FLUORODEOXYGLUCOSE PET: FUNCTIONAL AND MOLECULAR IMAGING WITH NOVEL PET TRACERS

Although $^{18}$F-FDG is the most commonly used PET tracer in the routine oncology imaging, there is an increasing interest for testing novel PET tracers to address biological tumor behavior beyond glucose metabolism, including targeting molecules, cell proliferation, hypoxia, and angiogenesis. In this section, we review some of the applications of these novel PET tracers, focusing on lung cancer management.

### *Imaging of Molecular Targets*

Molecularly targeted agents could provide clinical benefits in NSCLC patients with specific molecular

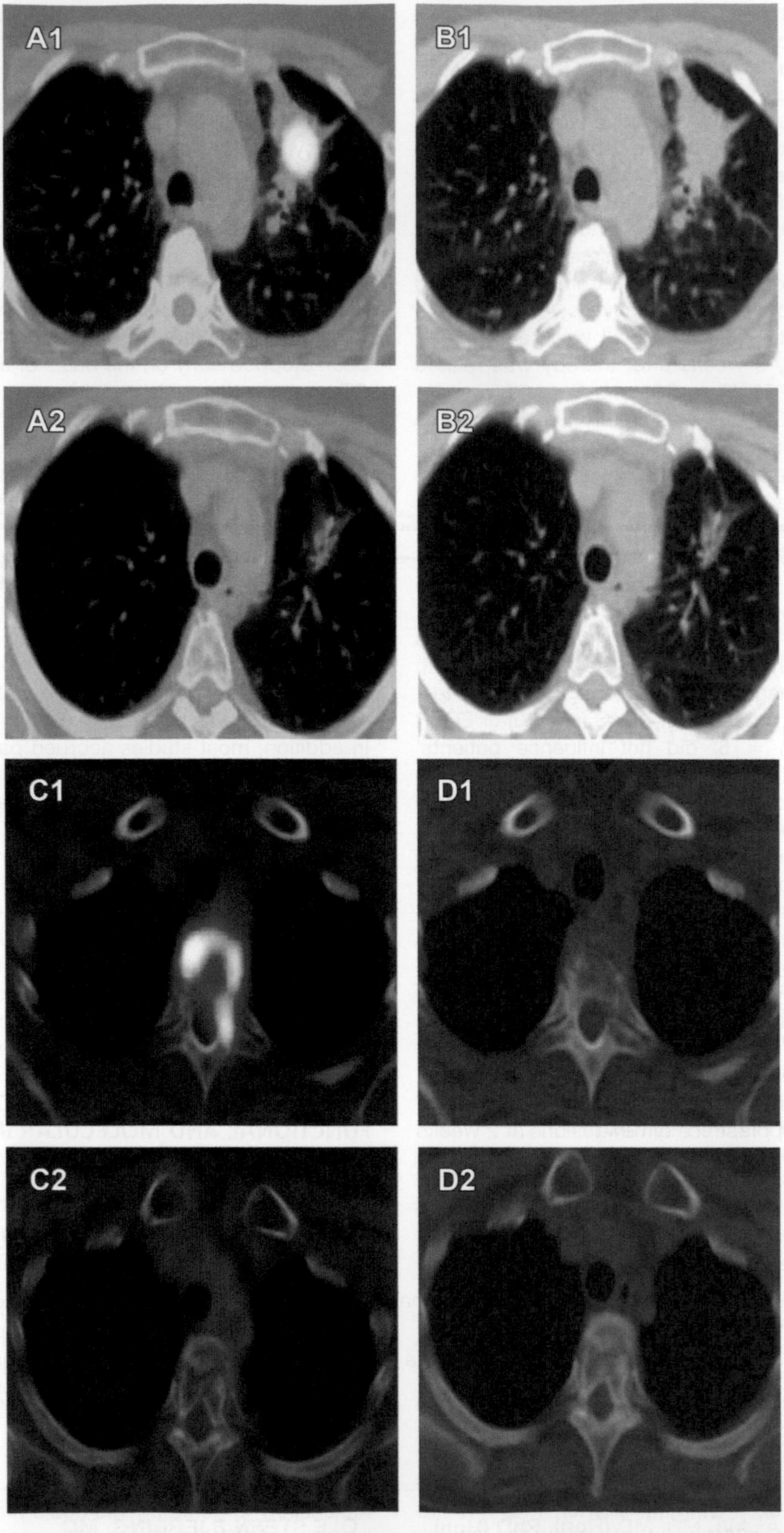
A1
B1
A2
B2
C1
D1
C2
D2

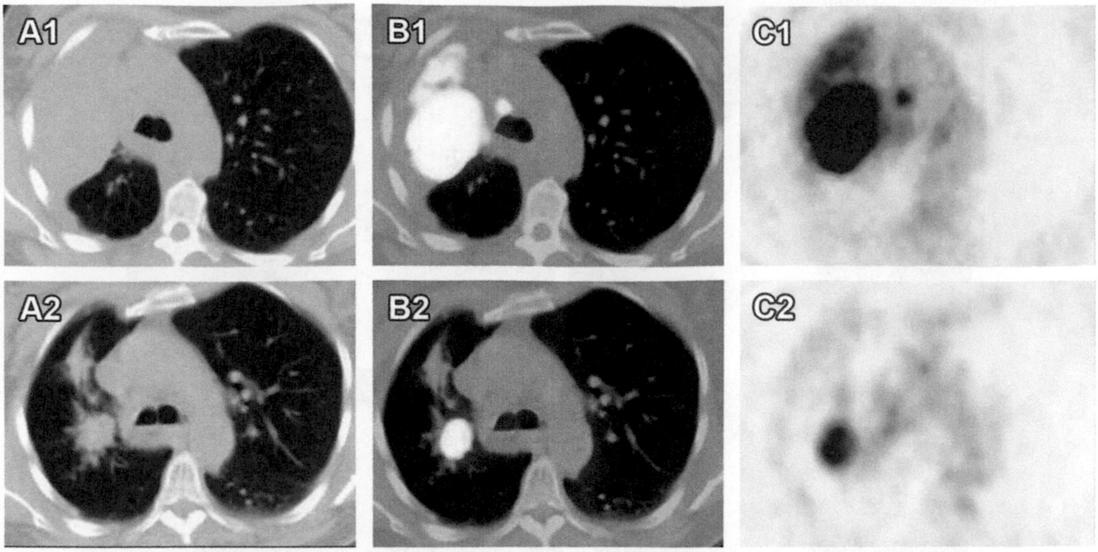


**Fig. 5.** A 58-year-old woman with a history of negative epidermal growth factor receptor (EGFR) and KRAS mutations T4N2M0, stage IIIB right upper lung lobe moderate to poorly differentiated adenocarcinoma. Baseline computed tomography (CT; *A1*), fused PET/CT (*B1*), and PET (*C1*) images demonstrated an intense hypermetabolic activity fusing to a large lung mass (maximum standardized uptake value [$SUV_{max}$], 12.6) within the right upper lobe associated with collapse of the right middle and upper lobe, and an $^{18}$F-fluorodeoxyglucose (FDG)-avid mediastinal node. After receiving chemotherapy with chemotherapy with pemetrexed and carboplatin, CT (*A2*), fused PET/CT (*B2*), and PET (*C2*) images demonstrated partial metabolic tumor response ($SUV_{max}$, 5.5) The patient received subsequent radiotherapy to the lung and she remains free of disease 2 years after treatment.

features or particular mutations. Using PET imaging based on radiolabeling monoclonal antibodies or small antibody fragments (immunoPET), or small-molecule inhibitors (TKI PET) that target this protein could aid to visualize tumor EGFR expression. ImmunoPET approaches to image EGFR expression have been investigated in several malignancies by using radiolabeled monoclonal antibodies, such as 89Zr-cetuximab and 89Zr-panitumumab,[67] and these studies remain under clinical trials. Challenges related to immunoPET approaches include unfavorable pharmacokinetics, owing to the relatively slow clearance of these radiotracers from the blood, and high physiologic uptake within the liver and kidneys.[67] The approach of labeling an EGFR receptor as drug therapy using PET was assessed by Memon and colleagues[68] in patients with NSCLC reporting that 11C-erlotinib could differentiate responders from nonresponders to erlotinib therapy. Meng and colleagues[69] assessed patients with advanced NSCLC of adenocarcinoma or squamous histology by using 11C-PD153035, an EGFR TKI analog PET imaging biomarker, which was able identify patients who were likely to respond to erlotinib treatment based on the uptake of 11C-PD153035 at the baseline scan.

## *Assessing Cell Proliferation*

DNA synthesis is a direct indicator of cellular proliferation, which can be measured using radiolabeled thymidine or its analog PET tracers. The most extensively studied PET tracer to image tumor proliferation is FLT, an analog of thymidine that gets phosphorylated by thymidine kinase 1,

**Fig. 4.** A 66-year-old woman with a history of epidermal growth factor receptor (EGFR) mutation (+) left upper lung lobe well-differentiated adenocarcinoma with osteolytic bony lesions at diagnosis. Baseline fused PET/computed tomography (CT; *A1*) scan and CT scan (*B1*) images demonstrated an intense hypermetabolic activity fusing to a 5 × 3-cm spiculated lung mass within the left upper lobe (maximum standardized uptake value [$SUV_{max}$], 4.6) with an intense $^{18}$F-fluorodeoxyglucose (FDG)-avid destructive bony lytic lesion in T3 vertebra body, seen in the fused PET/CT (*C1*) and CT (*D1*) images. After receiving combination of treatment with erlotinib plus bevacizumab and radiation therapy to the vertebra mass, posttreatment PET/CT scan demonstrated minimal linear FDG avidity within the left upper lobe ($SUV_{max}$ of 1.5; *A2, B2*), most likely inflammatory and complete metabolic response within the vertebra body (*C2, D2*).

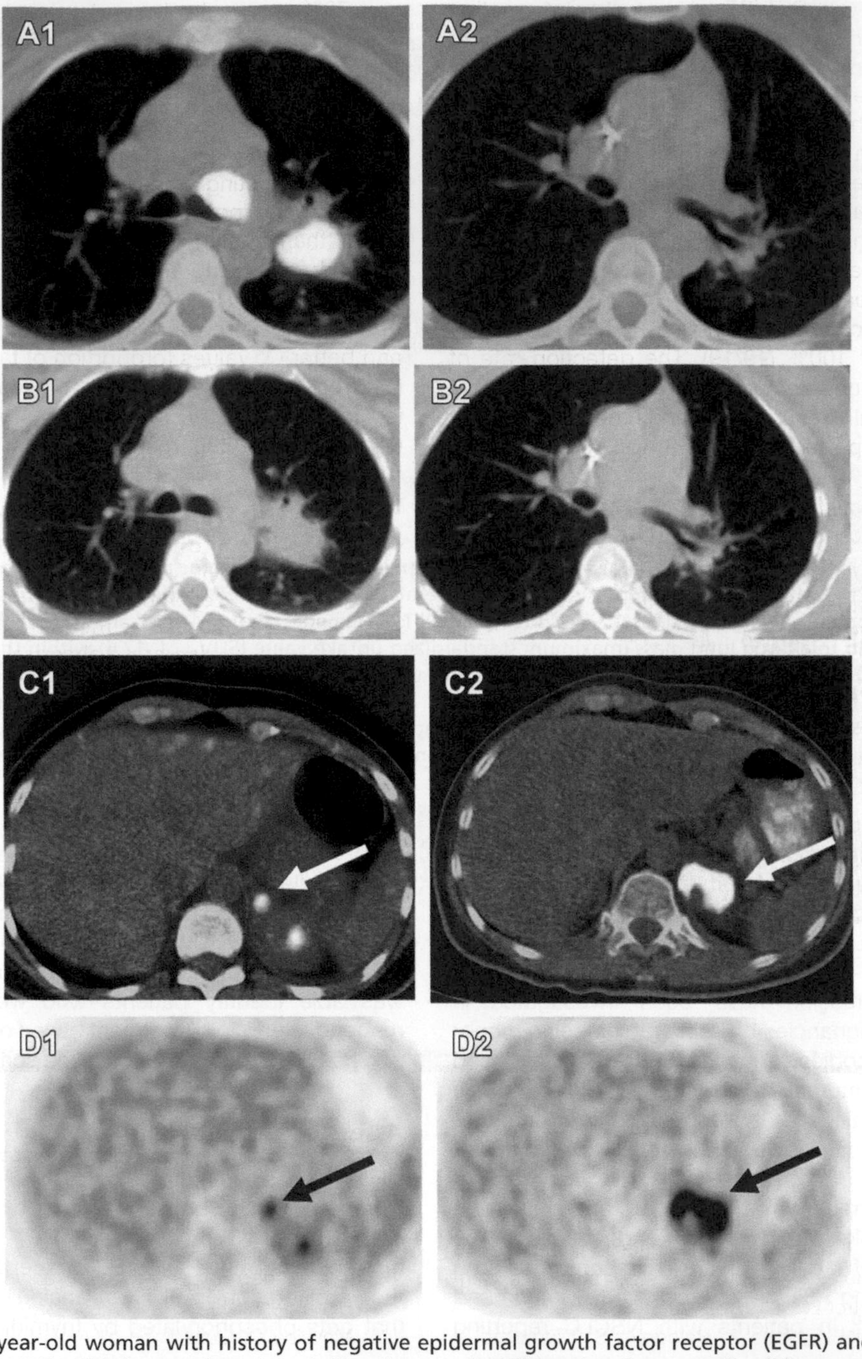


**Fig. 6.** A 52-year-old woman with history of negative epidermal growth factor receptor (EGFR) and ALK mutations, stage IV (T2bN2) left upper lung lobe infiltrating poorly differentiated non–small cell lung cancer (NSCLC). Baseline fused PET/computed tomography (*CT*; *A1*) and CT (*B1*) images demonstrated an intense hypermetabolic activity fusing to a left upper lung mass (maximum standardized uptake value [$SUV_{max}$], 10.4), and intense FDG-avid large anteroposterior window lymphadenopathy. Fused PET/CT (*C1*) and PET (*D1*) images at baseline also showed a small FDG-avid focus within the left adrenal gland ($SUV_{max}$, 2.8) concerning for a metastatic lesion (*arrow*). After receiving chemotherapy with paclitaxel and carboplatinum with associated radiation therapy to the lung, fused PET/CT (*A2*), and CT (*B2*) images demonstrated complete metabolic tumor response with the lung and mediastinum. However, there is interval metabolic progression of the left adrenal mass ($SUV_{max}$, 4.9), as seen in the fused PET/CT (*C2*) and PET (*D2*) images (*arrow*), which was proven by biopsy to be a metastasis. Patient received subsequent radiotherapy to the adrenal mass, and another 4 cycles of cisplatin and docetaxel with good partial response.

**Table 1**
**Prospective and retrospective studies evaluating $^{18}$F-FDG-PET imaging for therapeutic response and clinical outcome in NSCLC patients treated with EGFR-TKI**

| Study and Year | Design | No of Patients | EGFR Mutation | Anticancer Drugs | Criteria for PET Response | Outcome | HR and *P* Value |
|---|---|---|---|---|---|---|---|
| Bengtsson et al,[62] 2012 | Prospective | 125 | Tested (10/100) | Erlotinib | Presence/absence of new lesion at PET at 2 wk | OS | HR, NR; $P<4.4 \times 10^{-4}$ |
| Kahraman et al,[58] 2011 | Prospective | 30 | Tested (5/23) | Erlotinib | Reduction of 30% $SUV_{max}$ at 1 wk after treatment | PFS | HR, NR; *P* = .003 |
| Kobe et al,[61] 2012 | Retrospective | 30 | — | Erlotinib | ROC analysis of progression/ nonprogression at 6 wk | PFS (282 vs 118 d) | *P* = .022 |
| Mileshkin et al,[63] 2011 | Prospective | 51 | Tested (4/35) | Erlotinib | 15% reduction in $SUV_{max}$ at days 14 and 56 | PFS<br>OS | HR, 0.28; *P* = .001 (day 14)<br>HR, 0.32; *P* = .01 (day 56)<br>HR, 0.44; *P* = .03 (day 14)<br>HR, 0.49; *P* = .13 (day 56) |
| de Langen et al,[59] 2011 | Prospective | 40 | NR | Bevacizumab and erlotinib | 20% reduction in SUV at 3 wk | PFS (9.7 vs 2.8 mo) | HR, 0.38; *P* = .01 |
| Benz et al,[64] 2011 | Prospective | 22 | Tested (4/5) | Erlotinib | 30% reduction $SUV_{max}$ at 2 wk by PERCIST criteria. | PFS (47 vs 119 d)<br>OS (87 vs 828 d) | HR, NR; *P*<.001<br>HR, NR; *P* = .01 |
| Dingemans et al,[60] 2011 | Prospective | 40 | Tested (5/24) | Erlotinib and bevacizumab | 20% decrease in SUV at 3 wk | PFS | HR, NR; *P* = .01 |
| O'Brien et al,[65] 2012 | Prospective | 38 | Tested (34/47) | Erlotinib | 25% decrease in the mean weighted SUV at 6 wk | OS | HR, NR; *P* = .0021 |
| Aukema et al,[66] 2010 | Prospective | 23 | NR | Erlotinib | >25% reduction in SUV after 1 wk | Predict treatment response | Responders: >25% reduction<br>Nonresponders: <25% reduction |
| Zander et al,[73] 2011 | Prospective | 34 | Tested (4/28) | Erlotinib | 30% decrease in peak SUV at 1 wk | PFS<br>OS | HR, 0.23; *P* = .002<br>HR, 0.36; *P* = .04 |

*Abbreviations:* EGFR, epidermal growth factor receptor; HR, hazard ratio; PFS, progression-free survival; ROC, receiver operating characteristic; $SUV_{max}$, maximum standardized uptake value.

the key enzyme of the salvage pathway of DNA synthesis.[70] Indeed, intratumoral $^{18}$F-FLT uptake is strongly correlated with in vitro measurements of proliferation in biopsy specimens.[71] Because uptake of FLT depends on cell proliferation, it may be useful for assessing anticancer activity of cytostatic molecular targeting agents. In preclinical models, Sohn and colleagues[72] evaluated the usefulness of FLT PET at 7 days after gefitinib therapy in 28 nonsmoking patients with stage IV NSCLC. FLT PET imaging was able to predict response to gefinitib by using a decrease of greater than 10.9% in $SUV_{max}$ as a criterion for predicting response, which was associated with longer time to progression in responders as compared with nonresponders (7.9 vs 1.2 months; $P = .004$).[72,73] Similarly, Zander and colleagues[73] concluded that FLT scans after 1 week of erlotinib therapy were able to predict significantly prolonged PFS (hazard ratio [HR], 0.31; $P = .04$) in NSCLC patients. Likewise, in erlotinib-treated NSCLC patients, early PET FDG and FLT at 14 days for treatment showed a partial metabolic response, which positively correlated with improved PFS. Conversely, only the FDG PET day 14 partial metabolic response was significantly associated with improved OS (HR, 0.44; $P = .03$).[63] More recently, baseline FDG and FLT $SUV_{max}$ values of less than 6.6 and less than 3, respectively, were shown to be prognostic indicators (HR, 4.3 [$P<.001$] and HR, 2.2 [$P = .027$], respectively), correlating significantly with longer survival in metastatic NSCLC treated with erlotinib.[74–77] However, in another recent phase II trial of erlotinib with 34 stage IV NSCLC patients, FLT response at 1 week of therapy (defined as 30% reduction of peak SUV) predicted significantly longer PFS, although it did not predict OS or nonprogression by using CT after 6 weeks of therapy. The differences in results between studies may be owing to differences in the patient cohorts, that is, Asian versus European populations, which differ in EGFR mutations prevalence. Larger patient cohorts are needed to assess the potential benefit of FLT PET as an early predictor for response to therapy and survival with specifically defined EGFR mutation status.

### *Imaging Hypoxia*

Hypoxia is an important contributing factor for various changes exhibited by cancer cells, like angiogenesis, invasiveness, metastasis, genomic instability, and treatment resistance. The presence of tumor hypoxia is associated with negative patient prognosis and worse outcomes. Tumor hypoxia arises from inadequate blood supply owing to an imbalance between oxygen consumption and delivery. It serves as a powerful stimulus for the upregulation of genes involved in causing cancer and its metastasis. Although FDG is the most commonly used PET tracer, the results on FDG to image hypoxia are conflicting with lacking significant correlation and decreased ability to differentiate hypoxic and nonhypoxic areas compared with other techniques that are available to image hypoxia.[78–80] Multiple other PET tracers, including $^{18}$F-fluoromisonidazole (FMISO), $^{18}$F-fluoroazomycinarabinofuranoside ($^{18}$F-FAZA), $^{18}$F-flortanidazole ($^{18}$F-HX4), Copper (II; diacetyl-bis (N4-methylthiosemicarbazone); Cu-ATSM) have been developed to image and quantify tumor hypoxia.[81]

Most solid cancers, including lung cancer, exhibit some degree of hypoxia that is heterogeneously distributed within the tumor mass.[82,83] Hypoxia imaging also permits to monitor treatment response and provide prognostic information in lung cancer patients. FMISO, owing to its lipophilic nature, accumulates in hypoxic tumors over a period of 4 hours and clears from normoxic tissues starts after 30 minutes after injection. Eschmann and colleagues[84] studied the role of FMISO PET in predicting treatment response and tumor recurrence in 14 patients with NSCLC treated with radiotherapy. Patients with an accumulation-type curve, an SUV of greater than 2, and tumor-to-mediastinum ratios of greater than 2 before undergoing radiotherapy were at greatest risk of incomplete response to treatment with high chance of recurrence. Therefore, FMISO seems to aid in treatment decision making.[83,84] FMISO PET can also detect changes in hypoxia levels after EGFR-directed therapy in EGFR-mutant NSCLC. Arvold and associates[85] assessed this concept in patients with EGFR-mutant metastatic NSCLC in a small correlative pilot human study. FMISO PET scans were performed at 10 to 12 days after erlotinib initiation, reporting lower $SUV_{mean}$ values among the posterlotinib group with near-complete disappearance of FMISO uptake after erlotinib initiation.[85]

The other common PET tracers that are being evaluated in studies to image hypoxia in lung cancer include $^{18}$F-FAZA, $^{18}$F-HX4, and $^{62}$Cu-ATSM. $^{18}$F-FAZA is a hydrophilic PET tracer with improved diffusion into cells and faster clearance from body organs compared with $^{18}$F-FMISO, with significantly higher tumor-to-background ratios.[86,87] Trinkaus and colleagues[87] evaluated the role of $^{18}$F-FAZA PET scans in tumor hypoxia in 17 patients with locally advanced NSCLC, reporting that 65% of these patients showed tumor hypoxia on pretreatment PET scans, which was resolved in the majority after undergoing chemoradiation therapy.[88] The optimal time for the integration of hypoxia $^{18}$F-FAZA PET/CT information into radiotherapy treatment planning to benefit from hypoxia modification or dose escalation treatment in NSCLC patients was found to be after 2 weeks of radiotherapy. This timing was assessed in a small prospective study by Bollineni and colleagues,[83] and they reported that a stable change in fractional hypoxic volumes was identified on FAZA PET scans at 2 weeks after radiotherapy and nondetectable hypoxia levels at 4 weeks. However, the organ distribution of $^{18}$F-FAZA varies greatly with low uptake in lung tissue and its feasibility in lung cancer needs further evaluation in larger clinical trials.[81,89,90] $^{18}$F-HX4 is a hydrophilic molecule designed for better water solubility and faster clearance. It was shown to be safe and median tumor to muscle ratio 120 minutes after injection was 1.40 (range, 0.63–1.98) in NSCLC.[91] The uptake of $^{18}$F-HX4 among various tumors including lung cancer is highly reproducible, with spatially stable results.[92] Zegers and colleagues[91] compared the tumor metabolism using FDG-PET and hypoxia using HX4-PET imaging in 25 patients with NSCLC. They reported that hypoxic tumor volumes were found to be smaller than metabolic active volumes, with a significant correlation between FDG and HX4 parameters concluding that HX4 PET imaging addition could have the potential to individualize patient treatment in NSCLC. The uptake of Cu-ATSM in vivo in tissues was dependent on the tissue oxygen concentration with significantly higher uptake and retention in hypoxic tumor tissue.[93,94] Various positron-emitting isotopes of copper can be used $^{60}$Cu, $^{61}$Cu, $^{62}$Cu, and $^{64}$Cu had been studied. The advantages of using Cu-ATSM over 2-nitroimidazole derivatives are the higher tumor-to-background ratio and the shorter imaging times despite of its relatively lipophilic nature. Dehdashti and colleagues[95] assessed the treatment response by imaging hypoxia with $^{60}$Cu-ATSM in 14 patients with NSCLC. The mean tumor-to-muscle activity ratio was found to be significantly lower in responders (1.5 $\pm$ 0.4) compared with nonresponders (3.4 $\pm$ 0.8), concluding that $^{60}$Cu-ATSM could predict treatment response in lung cancer patients. Lopci and colleagues[94] assessed the PET parameters obtained by Cu-ATSM PET/CT in a prospective trial in various solid tumors including 7 patients with NSCLC, reporting that hypoxic tumor volume (HTV), and hypoxic burden (described as HB = HTV $\times$ $SUV_{mean}$) significant correlated with PFS. Larger studies are required to evaluate the prognostic significance of the presence and the resolution of hypoxia by using PET imaging in NSCLC.

### *Imaging Angiogenesis*

The visualization and quantification of tumor angiogenesis by using novel drugs targeting angiogenesis PET agents would be of great importance for patient selection and monitoring of response to antiangiogenic therapies. Several molecular targets for in vivo imaging of angiogenesis, such as metalloproteinases, $\alpha v\beta 3$ integrins, and vascular endothelial growth factor and its receptor, have been developed.[96] Promising PET angiogenesis radiotracers consisting of peptides containing arginine-glycine-aspartic acid (RGD) sequences, which bind to $\alpha v\beta 3$ integrins, are recently being evaluated in clinical trials. Most of the clinical experience in this setting has been obtained using $^{18}$F-galacto-RGD PET imaging, which is able to quantify $\alpha v\beta 3$ integrin expression within the tumors. In a study involving 10 patients with NSCLC, 18F-galacto-RGD uptake was found to strongly correlate with FDG uptake, suggesting that integrin expression imaging could provide complementary information to that of FDG imaging.[97] Whether this tracer could be useful for the purpose for stratification based on the risk of metastasis, monitoring therapy response, or adaptation of treatment remains to be established. Furthermore, although 18F-galacto-RGD uptake correlates well with $\alpha v\beta 3$ expression and microvessel density, the specificity of 18F-galacto-RGD PET is limited owing to $\alpha v\beta 3$ expression on cancer cells and in benign pathologies.

## SUMMARY

Recent applications of molecular targeting agents for genomically defined lung cancer patients have brought a new exciting approach in the response assessment of lung cancer. Future research directions will involve incorporation of molecular characteristics and next generation probes into new strategies to improve early tumor to enrich the target population.

Although targeted therapies have already revolutionized the field of lung cancer, next steps will involve strategies for using PET imaging to identify and manage secondary resistances to targeted therapies. Newer generation inhibitors and/or combination strategies to inhibit multiple pathways may ultimately overcome the issue of acquired resistance. Finally, new strategies against previously elusive targets, such as K-RAS, will most likely be developed and FDG as well as novel PET tracer will be used to diagnose and assess therapy.

In the era of personalized medicine, the development of highly advanced imaging will highlight and integrate molecular markers into the discussion for optimal patient care and clinical outcome.

## REFERENCES


1. Siegel R, Naishadham D, Jemal A. Cancer statistics, 2012. CA Cancer J Clin 2012;62(1):10–29.
2. Ginsberg MS, Grewal RK, Heelan RT. Lung cancer. Radiol Clin North Am 2007;45(1):21–43.
3. Larsen JE, Minna JD. Molecular biology of lung cancer: clinical implications. Clin Chest Med 2011; 32(4):703–40.
4. Maemondo M, Inoue A, Kobayashi K, et al. Gefitinib or chemotherapy for non-small-cell lung cancer with mutated EGFR. N Engl J Med 2010;362(25):2380–8.
5. Giaccone G, Herbst RS, Manegold C, et al. Gefitinib in combination with gemcitabine and cisplatin in advanced non-small-cell lung cancer: a phase III trial–INTACT 1. J Clin Oncol 2004;22(5):777–84.
6. Herbst RS, Giaccone G, Schiller JH, et al. Gefitinib in combination with paclitaxel and carboplatin in advanced non-small-cell lung cancer: a phase III trial–INTACT 2. J Clin Oncol 2004;22(5):785–94.
7. Grootjans W, Hermsen R, der Heijden EH, et al. The impact of respiratory gated positron emission tomography on clinical staging and management of patients with lung cancer. Lung Cancer 2015;90(2): 217–23.
8. Cooper WA, O'Toole S, Boyer M, et al. What's new in non-small cell lung cancer for pathologists: the importance of accurate subtyping, EGFR mutations and ALK rearrangements. Pathology 2011;43(2): 103–15.
9. Beer DG, Kardia SL, Huang CC, et al. Gene-expression profiles predict survival of patients with lung adenocarcinoma. Nat Med 2002;8(8):816–24.
10. Tam IY, Chung LP, Suen WS, et al. Distinct epidermal growth factor receptor and KRAS mutation patterns in non-small cell lung cancer patients with different tobacco exposure and clinicopathologic features. Clin Cancer Res 2006;12(5):1647–53.
11. Sherwood J, Dearden S, Ratcliffe M, et al. Mutation status concordance between primary lesions and metastatic sites of advanced non-small-cell lung cancer and the impact of mutation testing methodologies: a literature review. J Exp Clin Cancer Res 2015;34(1):92.
12. Basu S. The scope and potentials of functional radionuclide imaging towards advancing personalized medicine in oncology: emphasis on PET-CT. Discov Med 2012;13(68):65–73.
13. Basu S, Kwee TC, Gatenby R, et al. Evolving role of molecular imaging with PET in detecting and characterizing heterogeneity of cancer tissue at the primary and metastatic sites, a plausible explanation for failed attempts to cure malignant disorders. Eur J Nucl Med Mol Imaging 2011;38(6):987–91.
14. Bural G, Torigian DA, Houseni M, et al. Tumor metabolism measured by partial volume corrected standardized uptake value varies considerably in primary and metastatic sites in patients with lung cancer. A new observation. Hell J Nucl Med 2009; 12(3):218–22.
15. van Velden FH, Cheebsumon P, Yaqub M, et al. Evaluation of a cumulative SUV-volume histogram method for parameterizing heterogeneous intratumoural FDG uptake in non-small cell lung cancer PET studies. Eur J Nucl Med Mol Imaging 2011; 38(9):1636–47.
16. Kidd EA, Grigsby PW. Intratumoral metabolic heterogeneity of cervical cancer. Clin Cancer Res 2008;14(16):5236–41.
17. Hatt M, Tixier F, Cheze Le Rest C, et al. Robustness of intratumour (1)(8)F-FDG PET uptake heterogeneity quantification for therapy response prediction in oesophageal carcinoma. Eur J Nucl Med Mol Imaging 2013;40(11):1662–71.
18. Salamon J, Derlin T, Bannas P, et al. Evaluation of intratumoural heterogeneity on (1)(8)F-FDG PET/CT for characterization of peripheral nerve sheath tumours in neurofibromatosis type 1. Eur J Nucl Med Mol Imaging 2013;40(5):685–92.
19. Bradshaw TJ, Bowen SR, Jallow N, et al. Heterogeneity in intratumor correlations of 18F-FDG, 18F-FLT, and 61Cu-ATSM PET in canine sinonasal tumors. J Nucl Med 2013;54(11):1931–7.
20. Willaime JM, Turkheimer FE, Kenny LM, et al. Quantification of intra-tumour cell proliferation heterogeneity using imaging descriptors of 18F fluorothymidine-positron emission tomography. Phys Med Biol 2013; 58(2):187–203.
21. Saunders NA, Simpson F, Thompson EW, et al. Role of intratumoural heterogeneity in cancer drug resistance: molecular and clinical perspectives. EMBO Mol Med 2012;4(8):675–84.
22. Ganeshan B, Panayiotou E, Burnand K, et al. Tumour heterogeneity in non-small cell lung carcinoma assessed by CT texture analysis: a potential marker of survival. Eur Radiol 2012;22(4):796–802.
23. Win T, Miles KA, Janes SM, et al. Tumor heterogeneity and permeability as measured on the CT component of PET/CT predict survival in patients with non-small cell lung cancer. Clin Cancer Res 2013;19(13): 3591–9.
24. Soussan M, Orlhac F, Boubaya M, et al. Relationship between tumor heterogeneity measured on FDG-PET/CT and pathological prognostic factors in invasive breast cancer. PLoS One 2014;9(4):e94017.
25. Tixier F, Hatt M, Valla C, et al. Visual versus quantitative assessment of intratumor 18F-FDG PET uptake heterogeneity: prognostic value in non-small cell lung cancer. J Nucl Med 2014;55(8):1235–41.
26. Tixier F, Le Rest CC, Hatt M, et al. Intratumor heterogeneity characterized by textural features on

baseline 18F-FDG PET images predicts response to concomitant radiochemotherapy in esophageal cancer. J Nucl Med 2011;52(3):369–78.
27. van Gomez Lopez O, Garcia Vicente AM, Honguero Martinez AF, et al. Heterogeneity in [18F]fluorodeoxyglucose positron emission tomography/computed tomography of non-small cell lung carcinoma and its relationship to metabolic parameters and pathologic staging. Mol Imaging 2014;13.
28. Soussan M, Chouahnia K, Maisonobe JA, et al. Prognostic implications of volume-based measurements on FDG PET/CT in stage III non-small-cell lung cancer after induction chemotherapy. Eur J Nucl Med Mol Imaging 2013;40(5):668–76.
29. Gazdar AF. Personalized medicine and inhibition of EGFR signaling in lung cancer. N Engl J Med 2009;361(10):1018–20.
30. Brabender J, Danenberg KD, Metzger R, et al. Epidermal growth factor receptor and HER2-neu mRNA expression in non-small cell lung cancer Is correlated with survival. Clin Cancer Res 2001; 7(7):1850–5.
31. Naderi S, Ghorra C, Haddad F, et al. EGFR mutation status in Middle Eastern patients with non-squamous non-small cell lung carcinoma: a single institution experience. Cancer Epidemiol 2015; 39(6):1099–102.
32. Keedy VL, Temin S, Somerfield MR, et al. American Society of Clinical Oncology provisional clinical opinion: epidermal growth factor receptor (EGFR) Mutation testing for patients with advanced non-small-cell lung cancer considering first-line EGFR tyrosine kinase inhibitor therapy. J Clin Oncol 2011; 29(15):2121–7.
33. Hirsh V. Next-generation covalent irreversible Kinase inhibitors in NSCLC: focus on Afatinib. BioDrugs 2015;29(3):167–83.
34. Suda K, Tomizawa K, Mitsudomi T. Biological and clinical significance of KRAS mutations in lung cancer: an oncogenic driver that contrasts with EGFR mutation. Cancer Metastasis Rev 2010; 29(1):49–60.
35. Kumar A, Petri ET, Halmos B, et al. Structure and clinical relevance of the epidermal growth factor receptor in human cancer. J Clin Oncol 2008;26(10): 1742–51.
36. Zhou C, Wu YL, Chen G, et al. Erlotinib versus chemotherapy as first-line treatment for patients with advanced EGFR mutation-positive non-small-cell lung cancer (OPTIMAL, CTONG-0802): a multicentre, open-label, randomised, phase 3 study. Lancet Oncol 2011;12(8):735–42.
37. Dziadziuszko R, Witta SE, Cappuzzo F, et al. Epidermal growth factor receptor messenger RNA expression, gene dosage, and gefitinib sensitivity in non-small cell lung cancer. Clin Cancer Res 2006;12(10):3078–84.
38. Dahabreh IJ, Linardou H, Kosmidis P, et al. EGFR gene copy number as a predictive biomarker for patients receiving tyrosine kinase inhibitor treatment: a systematic review and meta-analysis in non-small-cell lung cancer. Ann Oncol 2011;22(3):545–52.
39. Na II, Byun BH, Kim KM, et al. 18F-FDG uptake and EGFR mutations in patients with non-small cell lung cancer: a single-institution retrospective analysis. Lung Cancer 2010;67(1):76–80.
40. Huang CT, Yen RF, Cheng MF, et al. Correlation of F-18 fluorodeoxyglucose-positron emission tomography maximal standardized uptake value and EGFR mutations in advanced lung adenocarcinoma. Med Oncol 2010;27(1):9–15.
41. Lee SM, Bae SK, Jung SJ, et al. FDG uptake in non-small cell lung cancer is not an independent predictor of EGFR or KRAS mutation status: a retrospective analysis of 206 patients. Clin Nucl Med 2015;40(12): 950–8.
42. Mak RH, Digumarthy SR, Muzikansky A, et al. Role of 18F-fluorodeoxyglucose positron emission tomography in predicting epidermal growth factor receptor mutations in non-small cell lung cancer. Oncologist 2011;16(3):319–26.
43. Lee EY, Khong PL, Lee VH, et al. Metabolic phenotype of stage IV lung adenocarcinoma: relationship with epidermal growth factor receptor mutation. Clin Nucl Med 2015;40(3):e190–5.
44. Jackman DM, Miller VA, Cioffredi LA, et al. Impact of epidermal growth factor receptor and KRAS mutations on clinical outcomes in previously untreated non-small cell lung cancer patients: results of an online tumor registry of clinical trials. Clin Cancer Res 2009;15(16):5267–73.
45. Roberts PJ, Stinchcombe TE. KRAS mutation: should we test for it, and does it matter? J Clin Oncol 2013;31(8):1112–21.
46. Kim WY, Prudkin L, Feng L, et al. Epidermal growth factor receptor and K-Ras mutations and resistance of lung cancer to insulin-like growth factor 1 receptor tyrosine kinase inhibitors. Cancer 2012;118(16): 3993–4003.
47. Linardou H, Dahabreh IJ, Kanaloupiti D, et al. Assessment of somatic k-RAS mutations as a mechanism associated with resistance to EGFR-targeted agents: a systematic review and meta-analysis of studies in advanced non-small-cell lung cancer and metastatic colorectal cancer. Lancet Oncol 2008;9(10):962–72.
48. Wang S, Wang Z. Meta-analysis of epidermal growth factor receptor and KRAS gene status between primary and corresponding metastatic tumours of non-small cell lung cancer. Clin Oncol (R Coll Radiol) 2015;27(1):30–9.
49. Ihle NT, Byers LA, Kim ES, et al. Effect of KRAS oncogene substitutions on protein behavior: implications for signaling and clinical outcome. J Natl Cancer Inst 2012;104(3):228–39.

50. Caicedo C, Garcia-Velloso MJ, Lozano MD, et al. Role of [(1)(8)F]FDG PET in prediction of KRAS and EGFR mutation status in patients with advanced non-small-cell lung cancer. Eur J Nucl Med Mol Imaging 2014;41(11):2058–65.
51. Brady AK, McNeill JD, Judy B, et al. Survival outcome according to KRAS mutation status in newly diagnosed patients with stage IV non-small cell lung cancer treated with platinum doublet chemotherapy. Oncotarget 2015;6(30):30287–94.
52. Roberts PJ, Stinchcombe TE, Der CJ, et al. Personalized medicine in non-small-cell lung cancer: is KRAS a useful marker in selecting patients for epidermal growth factor receptor-targeted therapy? J Clin Oncol 2010;28(31):4769–77.
53. Soda M, Choi YL, Enomoto M, et al. Identification of the transforming EML4-ALK fusion gene in non-small-cell lung cancer. Nature 2007;448(7153):561–6.
54. Kwak EL, Bang YJ, Camidge DR, et al. Anaplastic lymphoma kinase inhibition in non-small-cell lung cancer. N Engl J Med 2010;363(18):1693–703.
55. Shaw AT, Kim DW, Nakagawa K, et al. Crizotinib versus chemotherapy in advanced ALK-positive lung cancer. N Engl J Med 2013;368(25):2385–94.
56. Shaw AT, Ou SH, Bang YJ, et al. Crizotinib in ROS1-rearranged non-small-cell lung cancer. N Engl J Med 2014;371(21):1963–71.
57. Cook GJ, O'Brien ME, Siddique M, et al. Non-small cell lung cancer treated with erlotinib: heterogeneity of (18)F-FDG uptake at pet-association with treatment response and prognosis. Radiology 2015;276(3):883–93.
58. Kahraman D, Scheffler M, Zander T, et al. Quantitative analysis of response to treatment with erlotinib in advanced non-small cell lung cancer using 18F-FDG and 3'-deoxy-3'-18F-fluorothymidine PET. J Nucl Med 2011;52(12):1871–7.
59. de Langen AJ, van den Boogaart V, Lubberink M, et al. Monitoring response to antiangiogenic therapy in non-small cell lung cancer using imaging markers derived from PET and dynamic contrast-enhanced MRI. J Nucl Med 2011;52(1):48–55.
60. Dingemans AM, de Langen AJ, van den Boogaart V, et al. First-line erlotinib and bevacizumab in patients with locally advanced and/or metastatic non-small-cell lung cancer: a phase II study including molecular imaging. Ann Oncol 2011;22(3):559–66.
61. Kobe C, Scheffler M, Holstein A, et al. Predictive value of early and late residual 18F-fluorodeoxyglucose and 18F-fluorothymidine uptake using different SUV measurements in patients with non-small-cell lung cancer treated with erlotinib. Eur J Nucl Med Mol Imaging 2012;39(7):1117–27.
62. Bengtsson T, Hicks RJ, Peterson A, et al. 18F-FDG PET as a surrogate biomarker in non-small cell lung cancer treated with erlotinib: newly identified lesions are more informative than standardized uptake value. J Nucl Med 2012;53(4):530–7.
63. Mileshkin L, Hicks RJ, Hughes BG, et al. Changes in 18F-fluorodeoxyglucose and 18F-fluorodeoxythymidine positron emission tomography imaging in patients with non-small cell lung cancer treated with erlotinib. Clin Cancer Res 2011;17(10):3304–15.
64. Benz MR, Herrmann K, Walter F, et al. (18)F-FDG PET/CT for monitoring treatment responses to the epidermal growth factor receptor inhibitor erlotinib. J Nucl Med 2011;52(11):1684–9.
65. O'Brien ME, Myerson JS, Coward JI, et al. A phase II study of (1)(8)F-fluorodeoxyglucose PET-CT in non-small cell lung cancer patients receiving erlotinib (Tarceva); objective and symptomatic responses at 6 and 12 weeks. Eur J Cancer 2012;48(1):68–74.
66. Aukema TS, Kappers I, Olmos RA, et al. Is 18F-FDG PET/CT useful for the early prediction of histopathologic response to neoadjuvant erlotinib in patients with non-small cell lung cancer? J Nucl Med 2010;51(9):1344–8.
67. van de Watering FC, Rijpkema M, Perk L, et al. Zirconium-89 labeled antibodies: a new tool for molecular imaging in cancer patients. Biomed Res Int 2014;2014:203601.
68. Memon AA, Weber B, Winterdahl M, et al. PET imaging of patients with non-small cell lung cancer employing an EGF receptor targeting drug as tracer. Br J Cancer 2011;105(12):1850–5.
69. Meng X, Loo BW Jr, Ma L, et al. Molecular imaging with 11C-PD153035 PET/CT predicts survival in non-small cell lung cancer treated with EGFR-TKI: a pilot study. J Nucl Med 2011;52(10):1573–9.
70. Shields AF, Grierson JR, Dohmen BM, et al. Imaging proliferation in vivo with [F-18]FLT and positron emission tomography. Nat Med 1998;4(11):1334–6.
71. Chalkidou A, Landau DB, Odell EW, et al. Correlation between Ki-67 immunohistochemistry and 18F-fluorothymidine uptake in patients with cancer: a systematic review and meta-analysis. Eur J Cancer 2012;48(18):3499–513.
72. Sohn HJ, Yang YJ, Ryu JS, et al. [18F]Fluorothymidine positron emission tomography before and 7 days after gefitinib treatment predicts response in patients with advanced adenocarcinoma of the lung. Clin Cancer Res 2008;14(22):7423–9.
73. Zander T, Scheffler M, Nogova L, et al. Early prediction of nonprogression in advanced non-small-cell lung cancer treated with erlotinib by using [(18)F]fluorodeoxyglucose and [(18)F]fluorothymidine positron emission tomography. J Clin Oncol 2011;29(13):1701–8.
74. Scheffler M, Zander T, Nogova L, et al. Prognostic impact of [18F]fluorothymidine and [18F]fluoro-D-glucose baseline uptakes in patients with lung cancer treated first-line with erlotinib. PLoS One 2013;8(1):e53081.

75. Wilson WR, Hay MP. Targeting hypoxia in cancer therapy. Nat Rev Cancer 2011;11(6):393–410.
76. Yip C, Blower P, Goh V, et al. Molecular imaging of hypoxia in non-small-cell lung cancer. Eur J Nucl Med Mol Imaging 2015;42(6):956–76.
77. Graves EE, Maity A, Le QT. The tumor microenvironment in non-small-cell lung cancer. Semin Radiat Oncol 2010;20(3):156–63.
78. Cherk MH, Foo SS, Poon AM, et al. Lack of correlation of hypoxic cell fraction and angiogenesis with glucose metabolic rate in non-small cell lung cancer assessed by 18F-Fluoromisonidazole and 18F-FDG PET. J Nucl Med 2006;47(12):1921–6.
79. Zimny M, Gagel B, DiMartino E, et al. FDG–a marker of tumour hypoxia? A comparison with [18F]fluoromisonidazole and pO2-polarography in metastatic head and neck cancer. Eur J Nucl Med Mol Imaging 2006;33(12):1426–31.
80. Muzi M, Peterson LM, O'Sullivan JN, et al. 18F-Fluoromisonidazole quantification of hypoxia in human cancer patients using image-derived blood surrogate tissue reference regions. J Nucl Med 2015; 56(8):1223–8.
81. Walsh JC, Lebedev A, Aten E, et al. The clinical importance of assessing tumor hypoxia: relationship of tumor hypoxia to prognosis and therapeutic opportunities. Antioxid Redox Signal 2014;21(10): 1516–54.
82. Gaertner FC, Souvatzoglou M, Brix G, et al. Imaging of hypoxia using PET and MRI. Curr Pharm Biotechnol 2012;13(4):552–70.
83. Bollineni VR, Wiegman EM, Pruim J, et al. Hypoxia imaging using Positron Emission Tomography in non-small cell lung cancer: implications for radiotherapy. Cancer Treat Rev 2015;38(8):1027–32.
84. Eschmann SM, Paulsen F, Reimold M, et al. Prognostic impact of hypoxia imaging with 18F-misonidazole PET in non-small cell lung cancer and head and neck cancer before radiotherapy. J Nucl Med 2005; 46(2):253–60.
85. Arvold ND, Heidari P, Kunawudhi A, et al. Tumor hypoxia response after targeted therapy in EGFR-mutant non-small cell lung Cancer: proof of concept for FMISO-PET. Technol Cancer Res Treat 2015. [Epub ahead of print].
86. Reischl G, Dorow DS, Cullinane C, et al. Imaging of tumor hypoxia with [124I]IAZA in comparison with [18F]FMISO and [18F]FAZA–first small animal PET results. J Pharm Pharm Sci 2007;10(2):203–11.
87. Trinkaus ME, Blum R, Rischin D, et al. Imaging of hypoxia with 18F-FAZA PET in patients with locally advanced non-small cell lung cancer treated with definitive chemoradiotherapy. J Med Imaging Radiat Oncol 2013;57(4):475–81.
88. Bollineni VR, Koole MJ, Pruim J, et al. Dynamics of tumor hypoxia assessed by 18F-FAZA PET/CT in head and neck and lung cancer patients during chemoradiation: possible implications for radiotherapy treatment planning strategies. Radiother Oncol 2014;113(2):198–203.
89. Souvatzoglou M, Grosu AL, Roper B, et al. Tumour hypoxia imaging with [18F]FAZA PET in head and neck cancer patients: a pilot study. Eur J Nucl Med Mol Imaging 2007;34(10):1566–75.
90. van Loon J, Janssen MH, Ollers M, et al. PET imaging of hypoxia using [18F]HX4: a phase I trial. Eur J Nucl Med Mol Imaging 2010;37(9):1663–8.
91. Zegers CM, van Elmpt W, Szardenings K, et al. Repeatability of hypoxia PET imaging using [(18)F] HX4 in lung and head and neck cancer patients: a prospective multicenter trial. Eur J Nucl Med Mol Imaging 2015;42(12):1840–9.
92. Zegers CM, van Elmpt W, Reymen B, et al. In vivo quantification of hypoxic and metabolic status of NSCLC tumors using [18F]HX4 and [18F]FDG-PET/CT imaging. Clin Cancer Res 2014;20(24):6389–97.
93. Lewis JS, Sharp TL, Laforest R, et al. Tumor uptake of copper-diacetyl-bis(N(4)-methylthiosemicarbazone): effect of changes in tissue oxygenation. J Nucl Med 2001;42(4):655–61.
94. Lopci E, Grassi I, Rubello D, et al. Prognostic evaluation of disease outcome in solid tumors investigated with 64Cu-ATSM PET/CT. Clin Nucl Med 2016;41(2):e87–92.
95. Dehdashti F, Mintun MA, Lewis JS, et al. In vivo assessment of tumor hypoxia in lung cancer with 60Cu-ATSM. Eur J Nucl Med Mol Imaging 2003; 30(6):844–50.
96. Gaertner FC, Kessler H, Wester HJ, et al. Radiolabelled RGD peptides for imaging and therapy. Eur J Nucl Med Mol Imaging 2012;39(Suppl 1):S126–38.
97. Beer AJ, Lorenzen S, Metz S, et al. Comparison of integrin alphaVbeta3 expression and glucose metabolism in primary and metastatic lesions in cancer patients: a PET study using 18F-galacto-RGD and 18F-FDG. J Nucl Med 2008;49(1):22–9.

# PET Imaging Toward Individualized Management of Urologic and Gynecologic Malignancies

Ida Sonni, MD*, Andrei Iagaru, MD

**KEYWORDS**

• PET • Endometrial cancer • Cervical cancer • Ovarian cancer • Prostate cancer • Renal cancer • Bladder cancer • Targeted therapy

**KEY POINTS**

- A deeper understanding of cancer cell biology has paved the way to developing new targeted therapies and, in parallel, new imaging probes to guide their use.
- Several PET radiopharmaceuticals have been developed with the specific purpose of guiding individualized management of patients with cancer (selection of suitable patients and monitor response to targeted therapies).
- In urologic and gynecologic malignancies, the most promising PET radiopharmaceuticals are those targeting angiogenesis, hormone receptors (androgen receptor in prostate cancer, estrogen receptor in endometrial and ovarian cancer), and cell surface antigens (prostate-specific membrane antigen in prostate cancer, girentuximab in renal cell cancer).
- Only a few of these PET radiopharmaceuticals are used in routine clinical setting, while most are still to be evaluated in clinical trials to define their clinical role.

## INTRODUCTION

PET is becoming an indispensable tool in oncology.[1–3] Molecular imaging with PET relies on the use of specifically designed radiopharmaceuticals that target cell characteristics and therefore enable their in vivo visualization. The advent of multimodality imaging more than a decade ago, with the hybrid functional/anatomic imaging PET/computed tomography (PET/CT), and more recently PET/MR imaging, has led to an increased utility of such imaging technique, which is now a well-established tool in the detection and assessment of several types of cancer.

In an era characterized by continuous advancement in the understanding of the cellular and molecular basis of neoplastic progression, the role of molecular imaging with PET is proportionally increasing. A deeper understanding of cancer cell biology has paved the way to developing new targeted therapies and, in parallel, new imaging probes to guide their use.

The focus of this review is directed toward the role of PET imaging in the individualized management of patients affected by urologic and gynecologic malignancies, with special attention to the identification of promising PET radioligands used in this perspective (**Table 1**).

## PET IN UROLOGIC MALIGNANCIES

### *Renal Cell Carcinoma*

Renal cell carcinoma (RCC) is the most frequent type of renal tumors, accounting for approximately

The authors have nothing to disclose.
Division of Nuclear Medicine and Molecular Imaging, Department of Radiology, Stanford University, 300 Pasteur Drive, Stanford, CA 94305, USA
* Corresponding author.
*E-mail address:* isonni@stanford.edu

PET Clin 11 (2016) 261–272
http://dx.doi.org/10.1016/j.cpet.2016.02.007

**Table 1**
**Brief overview of PET radiopharmaceuticals used in the individualized management of urologic and gynecologic malignancies**

| Target | PET Radiopharmaceutical | Tumor | Reference |
|---|---|---|---|
| *Angiogenesis* | | | |
| VEGFR | $^{89}$Zr-Bevacizumab | RCC | 11 |
| Integrin $\alpha_3\beta_v$ | $^{18}$F-FPRGD$_2$ | RCC | 12 |
| | $^{18}$F-FPPRGD$_2$ | Cervical and OC | 77 |
| *Cell-surface antigens* | | | |
| Carbonic anhydrase IX | $^{124}$I-cG250 | RCC | 8,15 |
| PSMA | $^{18}$F-DCFBC | PCa | 24,25 |
| | $^{68}$Ga-PSMA-HBED-CC | | 26–33 |
| | $^{68}$Ga-PSMA-617 | | 34 |
| | $^{68}$Ga-PSMA-I&T | | 37–39 |
| | $^{124}$I-MIP-1095 | | 40 |
| *Hypoxia* | $^{18}$F-FMISO | RCC | 14 |
| *Hormone receptors* | | | |
| AR | $^{18}$F-FDHT | PCa | 44–46 |
| ER | $^{18}$F-FES | EC | 62,63 |
| | | OC | 64 |

90% of renal malignancies and 2% of all malignant tumors. At diagnosis, RCC presents as a metastatic disease (mRCC) in about one-third of patients, whereas about 50% of patients will develop local relapse or metastases during follow-up after nephrectomy.[4–6]

Among RCC, the clear-cell subtype (ccRCC) is the most diffuse variant (nearly 60% of RCC)[7] and is characterized by poor prognosis, mainly because of the high metastatic potential. Indeed, around 90% of patients who present mRCC at diagnosis, or who will later develop metastases at a later stage, have the clear-cell histologic subtype.[8] The poor prognosis in patients with mRCC can be partly explained by limited therapeutic options, because mRCC is resistant to conventional cytotoxic therapy and chemotherapy.[4] These data highlight the great need to find more effective therapies for advanced RCC.

### *Targeting angiogenesis in renal cell carcinoma*

Tumor angiogenesis is a key factor in tumor growth, disease progression, and distant dissemination for many types of cancer, including RCC. In the past few years, the introduction of therapies targeted against tumor vessels (antiangiogenesis) for the treatment of mRCC represented a major breakthrough. New antiangiogenesis therapies include vascular endothelial growth factor (VEGF) and mammalian target of rapamycin (mTOR) inhibitors. Sorafenib was the first of the family receiving US Food and Drug Administration (FDA) approval for cytokine-refractory mRCC in 2005, followed by sunitnib, temsirolimus, everolimus, bevacizumab, and more recently, pazopanib.[9] These new therapeutic agents have substantially increased progression-free and overall survival in mRCC patients.[10] However, not all patients respond to this therapies, which are expensive and associated with side effects.

Imaging tumor angiogenesis could be a useful approach for evaluating appropriateness and efficacy of such targeted therapies, and the 2 mainly investigated pathways regulating angiogenesis investigated by PET imaging are the VEGF/vascular endothelial growth factor receptor (VEGFR) pathway and vascular integrins, such as $\alpha_v\beta_3$.

Bevacizumab is a monoclonal antibody that binds to all isoforms of VEGFR and inhibits its proangiogenic function. Oosting and colleagues[11] used $^{89}$Zr-Bevacizumab in a pilot study involving 22 patients with mRCC. Patients were divided into 2 groups, one treated with bevacizumab plus interferon-$\alpha$ and the other treated with sunitinib, both standard antiangiogenic treatments for mRCC. Results of the study showed that the radiopharmaceutical visualizes tumor lesions, that antiangiogenic treatment alters tumor $^{89}$Zr-Bevacizumab uptake, and that patients with intense tumor uptake at baseline had a longer time to disease progression.

Withofs and colleagues[12] used $^{18}$F-FB-mini-PEG-E[c(RGDyK)]2 ($^{18}$F-FPRGD$_2$) in 27 patients with renal mass before surgical resection to investigate the correlation of radioligand's uptake with $\alpha_v\beta_3$ integrin expression and angiogenesis in renal masses, in particular in RCC. $^{18}$F-FPRGD$_2$ is a radioligand targeting $\alpha_v\beta_3$ integrin, a cell surface receptor overexpressed in proliferating vessels that plays a significant role in angiogenesis. Results of the study showed that $^{18}$F-FPRGD$_2$ reliably estimates $\alpha_v\beta_3$ integrin expression in renal tumors, but represents angiogenesis only when tumor cells do not express the integrin. The investigators conclude stating that imaging angiogenesis using $^{18}$F-FPRGD$_2$, and most likely all other RGD-based radiotracers, can be useful in a research setting when investigating $\alpha_v\beta_3$ integrin as a prognostic factor, but may be inadequate for assessing angiogenesis in RCC and other tumor types, and therefore, they do not see future developments of this family of angiogenesis PET imaging probes. Further studies involving larger populations are needed to confirm the conclusions of the study.

The authors' group also used a PET radiopharmaceutical targeting $\alpha_v\beta_3$ integrin, namely PEG3-E[c(RGDyk)]2 ($^{18}$F-FPPRGD$_2$), in RCC patients, and an image of the preliminary experience is shown in **Fig. 1**.

Sunitinib (SU11248) is a tyrosine kinase inhibitor targeting VEGFRs and PDGFRs (platelet-derived growth factor receptor), FDA approved as a therapeutic agent for mRCC. In the case that treatment with the drug is taken into consideration, radiolabeling sunitinib with $\beta^+$ emitting radioisotopes would represent an ideal approach to individualized patients management, because it could enable high accuracy in therapy planning, with selection only of those patients who could benefit from the treatment, therapy monitoring, and response evaluation. Therefore, sunitinib has been radiolabeled with $^{18}$F for PET imaging ($^{18}$F-SU11248),[13] but results of its use in clinical trials have not been published yet.

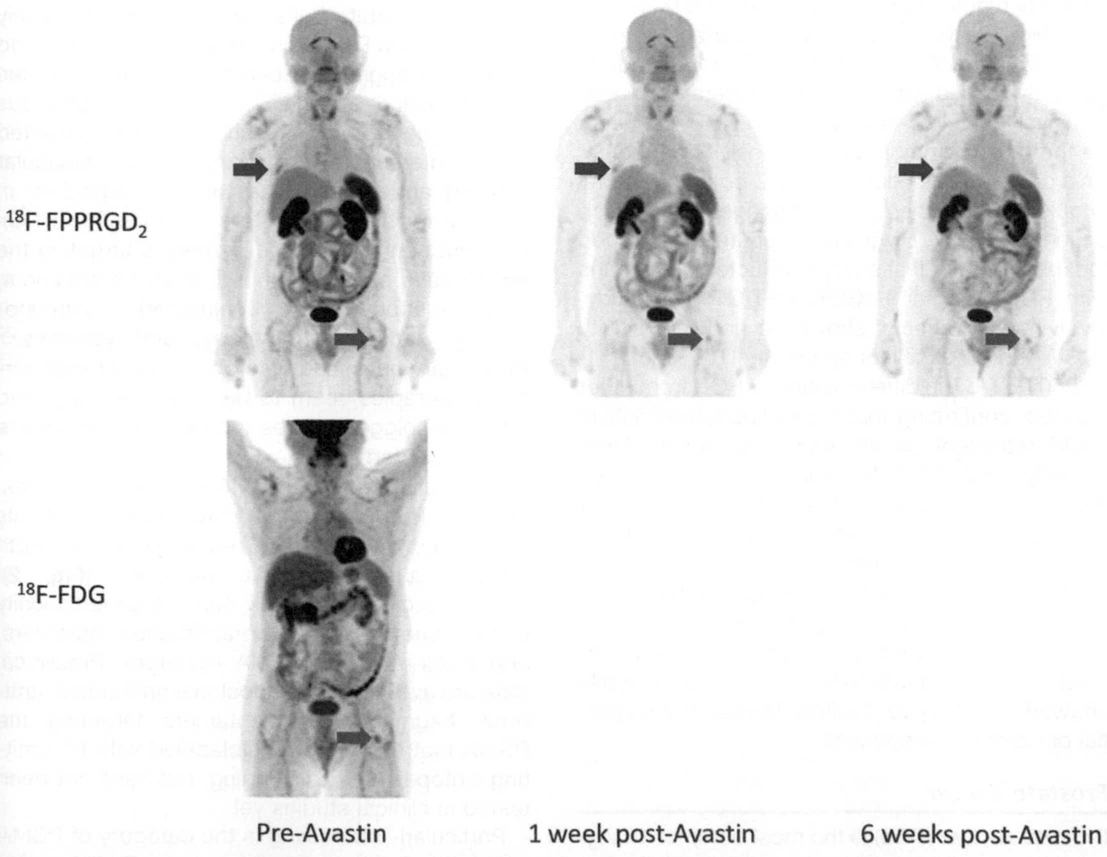


**Fig. 1**. A 77-year-old man with RCC. $^{18}$F-FPPRGD$_2$ was done before bevacizumab, as well as at 1 week and 6 weeks after starting bevacizumab, showing no changes in uptake. $^{18}$F-FDG was only done before bevacizumab. Both $^{18}$F-FPPRGD$_2$ and $^{18}$F-FDG show left femur metastasis (*blue arrows*), but a rib metastasis is only identified on $^{18}$F-FPPRGD$_2$ (*red arrows*). The patient had disease progression on clinical follow-up.

### Targeting hypoxia in renal cell carcinoma

Tumor hypoxia is known to confer resistance to radiation therapy and chemotherapy. $^{18}$F-Fluoromisonidazole ($^{18}$F-FMISO) is the most frequently used PET radiopharmaceutical to assess in vivo tumor hypoxia. Because a key factor in most RCC is the loss of function of the von Hippel-Lindau protein, with consequent overexpression of hypoxia-inducible factor and increased secretion of VEGF, $^{18}$F-FMISO has been investigated in RCC. Hugonnet and colleagues[14] used $^{18}$F-FMISO to assess efficacy of sunitinib in a population of 53 patients with mRCC. Results of the study showed that antiangiogenic therapy with sunitinib reduces tumor hypoxia on target lesions. Tumor hypoxia seems therefore to be linked to a higher risk of progression in patients treated with sunitinib for mRCC, and monitoring antiangiogenic therapy with this radioligand may be considered for future clinical applications.

### Targeting carbonic anhydrase IX in renal cell carcinoma

cG250 (girentuximab) is a chimeric monoclonal antibody binding to carbonic anhydrase IX, an antigen highly expressed on the cell surface of more than 95% of ccRCC. $^{124}$I-cG250 is a PET radioligand developed with the intent of identifying noninvasively the clear-cell subtype of RCC, known to be the most common and aggressive phenotype. An a priori identification of ccRCC could be helpful in guiding initial therapeutic management of such patients. In 2007, Divgi and colleagues[8] published the results of the first study conducted on humans with RCC using $^{124}$I-cG250 PET/CT. The study, involving 26 patients, showed a good sensitivity (94%) and an excellent specificity (100%) of $^{124}$I-cG250 PET/CT in differentiating ccRCC from other masses, confirming that the radiopharmaceutical could represent an alternative to biopsy. More recently, in 2013,[15] the same group confirmed the promising initial results in a larger multicenter trial involving 226 patients. cG250 has also been radiolabeled with $\beta^-$ emitting isotopes for therapeutic purposes with radioimmunotherapy.[16] Several phase I and II studies have been carried out on patients with advanced RCC using $^{131}$I-labeled and $^{177}$Lu-labeled cG250,[16–20] and results showed the ability to stabilize disease, but no partial or complete responses.

## Prostate Cancer

Prostate cancer (PCa) is the most common malignancy and a major cause of cancer death in men worldwide.[21] Incidence varies between countries, and prevalence seems to be higher in western countries and in migrant populations, suggesting an influence of environmental factors and lifestyle. Therapeutic management of patients with PCa relies on their accurate classification into 3 risk groups (low, intermediate, and high risk) at diagnosis; however, accurate staging and restaging of PCa remain a challenge. Imaging plays an important role in providing physicians with noninvasive biomarkers of disease, but given the lack of specificity of many conventional imaging techniques, functional and molecular imaging with PET represents an interesting solution. Several cell surface proteins, receptors, enzymes, and peptides have been studied as potential targets for PCa imaging, but in this review, only those who could play a role in personalized treatment design, that is, those targets suitable for treatment and functional imaging of PCa, are described.

### Targeting the prostate-specific membrane antigen in prostate cancer

Prostate-specific membrane antigen (PSMA) is undoubtedly one of the most attracting targets for imaging and therapeutic purposes in PCa. PSMA is a cell surface enzyme expressed on epithelial prostate cells and other tissues, highly upregulated in PCa cells.[22] PSMA levels are linked to a more aggressive behavior and to androgen independence of PCa.[23] Because of numerous advantageous characteristics, it has attracted large interest as a target for molecular imaging and radionuclide therapy, especially in castrate-resistant prostate cancer (CRPC). Different new therapeutic strategies targeting the PSMA have been developed, such as aptamers, PSMA-antibody-drug conjugated, immunotherapy, radioimmunotherapy, and vaccines.[22] Preliminary published data on the use of such targeted therapies seem to be very promising, and results of bigger studies recently completed are to be expected soon.

In parallel to new PSMA-targeted therapies, several PSMA-targeting radiopharmaceuticals have been developed in recent years, for both imaging and therapeutic purposes (**Fig. 2**). PSMA-specific molecules can be schematically divided into 3 categories: antibodies, aptamers, and small-molecule PSMA inhibitors. Preclinical data are available on monoclonal antibodies, antibody fragments, and aptamers targeting the PSMA that have been radiolabeled with $\beta^+$ emitting isotopes for PET imaging, but have not been tested in clinical studies yet.

Particularly interesting is the category of PSMA inhibitors of low molecular weight. These molecules have been radiolabeled with different $\beta^+$ emitting isotopes, such as $^{68}$Ga-, $^{11}$C-, $^{18}$F-, $^{64}$Cu-, $^{89}$Zr-, and $^{86}$Y-, for PET imaging, and

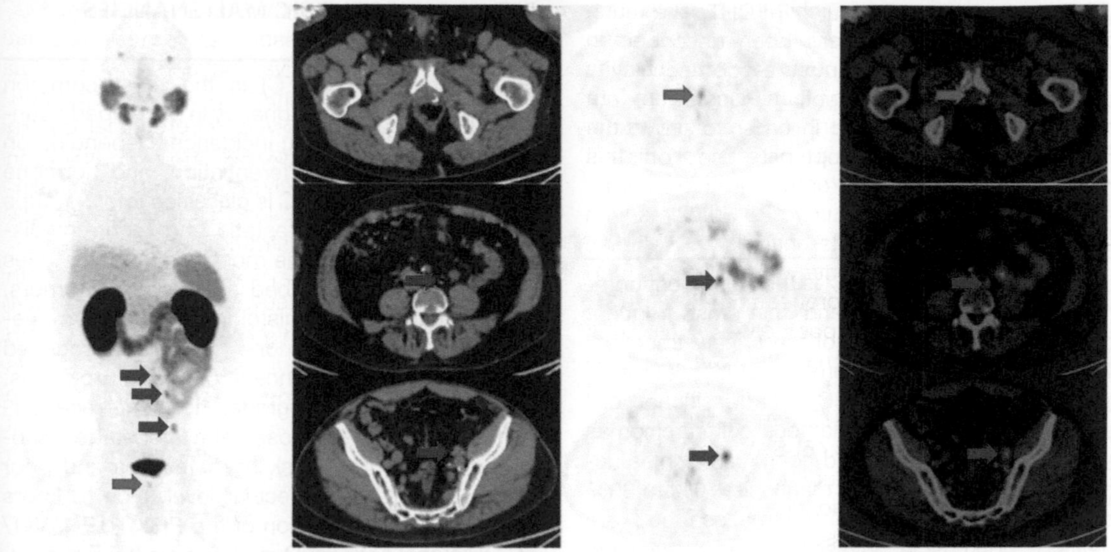

**Fig. 2.** A 71-year-old man with history of PCa (Gleason 4 + 3) treated with prostatectomy and radiation therapy, presenting with increasing PSA (4.76 ng/mL). $^{68}$Ga-PSMA-HBED-CC shows uptake in the prostate bed (*blue arrows*) as well as in multiple pelvic and retroperitoneal lymph nodes (*red arrows*).

some showed very promising results in clinical studies.

$^{18}$F-DCFBC is currently being evaluated in clinical studies, and already published data[24,25] showed a potential utility in the localization of early bone metastases as well as the ability to detect primary PCa, especially high-grade and larger-sized tumors (Gleason 8 and 9, <1.1 mL).

Several $^{68}$Ga-labeled PSMA inhibitors have been developed, the most clinically used so far being $^{68}$Ga-PSMA-HBED-CC (or PSMA-11).[26–33] This compound showed strong binding affinity to the PSMA as well as efficient internalization in PCa cells and superiority to other well-established imaging modalities, that is, PET with $^{18}$F-fluoromethylcholine.

Recently, from the modification of PSMA-11, a new small molecule was developed, namely PSMA-617, and it showed the highest binding affinity to PSMA obtained so far.[34] PSMA-617 has also been radiolabeled with $^{177}$Lu- for therapeutic purposes and showed encouraging results.[35,36]

Another promising compound evaluated for theranostics in PCa patients is [$^{68}$Ga/$^{177}$Lu] DOTAGA-(I-y)fk(Sub-KuE), termed PSMA I&T (imaging and therapy).[37–39] The $^{68}$Ga-PSMA I&T tracer showed high potential for detection of metastatic PCa, whereas $^{177}$Lu-PSMA I&T radionuclide therapy, in a proof-of-concept study, has been proven feasible, safe, and effective in the same population of patients.

Other groups evaluated PSMA-targeting monoclonal antibodies for theranostics. Zechmann and colleagues[40] radiolabeled MIP-1095 with $^{124}$I-, for PET imaging, and with $^{131}$I-, for radionuclide therapy in metastatic CRPC patients obtaining promising results, and Baur and colleagues[41] radiolabeled CHX-A″-DTPA-DUPA-Pep with $^{68}$Ga-, $^{90}$Y-, and $^{177}$Lu-, but it has not been tested in humans yet.

Another monoclonal antibody targeting the PSMA, namely J591, was radiolabeled with $^{177}$Lu-, and used by Tagawa and colleagues[42] in a phase II study including 47 patients with metastatic CRPC. The study showed that a single dose of $^{177}$Lu-J591 is well tolerated by patients, determining a reversible myelosuppression. Reduction of PSA was seen in most patients, but further studies are needed, and the authors confirmed that a randomized phase III study is planned.

### *Targeting the androgen receptor in prostate cancer*

The androgen receptor (AR) plays a key role in the development and progression of PCa, which is defined as an androgen-dependent malignant disease. Standard treatment of patients with PCa with hormone-sensitive metastatic disease is indeed based on the use of gonadotropin-releasing hormone (GnRH) analogues, either alone or in combination with an antiandrogen.[43] Imaging the AR with PET could therefore represent an interesting approach to guide the therapeutic management of patients with PCa. The most extensively evaluated PET radiopharmaceutical targeting the AR is an analogue of 5α-dihydrotestosterone

(DHT) radiolabeled with $^{18}F$, $^{18}F$-FDHT. The feasibility of $^{18}F$-FDHT PET has been described in 2004[44]; later studies confirmed a good sensitivity of the radioligand in detecting PCa lesion, but further efforts are needed in order to prove the real utility and the optimal use of this radioligand.[45,46]

### *Urinary Bladder Cancer*

Urinary bladder cancer (BC) is the ninth most common cancer worldwide and the most frequent between all malignancies of the urinary tract.[47,48] The vast majority of BC (more than 90%) are urothelial cell carcinomas (UCC, or transitional cell carcinomas), whereas squamous cell carcinomas account for nearly 5%, and adenocarcinomas account for less than 2%. At diagnosis, 70% to 80% of UCC are confined to the mucosa and are defined nonmuscle invasive bladder cancers, treated with transurethral tumor resection, followed by intravesical chemotherapy or immunotherapy (bacillus Calmette-Guerin immunotherapy). Muscle-invasive bladder cancer accounts for 20% to 30% of newly diagnosed BCa and represents a therapeutic challenge, mostly because of the aggressive behavior, chemoresistance, and rapid metastatization.[47]

#### *Targeting angiogenesis in bladder cancer*

New promising therapeutic approaches for BC include antibody-based strategies. Among them, an interesting target is undoubtedly angiogenesis, and VEGF in particular. Many of the antiangiogenesis therapies investigated showed encouraging results in preclinical and clinical phase I and II studies, but only a few phase III trials are currently being conducted.[47,49] Considering the potential role of new antiangiogenesis treatments, functional imaging of angiogenesis with PET could be a useful tool in the selection of good candidates to therapy as well as monitoring response and follow-up, but unfortunately, to the authors' knowledge, no study assessing the utility of angiogenesis PET in such patients has been published. The role of PET imaging in the evaluation of urologic malignancies has always been limited by the physiologic excretion of many radiopharmaceuticals via the urinary system. This important aspect has diverted attention to those PET radiopharmaceuticals not excreted in the urine, such as, $^{11}C$-methionine, $^{11}C$-choline, and $^{11}C$-acetate, but none of them is yet recommended by international guidelines. Urinary excretion of most PET radiopharmaceuticals undoubtedly represents a limiting factor, and developing ideal PET ligands for imaging BC still remains a challenge.

## PET IN GYNECOLOGIC MALIGNANCIES

### *Endometrial Cancer*

Endometrial cancer (EC) is the most common pelvic gynecologic malignancy in developed countries, with an increasing incidence. Depending on histology, grade of differentiation, and hormone receptor expression, EC is classified into 2 groups to assess risk for metastatic and recurrent disease: type I ECs are the most common subtypes and are usually described as low-grade tumors, with endometrioid histology and hormone-receptor-positivity tumors, usually associated with low risk of recurrence and a good prognosis; type II ECs are high-grade, hormone-receptor-negative tumors, diagnosed at a later stage, associated with a higher risk of metastasis and poor prognosis.[50] On a molecular level, type I tumors frequently have alteration of the PI3K/PTEN/AKT/mTOR signal pathway; type II tumors have overexpression of HER2, whereas upregulation of epidermal growth factor (EGFR) and VEGFR seem to be involved in oncogenesis and progression of both types of EC.[51,52] Alteration of these pathways has a key role in promoting EC growth and metastases; therefore, new therapies targeting the dysfunctional pathways have been investigated. Unfortunately, despite the vast evidence supporting the heterogeneity of the 2 types of EC, most of the clinical trials conducted so far have not taken this aspect into consideration and have not stratified patients according to the type of cancer. This finding could partially explain the disappointing results obtained so far in clinical trials investigating efficacy of mTOR inhibitors, EGFR/HER2 inhibitors, and antiangiogenic agents.[50] New targeted therapies however hold a great potential for further investigation and implementation.

### *Ovarian Cancer*

Ovarian cancer (OC) is the second most common pelvic gynecologic malignancy after EC, representing 3% of all female malignancies, but among the gynecologic tumors, it is the one with the highest mortality.[53] Approximately 10% of OC are inherited autosomal forms caused by genetic mutations, in the vast majority due to mutation of BRCA-1 and BRCA-2 genes (90%) and in a lower percentage caused by Lynch syndrome (10%).[54] Around 90% of OC are epithelial OCs and can be histologically divided into serous, mucinous, endometrioid, clear cell, and nondifferentiated.[55] Because of the lack of specific symptoms in early phases and of accurate screening methods, OC is often diagnosed at an advanced stage and therefore is associated with poor prognosis and high mortality. Early diagnosis and appropriate initial tumor staging are essential factors to ensure a better prognosis; indeed, OC diagnosed at an early stage (stage I) has a significantly better prognosis and a better 5-year survival rate than later diagnosed cancers (stage III and IV), at 25% and 90%, respectively.[56] Standard management of OC includes cytoreductive surgery, to reduce the burden of disease, and platinum-based plus taxane chemotherapy. Unfortunately, only a small proportion of patients will have a complete response to initial therapy, whereas the rest of the patients will relapse and die of disease.

## *Cervical Cancer*

Cervical cancer is the third most common cancer in women and the fourth cause of death due to cancer worldwide, with more than 85% of deaths occurring in developing countries.[57] The mortality of cervical cancer has notably decreased in industrialized countries because of the wide use of screening with cytology (Papanicolaou smear test) and human papillomavirus DNA testing in high-risk populations. Screening methods allow detection of precancerous lesions and early stage cancer, but unfortunately, are still lacking in developing countries. When diagnosed at early stages, cervical cancer can be cured by radical surgery, and when locally advanced, can be controlled by chemoradiotherapy, but advanced metastatic and nonoperable disease have few therapeutic options, and prognosis is poor. Novel therapies are therefore needed for cervical cancer, and several strategies, such as anti-VEGF, anti-EGFR, or mTOR inhibitors, have been already investigated with promising results.

### *Targeting estrogen receptor in endometrial and ovarian cancer*

Estrogen receptors (ERs), existing in the 2 isoforms ERα and Erβ, are responsible for mediating signaling of the sex hormone estrogen. ERs are intracellular receptors that play a key role in regulating proliferation and differentiation in normal tissues, but also in promoting development and progression of estrogen-dependent malignancies, like EC and OC. Targeted hormonal therapies aiming at either blocking the effects of estrogen or at reducing their circulating levels (such as selective estrogen receptor modulators, GnRH analogues, and aromatase inhibitors), represent effective treatments for recurrent EC.[58] However, it is clear that only patients with ER-dependent tumors would benefit from such targeted therapies; therefore, a previous careful and appropriate selection of patients to be treated would be needed. ER expression on cancer cells can change during the course of disease, and it is not uncommon to have a discrepancy in ER expression between primary tumor and its metastases, as it has been largely described in breast cancer and recently also in OC.[59,60] Imaging ER expression using PET could represent a predictive biomarker and could help selecting those patients who are most likely to benefit from hormonal therapy. Among the numerous potential radiopharmaceuticals targeting the ER, the most promising is $^{18}$F-FES, which targets ERα. $^{18}$F-FES PET has been more extensively used in patients with breast cancer, with good results,[61] and to a lesser extent in endometrial and OC.

The Japanese group guided by Tsujikawa[62] studied 22 patients affected by EC and 9 patients with endometrial hyperplasia using both $^{18}$F-FES and $^{18}$F-FDG PET to evaluate, noninvasively by means of PET, the correlation between ER expression, glucose metabolism, and their ratio (FDG-to-FES standardized uptake value [SUV] ratio) to the aggressiveness of tumors, in terms of staging and pathologic findings. The group demonstrated that SUV measured on $^{18}$F-FES is significantly different between low- and high-risk carcinoma, and that the FDG-to-FES SUV ratio is significantly higher in high-risk carcinoma than in low-risk carcinoma and hyperplasia.

In 2007, Yoshida and colleagues[63] in a case report showed the utility of $^{18}$F-FES PET in guiding hormonal therapy in EC patients.

The group from Groningen guided by van Kruchten[64] has recently published the results of the first feasibility study conducted using $^{18}$F-FES PET/CT on 14 patients affected by OC. The study showed that $^{18}$F-FES PET/CT can reliably assess ERα expression in OC noninvasively with good sensitivity (78%) and excellent specificity (100%) and could therefore represent an ideal biomarker for predicting response to endocrine therapy in OC patients.

### *Targeting folate receptor in endometrial and ovarian cancer*

Folic acid is an essential vitamin needed by all eukaryotic cells for DNA synthesis and exerts its actions via the folate receptors (FRs). The high-affinity FRs are cell membrane glycoproteins existing in 4 isoforms: FRα, FRβ, FRγ, and FRδ. FRα in particular shows limited expression in normal tissues and is highly expressed in several different types of epithelial carcinomas,[65,66] including EC and OC. The very high affinity of folic acid for the FRs, together with the upregulation of the latter in tumor cells, makes folate an ideal targeting agent for both imaging and therapeutic purposes. Folate has indeed been conjugated with other molecules, including drugs that are specifically delivered to FR-positive tumor cells (FR antisense oligonucleotides, FR-coupled immunotherapy, chemotherapy, and radiotherapy).[67] In parallel to FR targeted therapy, a variety of PET radiopharmaceuticals targeting the FR have been developed, either labeled with $^{124}$I-, $^{68}$Ga-, or $^{18}$F-, but have not been clinically used yet.[65,68–72]

***Targeting angiogenesis in endometrial, ovarian, and cervical cancer***

As already mentioned, angiogenesis plays a central role in the progression of several types of cancer, including EC, cervical, and OC. Increased VEGF expression is associated with a more aggressive behavior and a poorer prognosis, and this explains the interest directed toward new targeted therapies with antiangiogenic properties.

Response rates obtained using antiangiogenic drugs (sunitinib, sorafenib, thalidomide, bevacizumab, aflibercept) range from 5% to 15% in recurrent or persistent EC,[73] whereas results are much more encouraging in OC. Because of the progression-free survival improvements obtained by adding bevacizumab to chemotherapy in OC, the anti-VEGF drug has now been approved in Europe by the European Medicines Agency, in combination with standard chemotherapy for both newly diagnosed and relapsing OC, and in the United States by the FDA, when combined with chemotherapy for platinum-resistant relapse OC.[74]

As well as in OC, bevacizumab has been proven to improve overall survival and progression-free survival in patients with cervical cancer when associated with standard chemotherapy. Results of a phase III trial have recently been published and showed that the addition of bevacizumab in the treatment of advanced cervical cancer was not accompanied by any significant deterioration in health-related quality of life.[75]

Imaging angiogenesis using PET could be a precious tool when selecting patients to be treated with antiangiogenic drugs, because of the known undesired toxic effects collateral to these targeted

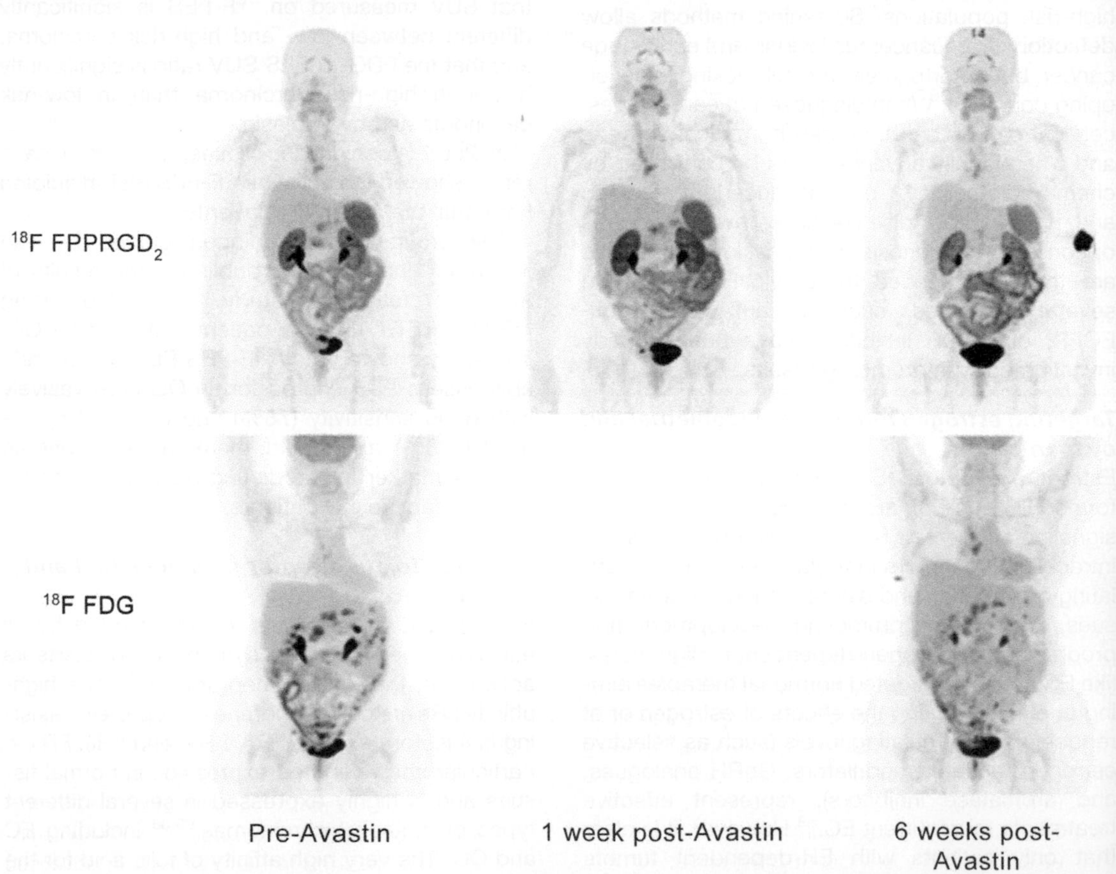


**Fig. 3.** A 59-year-old woman with OC. $^{18}$F-FPPRGD$_2$ was done before bevacizumab, as well as at 1 week and 6 weeks after starting bevacizumab, showing no changes in uptake. $^{18}$F-FDG was done before bevacizumab, as well as at 1 week after starting bevacizumab, also showing no changes in uptake. The patient had disease progression on clinical follow-up.

therapies.[76] No published data of clinical studies investigating angiogenesis imaging with PET in gynecologic malignancies are yet available. However, the authors' group recently conducted a study,[77] using the novel PET radiopharmaceutical $^{18}$F-FPPRGD$_2$, which targets the integrin $\alpha_v\beta_3$, in patients affected by ovarian and cervical cancer. Patients underwent $^{18}$F-FPPRGD$_2$ PET before and after antiangiogenic therapies. The pilot study showed encouraging results confirming that $^{18}$F-FPPRGD$_2$ may have the potential to predict early response to antiangiogenic therapy (**Fig. 3**).

## SUMMARY

Early diagnosis is the most critical factor influencing the clinical outcome in patients affected by cancer, including urologic and gynecologic malignancies. Standard therapeutic approaches often fail when diagnosis is identified at later stages. Many efforts have therefore been directed toward the development of new therapeutic approaches that could target specific characteristics of the tumor cells or of the microenvironment, and improve prognosis.

Angiogenesis represents one of the most promising targets for both therapeutic and imaging purposes in almost all urologic and gynecologic malignancies, but large studies investigating the clinical role of PET radiopharmaceuticals targeting angiogenesis are still needed.

Targeted hormonal therapies are effective treatments for those malignancies overexpressing the hormonal receptors (eg, PCa overexpressing AR and gynecologic malignancies overexpressing ER). Imaging AR and ER expression using PET could help in selecting patients who are most likely to benefit from hormonal therapy, and $^{18}$F-FES, imaging ER, and $^{18}$F-FDHT, imaging AR, appear to be very good candidates.

Several molecules targeting the PSMA have been developed as imaging agents in PCa, and some of them have also been radiolabeled with β- emitting isotopes for therapeutic purposes. Future investigations will define which one of the many radiopharmaceuticals will have the most significant impact.

## REFERENCES


1. Gallamini A, Zwarthoed C, Borra A. Positron emission tomography (PET) in oncology. Cancers (Basel) 2014;6(4):1821–89.
2. Nanni C, Rubello D, Al-Nahhas A, et al. Clinical PET in oncology: not only FDG. Nucl Med Commun 2006; 27(9):685–8.
3. Rice SL, Roney CA, Daumar P, et al. The next generation of positron emission tomography radiopharmaceuticals in oncology. Semin Nucl Med 2011;41(4): 265–82.
4. Lilleby W, Fossa SD. Chemotherapy in metastatic renal cell cancer. World J Urol 2005;23(3):175–9.
5. Cho E, Adami HO, Lindblad P. Epidemiology of renal cell cancer. Hematol Oncol Clin North Am 2011; 25(4):651–65.
6. Gupta K, Miller JD, Li JZ, et al. Epidemiologic and socioeconomic burden of metastatic renal cell carcinoma (mRCC): a literature review. Cancer Treat Rev 2008;34(3):193–205.
7. Cohen HT, McGovern FJ. Renal-cell carcinoma. N Engl J Med 2005;353(23):2477–90.
8. Divgi CR, Pandit-Taskar N, Jungbluth AA, et al. Preoperative characterisation of clear-cell renal carcinoma using iodine-124-labelled antibody chimeric G250 (124I-cG250) and PET in patients with renal masses: a phase I trial. Lancet Oncol 2007;8(4): 304–10.
9. Ammari S, Thiam R, Cuenod CA, et al. Radiological evaluation of response to treatment: application to metastatic renal cancers receiving anti-angiogenic treatment. Diagn Interv Imaging 2014;95(6):527–39.
10. Hutson TE. Targeted therapies for the treatment of metastatic renal cell carcinoma: clinical evidence. Oncologist 2011;16(Suppl 2):14–22.
11. Oosting SF, Brouwers AH, van Es SC, et al. 89Zr-bevacizumab PET visualizes heterogeneous tracer accumulation in tumor lesions of renal cell carcinoma patients and differential effects of antiangiogenic treatment. J Nucl Med 2015;56(1):63–9.
12. Withofs N, Signolle N, Somja J, et al. 18F-FPRGD2 PET/CT imaging of integrin αvβ3 in renal carcinomas: correlation with histopathology. J Nucl Med 2015;56(3):361–4.
13. Wang JQ, Miller KD, Sledge GW, et al. Synthesis of [18F]SU11248, a new potential PET tracer for imaging cancer tyrosine kinase. Bioorg Med Chem Lett 2005;15(19):4380–4.
14. Hugonnet F, Fournier L, Medioni J, et al. Metastatic renal cell carcinoma: relationship between initial metastasis hypoxia, change after 1 month's sunitinib, and therapeutic response: an 18F-fluoromisonidazole PET/CT study. J Nucl Med 2011;52(7): 1048–55.
15. Divgi CR, Uzzo RG, Gatsonis C, et al. Positron emission tomography/computed tomography identification of clear cell renal cell carcinoma: results from the REDECT trial. J Clin Oncol 2013;31(2): 187–94.
16. Brouwers AH, van Eerd JE, Frielink C, et al. Optimization of radioimmunotherapy of renal cell carcinoma: labeling of monoclonal antibody cG250 with 131I, 90Y, 177Lu, or 186Re. J Nucl Med 2004; 45(2):327–37.

17. Brouwers AH, Mulders PF, de Mulder PH, et al. Lack of efficacy of two consecutive treatments of radioimmunotherapy with 131I-cG250 in patients with metastasized clear cell renal cell carcinoma. J Clin Oncol 2005;23(27):6540–8.
18. Divgi CR, Bander NH, Scott AM, et al. Phase I/II radioimmunotherapy trial with iodine-131-labeled monoclonal antibody G250 in metastatic renal cell carcinoma. Clin Cancer Res 1998;4(11):2729–39.
19. Divgi CR, O'Donoghue JA, Welt S, et al. Phase I clinical trial with fractionated radioimmunotherapy using 131I-labeled chimeric G250 in metastatic renal cancer. J Nucl Med 2004;45(8):1412–21.
20. Stillebroer AB, Boerman OC, Desar IM, et al. Phase 1 radioimmunotherapy study with lutetium 177-labeled anti-carbonic anhydrase IX monoclonal antibody girentuximab in patients with advanced renal cell carcinoma. Eur Urol 2013;64(3):478–85.
21. Attard G, Parker C, Eeles RA, et al. Prostate cancer. Lancet 2016;387(10013):70–82.
22. Santoni M, Scarpelli M, Mazzucchelli R, et al. Targeting prostate-specific membrane antigen for personalized therapies in prostate cancer: morphologic and molecular backgrounds and future promises. J Biol Regul Homeost Agents 2014;28(4):555–63.
23. Mease RC, Foss CA, Pomper MG. PET imaging in prostate cancer: focus on prostate-specific membrane antigen. Curr Top Med Chem 2013;13(8):951–62.
24. Cho SY, Gage KL, Mease RC, et al. Biodistribution, tumor detection, and radiation dosimetry of 18F-DCFBC, a low-molecular-weight inhibitor of prostate-specific membrane antigen, in patients with metastatic prostate cancer. J Nucl Med 2012;53(12):1883–91.
25. Rowe SP, Gage KL, Faraj SF, et al. (1)(8)F-DCFBC PET/CT for PSMA-based detection and characterization of primary prostate cancer. J Nucl Med 2015;56(7):1003–10.
26. Afshar-Oromieh A, Avtzi E, Giesel FL, et al. The diagnostic value of PET/CT imaging with the (68)Ga-labelled PSMA ligand HBED-CC in the diagnosis of recurrent prostate cancer. Eur J Nucl Med Mol Imaging 2015;42(2):197–209.
27. Afshar-Oromieh A, Haberkorn U, Schlemmer HP, et al. Comparison of PET/CT and PET/MRI hybrid systems using a 68Ga-labelled PSMA ligand for the diagnosis of recurrent prostate cancer: initial experience. Eur J Nucl Med Mol Imaging 2014;41(5):887–97.
28. Afshar-Oromieh A, Malcher A, Eder M, et al. PET imaging with a [68Ga]gallium-labelled PSMA ligand for the diagnosis of prostate cancer: biodistribution in humans and first evaluation of tumour lesions. Eur J Nucl Med Mol Imaging 2013;40(4):486–95.
29. Afshar-Oromieh A, Zechmann CM, Malcher A, et al. Comparison of PET imaging with a (68)Ga-labelled PSMA ligand and (18)F-choline-based PET/CT for the diagnosis of recurrent prostate cancer. Eur J Nucl Med Mol Imaging 2014;41(1):11–20.
30. Eder M, Neels O, Muller M, et al. Novel preclinical and radiopharmaceutical aspects of [68Ga]Ga-PSMA-HBED-CC: a new PET tracer for imaging of prostate cancer. Pharmaceuticals (Basel) 2014;7(7):779–96.
31. Eder M, Schafer M, Bauder-Wust U, et al. 68Ga-complex lipophilicity and the targeting property of a urea-based PSMA inhibitor for PET imaging. Bioconjug Chem 2012;23(4):688–97.
32. Eiber M, Maurer T, Souvatzoglou M, et al. Evaluation of hybrid (6)(8)Ga-PSMA ligand PET/CT in 248 patients with biochemical recurrence after radical prostatectomy. J Nucl Med 2015;56(5):668–74.
33. Demirkol MO, Acar O, Ucar B, et al. Prostate-specific membrane antigen-based imaging in prostate cancer: impact on clinical decision making process. Prostate 2015;75(7):748–57.
34. Afshar-Oromieh A, Hetzheim H, Kratochwil C, et al. The novel theranostic PSMA-ligand PSMA-617 in the diagnosis of prostate cancer by PET/CT: biodistribution in humans, radiation dosimetry and first evaluation of tumor lesions. J Nucl Med 2015;56(11):1697–705.
35. Kratochwil C, Giesel FL, Eder M, et al. [(1)(7)(7)Lu]Lutetium-labelled PSMA ligand-induced remission in a patient with metastatic prostate cancer. Eur J Nucl Med Mol Imaging 2015;42(6):987–8.
36. Ahmadzadehfar H, Rahbar K, Kurpig S, et al. Early side effects and first results of radioligand therapy with (177)Lu-DKFZ-617 PSMA of castrate-resistant metastatic prostate cancer: a two-centre study. EJNMMI Res 2015;5(1):114.
37. Herrmann K, Bluemel C, Weineisen M, et al. Biodistribution and radiation dosimetry for a probe targeting prostate-specific membrane antigen for imaging and therapy. J Nucl Med 2015;56(6):855–61.
38. Weineisen M, Schottelius M, Simecek J, et al. 68Ga- and 177Lu-labeled PSMA I&T: optimization of a PSMA-targeted theranostic concept and first proof-of-concept human studies. J Nucl Med 2015;56(8):1169–76.
39. Weineisen M, Simecek J, Schottelius M, et al. Synthesis and preclinical evaluation of DOTAGA-conjugated PSMA ligands for functional imaging and endoradiotherapy of prostate cancer. EJNMMI Res 2014;4(1):63.
40. Zechmann CM, Afshar-Oromieh A, Armor T, et al. Radiation dosimetry and first therapy results with a (124)I/(131)I-labeled small molecule (MIP-1095) targeting PSMA for prostate cancer therapy. Eur J Nucl Med Mol Imaging 2014;41(7):1280–92.
41. Baur B, Solbach C, Andreolli E, et al. Synthesis, radiolabelling and in vitro characterization of the

gallium-68-, yttrium-90- and lutetium-177-labelled PSMA ligand, CHX-A″-DTPA-DUPA-Pep. Pharmaceuticals (Basel) 2014;7(5):517–29.
42. Tagawa ST, Milowsky MI, Morris M, et al. Phase II study of Lutetium-177-labeled anti-prostate-specific membrane antigen monoclonal antibody J591 for metastatic castration-resistant prostate cancer. Clin Cancer Res 2013;19(18):5182–91.
43. Chen Y, Clegg NJ, Scher HI. Anti-androgens and androgen-depleting therapies in prostate cancer: new agents for an established target. Lancet Oncol 2009;10(10):981–91.
44. Larson SM, Morris M, Gunther I, et al. Tumor localization of 16beta-18F-fluoro-5alpha-dihydrotestosterone versus 18F-FDG in patients with progressive, metastatic prostate cancer. J Nucl Med 2004; 45(3):366–73.
45. Beattie BJ, Smith-Jones PM, Jhanwar YS, et al. Pharmacokinetic assessment of the uptake of 16beta-18F-fluoro-5alpha-dihydrotestosterone (FDHT) in prostate tumors as measured by PET. J Nucl Med 2010;51(2):183–92.
46. Dehdashti F, Picus J, Michalski JM, et al. Positron tomographic assessment of androgen receptors in prostatic carcinoma. Eur J Nucl Med Mol Imaging 2005;32(3):344–50.
47. Azevedo R, Ferreira JA, Peixoto A, et al. Emerging antibody-based therapeutic strategies for bladder cancer: a systematic review. J Control Release 2015;214:40–61.
48. Witjes JA, Comperat E, Cowan NC, et al. EAU guidelines on muscle-invasive and metastatic bladder cancer: summary of the 2013 guidelines. Eur Urol 2014;65(4):778–92.
49. Mazzola CR, Chin J. Targeting the VEGF pathway in metastatic bladder cancer. Expert Opin Investig Drugs 2015;24(7):913–27.
50. Morice P, Leary A, Creutzberg C, et al. Endometrial cancer. Lancet 2015. [Epub ahead of print].
51. Dedes KJ, Wetterskog D, Ashworth A, et al. Emerging therapeutic targets in endometrial cancer. Nat Rev Clin Oncol 2011;8(5):261–71.
52. Dong P, Kaneuchi M, Konno Y, et al. Emerging therapeutic biomarkers in endometrial cancer. Biomed Res Int 2013;2013:130362.
53. Siegel R, Ma J, Zou Z, et al. Cancer statistics, 2014. CA Cancer J Clin 2014;64(1):9–29.
54. Mourits MJ, de Bock GH. Managing hereditary ovarian cancer. Maturitas 2009;64(3):172–6.
55. Benedet JL, Bender H, Jones H 3rd, et al. FIGO staging classifications and clinical practice guidelines in the management of gynecologic cancers. FIGO Committee on Gynecologic Oncology. Int J Gynaecol Obstet 2000;70(2): 209–62.
56. Barnholtz-Sloan JS, Schwartz AG, Qureshi F, et al. Ovarian cancer: changes in patterns at diagnosis and relative survival over the last three decades. Am J Obstet Gynecol 2003;189(4):1120–7.
57. Jemal A, Bray F, Center MM, et al. Global cancer statistics. CA Cancer J Clin 2011;61(2):69–90.
58. Carlson MJ, Thiel KW, Leslie KK. Past, present, and future of hormonal therapy in recurrent endometrial cancer. Int J Womens Health 2014;6:429–35.
59. Aurilio G, Disalvatore D, Pruneri G, et al. A meta-analysis of oestrogen receptor, progesterone receptor and human epidermal growth factor receptor 2 discordance between primary breast cancer and metastases. Eur J Cancer 2014;50(2):277–89.
60. van Kruchten M, van der Marel P, de Munck L, et al. Hormone receptors as a marker of poor survival in epithelial ovarian cancer. Gynecol Oncol 2015; 138(3):634–9.
61. Talbot JN, Gligorov J, Nataf V, et al. Current applications of PET imaging of sex hormone receptors with a fluorinated analogue of estradiol or of testosterone. Q J Nucl Med Mol Imaging 2015;59(1):4–17.
62. Tsujikawa T, Yoshida Y, Kudo T, et al. Functional images reflect aggressiveness of endometrial carcinoma: estrogen receptor expression combined with 18F-FDG PET. J Nucl Med 2009;50(10): 1598–604.
63. Yoshida Y, Kurokawa T, Sawamura Y, et al. The positron emission tomography with F18 17beta-estradiol has the potential to benefit diagnosis and treatment of endometrial cancer. Gynecol Oncol 2007;104(3): 764–6.
64. van Kruchten M, de Vries EF, Arts HJ, et al. Assessment of estrogen receptor expression in epithelial ovarian cancer patients using 16alpha-18F-fluoro-17beta-estradiol PET/CT. J Nucl Med 2015;56(1):50–5.
65. Ke CY, Mathias CJ, Green MA. Folate-receptor-targeted radionuclide imaging agents. Adv Drug Deliv Rev 2004;56(8):1143–60.
66. Muller C. Folate-based radiotracers for PET imaging–update and perspectives. Molecules (Basel) 2013;18(5):5005–31.
67. Brown Jones M, Neuper C, Clayton A, et al. Rationale for folate receptor alpha targeted therapy in "high risk" endometrial carcinomas. Int J Cancer 2008;123(7):1699–703.
68. Al Jammaz I, Al-Otaibi B, Amer S, et al. Rapid synthesis and in vitro and in vivo evaluation of folic acid derivatives labeled with fluorine-18 for PET imaging of folate receptor-positive tumors. Nucl Med Biol 2011;38(7):1019–28.
69. Aljammaz I, Al-Otaibi B, Al-Hokbany N, et al. Development and pre-clinical evaluation of new 68Ga-NOTA-folate conjugates for PET imaging of folate receptor-positive tumors. Anticancer Res 2014; 34(11):6547–56.
70. AlJammaz I, Al-Otaibi B, Al-Rumayan F, et al. Development and preclinical evaluation of new

(124)I-folate conjugates for PET imaging of folate receptor-positive tumors. Nucl Med Biol 2014; 41(6):457–63.

71. Mathias CJ, Lewis MR, Reichert DE, et al. Preparation of 66Ga- and 68Ga-labeled Ga(III)-deferoxamine-folate as potential folate-receptor-targeted PET radiopharmaceuticals. Nucl Med Biol 2003;30(7):725–31.
72. Schieferstein H, Ross TL. (18)F-labeled folic acid derivatives for imaging of the folate receptor via positron emission tomography. J Labelled Comp Radiopharm 2013;56(9–10):432–40.
73. Gadducci A, Sergiampietri C, Guiggi I. Antiangiogenic agents in advanced, persistent or recurrent endometrial cancer: a novel treatment option. Gynecol Endocrinol 2013;29(9):811–6.
74. Liu JF, Matulonis UA. Bevacizumab in newly diagnosed ovarian cancer. Lancet Oncol 2015;16(8): 876–8.
75. Penson RT, Hu ang HQ, Wenzel LB, et al. Bevacizumab for advanced cervical cancer: patient-reported outcomes of a randomised, phase 3 trial (NRG Oncology-Gynecologic Oncology Group protocol 240). Lancet Oncol 2015;16(3):301–11.
76. Stone RL, Sood AK, Coleman RL. Collateral damage: toxic effects of targeted antiangiogenic therapies in ovarian cancer. Lancet Oncol 2010;11(5): 465–75.
77. Minamimoto R, Hancock S, Schneider B, et al. Pilot comparison of 68Ga-RM2 PET and 68Ga-PSMA PET in patients with biochemically recurrent prostate cancer. J Nucl Med 2015. [Epub ahead of print].

# Personalized Clinical Decision Making in Gastrointestinal Malignancies
## The Role of PET

Søren Hess, MD[a,b,c,*], Ole Steen Bjerring, MD[c,d],
Per Pfeiffer, MD, PhD[c,e],
Poul Flemming Høilund-Carlsen, MD, DMSc[a,c]

**KEYWORDS**

• PET • FDG • Pancreatic cancer • Gastric cancer • Colorectal cancer • GIST

**KEY POINTS**

- The routine application of fluorodeoxyglucose (FDG)-PET/CT in gastrointestinal (GI) malignancies remains controversial.
- FDG-PET/CT for pretherapeutic evaluation of local involvement or lymph node staging currently is not supported by the literature.
- FDG-PET/CT has a place for evaluating distant metastatic status in both upper and lower GI malignancies.
- Preoperative response evaluation seems promising, especially in gastric cancer, but further studies are needed.
- FDG-PET/CT is a valuable tool in GI stromal tumors (GISTs).

## INTRODUCTION

In a recent commentary in *The New England Journal of Medicine*, Jameson and Longo[1] outlined a personalized approach to cancer management. They consider personalized (or individualized or precision) medicine as a means to better patient selection for treatments targeted to the individual needs of patients based on unique features that separate them from other patients with similar characteristics. Such features include application of molecular profiles in the initial diagnostic process or later in the course of treatment, with the goal to improve clinical outcomes and obviate futile treatments for those less likely to benefit from any given standard regimen.[1]

Although clinical molecular imaging is not always considered part of personalized medicine, the use of FDG-PET/CT as part of clinical decision making is gaining momentum in various cancer settings.[1,2] FDG-PET/CT has limited space in the initial diagnostic work-up of GI malignancies and its use in staging and clinical decision of GI cancers remains controversial. It may have a role, however, in detecting otherwise unknown metastatic disease prior to surgery to avoid futile procedures, albeit there are challenges to its use,

The authors have nothing to disclose.
[a] Department of Nuclear Medicine, Odense University Hospital, Sdr. Boulevard 29, 5000 Odense C, Denmark; [b] Division of Nuclear Medicine, Department of Radiology and Nuclear Medicine, Hospital of South West Jutland, Finsensgade 10, 6700 Esbjerg, Denmark; [c] Department of Clinical Research, Faculty of Health Sciences, University of Southern Denmark, Winsløwsparken 19, 3, 5000 Odense C, Denmark; [d] Department of Gastrointestinal Surgery, Odense University Hospital, Sdr. Boulevard 29, 5000 Odense C, Denmark; [e] Department of Clinical Oncology, Odense University Hospital, Sdr. Boulevard 29, 5000 Odense C, Denmark
* Corresponding author.
*E-mail address:* Soeren.hess@rsyd.dk

PET Clin 11 (2016) 273–283
http://dx.doi.org/10.1016/j.cpet.2016.02.005

including physiologic uptake in the GI tract and benign inflammatory conditions in the stomach, colon, and rectum.[3]

Chemotherapy induces tumor regression in approximately half of patients with metastatic disease from GI cancer. One challenge regarding presurgical/neoadjuvant chemotherapy is that it is often not possible to predict which patients will experience progression during therapy. Neoadjuvant therapy may reduce tumor burden and increase 5-year survival by approximately 15% (from 20%–25% to 35%–40%), but this also means that a majority of patients do not gain benefit but only experience toxicity.[4] With FDG-PET/CT it may be possible to go beyond the morphologic Response Evaluation Criteria in Solid Tumors (RECIST) for separating patients who respond to neoadjuvant chemotherapy from nonresponders; the latter category should be switched to surgery upfront to reduce the risk of progression and toxicity-related deaths.[5,6]

This article outlines the potential use of FDG-PET/CT in clinical decision making in GI malignancies with special regard to preoperative evaluation and response assessment. Gastric cancer (including the gastroesophageal junction), pancreatic cancer (excluding neuroendocrine tumors), colorectal cancer (CRC), and GISTs are discussed.

## GASTRIC CANCER

The National Comprehensive Cancer Network has established the accuracy of PET/CT staging in a variety of malignancies.[7] In gastric cancer, PET/CT may lead to a change in management in one-third of patients by detecting distant metastases, whereas sensitivity is low for locally advanced disease and local lymph node metastases.[7] Compared with contrast-enhanced CT (ceCT) and endoscopic ultrasound (EUS), PET and PET/CT have consistently shown poorer accuracy (48%–72% vs 69%) for lymph node metastases, due to a lower sensitivity (22%–40% vs 83%), as opposed to a higher accuracy for distant metastases (86% vs 62%), whereas specificity has consistently been reported high (>95%).[3] These results have been corroborated by newer studies and a recent meta-analysis.[8–12] A single study has assessed EUS and FDG-PET/CT for primary and locoregional staging and found the combination superior to either imaging modality alone, that is, a combined detection rate of 99% compared with 97% and 90% with EUS alone and PET/CT alone, respectively, for primary tumor, and 68% (combined) versus 52% (EUS alone) and 44% (PET/CT alone) for the detection of locoregional lymph nodes. Thus, FDG-PET/CT alone or in combination with EUS was clearly superior to EUS alone for distant metastases.[13] For the demonstration of peritoneal dissemination of abdominal malignancies, Yang and colleagues[14] found PET/CT better than ceCT, with sensitivities of 74% and 39%, respectively, with similar specificities of 93% to 94%.

Gastric cancer was the subject of one of the earliest studies on PET for response assessment almost 2 decades ago,[15] but since the turn of the century, one group in particular has pioneered the use of PET for early response assessment of neoadjuvant treatment in adenocarcinomas of the gastroesophageal junction. The Munich group presented its first preliminary results in 2001: 40 patients underwent PET scans at baseline and 14 days after the first cycle of chemotherapy, and changes in FDG uptake were assessed semiquantitatively and compared with clinical response (reduction of tumor length and wall thickness determined by endoscopy and/or imaging) and histopathologic response. The investigators determined the optimal cutoff for differentiation between responders and nonresponders to be a greater than 35% reduction in the FDG uptake expressed as standard uptake value (SUV), although not further stated if it was maximum SUV (SUVmax), mean SUV (SUVmean), or some other SUV value. Using this cutoff they found sensitivity and specificity for clinical response of 93% and 95%, respectively. Furthermore, histopathologically complete or subtotal regression was achieved in 53% of responders compared with 5% of nonresponders, and progression-free survival (PFS) and overall survival were significantly shorter in nonresponders.[16]

The same group presented similar results in several subsequent neoadjuvant studies, including their so-called MUNICON (Metabolic response evalUatioN for Individualisation of neoadjuvant Chemotherapy in Esophageal and esophagogastric adeNocarcinoma) studies: histopathologic response rates were higher in metabolic responders compared with nonresponders (69% vs 17%), and median survival was not reached in responders, whereas it was 24 months in nonresponders. Nonresponders proceeded directly to surgery after response assessment as early as 14 days after the first series of neoadjuvant chemotherapy. Responders had longer PFS than nonresponders (29.7 months vs 14.1). When nonresponders were switched to salvage neoadjuvant chemotherapy, histopathologic response rates increased (from 0% to 26%). Survival was slightly higher in nonresponders who proceeded directly to surgery compared with historic controls completing 3 series of preoperative chemotherapy, possibly due to fewer toxicity-related deaths. The primary endpoint was an increase in R0 resections (74% to 94%), but this was not reached.[17–19]

## PANCREATIC CANCER

Shortcomings of PET/CT in the detection and especially for the assessment of resectability of pancreatic tumors prevent its use up-front. Due to the metabolic activity in the primary tumor, which may obscure peripancreatic structures, PET does not suffice for the latter purpose, even when coregistered with ceCT, and studies on PET for lymph node involvement in pancreatic cancer have also been disappointing due to sensitivities below 50%.[20,21] Instead, ceCT and EUS are the best validated methods and are considered the reference standards for assessing locoregional and lymph node involvement. PET may be superior to ceCT, however, for the detection of distant metastases and may via this influence patient management considerably (**Fig. 1**). Thus, in a study by Heinrich and colleagues[22] with 59 patients, PET detected 13 of 16 patients with distant metastases, and in 5 cases detection was only achieved by PET. Additional findings also led to changes, and overall management was changed in 16% (6/37) of patients initially deemed resectable by conventional imaging. Bang and colleagues[23] assessed staging generally and found higher accuracy of FDG-PET compared with ceCT with regard to liver metastases. Also, PET changed disease stage and resectability status in approximately one-quarter of patients, primarily due to previously undetected distant metastases. Subsequent studies failed to reproduce these results and instead found PET sensitivities that were inferior to ceCT for subcentimeter liver lesions.[3]

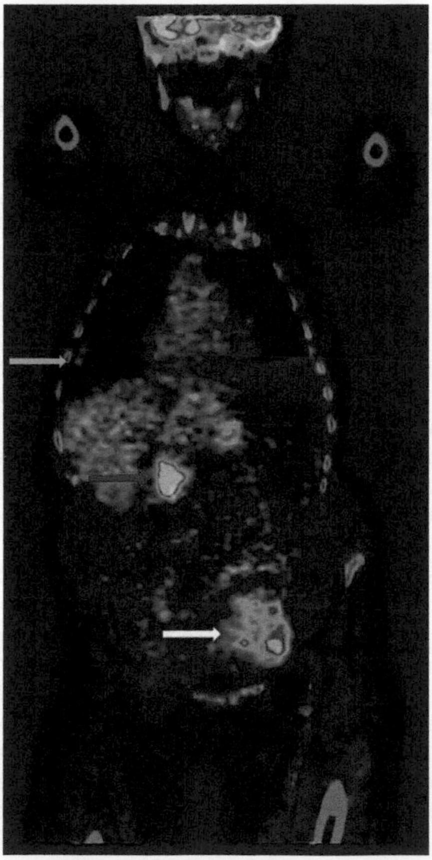

**Fig. 1.** Initial staging of a patient with pancreatic cancer. Fused coronal FDG-PET/CT shows increased uptake in the pancreatic mass (*red arrow*), multiple lung metastases (only one is shown [*blue arrow*]), and peritoneal carcinosis (*white arrow*).

Some studies have assessed the prognostic value of PET in pancreatic cancer and have in general found that high-baseline SUV values correspond with more widespread disease and poorer prognosis.[24–26] The clinical relevance of this is limited, however, and as with gastric cancer, it would be more valuable if early assessment of FDG uptake could predict response to preoperative/neoadjuvant chemotherapy, even if only a small fraction of patients received this type of treatment. Maemura and colleagues[27] found higher baseline SUVmax in metastatic pancreatic cancer than in localized tumors, and Sperti and colleagues[28] reported that an SUVmax greater than 4 was associated with shorter survival, that is, 2 observations suggest that early quantification by PET could serve as a marker of more aggressive disease with greater risk of progression during preoperative chemotherapy. Kittaka and colleagues[29] assessed treatment response in 40 patients treated with preoperative chemoradiotherapy and found generally higher baseline values and more pronounced decrease in SUVmax in responders than nonresponders (defined according to pathologic response). Despite statistical significance, there was considerable overlap of the cutoff values used: for baseline SUVmax, a chosen cutoff greater than 4.6 was found in 71% of responders and in 32% of nonresponders and, similarly, a chosen cutoff greater than 0.46 was found in 71% of responders and in 26% of nonresponders, all of which limits the clinical use.

## COLORECTAL CANCER

In general, PET has no role in primary tumor detection or characterization in CRC, although some studies have assessed the potential added value.[3] For instance, Mori and Oguchi[30] found 16 of 17 synchronous tumors proximal to an endoscopically nonpassable tumor, but only lesions larger than 8 mm were detectable, and it was not possible to distinguish between adenomas and carcinomas. Incidental focal bowel uptake, on the other hand, is often encountered on PET and also warrants further investigations in cases with no morphologic correlation on CT. Peng and colleagues[31] found focal colonic uptake in 1.3% of scans in a prospective study, including greater than 10,000 PET scans yielding cancerous and precancerous lesions in 21% and 24% of cases, respectively, confirmed by colonoscopy and pathology.

As with gastric and pancreatic cancers, N-staging of CRC with PET has been equally disappointing for the same reasons, that is, insufficient spatial resolution to detect small sized lymph-nodes and physiologic or tumor uptake obscuring activity in the intestine and urinary bladder or in other tissues adjacent to the primary tumor. This issue was summarized in a recent meta-analysis by Lu and colleagues[32] (n = 409, 10 studies) who found pooled sensitivity, specificity, and accuracy of FDG-PET/CT of 43%, 88%, and 71%, respectively, for lymph node staging in CRC.

In recent years, the treatment strategies for CRC metastatic disease have changed considerably compared with many other malignancies, because distant metastases in CRC do not exclude curative resection per se, although extrahepatic lesions limit the curative potential depending on number and location.[33] Niekel and colleagues[34] performed a meta-analysis of prospective studies comparing ceCT, MR imaging, and PET(/ceCT) in CRC from 1990 to 2010 (n = 3391, 39 studies). The pooled per-lesion sensitivities of the 3 approaches were 74%, 80%, and 81%, respectively, with nonsignificance between groups, whereas the corresponding pooled per-patient values were 84%, 88%, and 94%, respectively, with significant difference in favor of PET versus ceCT (*P* = .025). The pooled per-patient specificities were comparable for all modalities (>90%). The data were mainly obtained by stand-alone PET rather than PET/CT. Two earlier meta-analyses found comparable results.[35,36] A controversial issue is the detectable size of liver lesions. The study by Niekel and colleagues[34] found significantly higher sensitivity of MR imaging for subcentimeter lesions compared with CT but with too few PET data for comparison. Another study of 131 patients undergoing liver metastatectomy found comparable performance of ceCT and PET, that is, of the liver metastases identified during laparotomy, CT and PET detected only 16% of subcentimeter lesions but 72% to 75% of 1-cm to 2-cm lesions and 95% to 97% of lesions greater than 20 mm.[37] The significance of unexpected smaller hepatic metastases found by intraoperative ultrasound and palpation remains uncertain, and only 9 of the 131 patients (7%) were subsequently deemed noncurable. These findings may have implications for the indications for adjuvant chemotherapy but should be interpreted with caution, considering that the PET technique since then has improved significantly in terms of resolution and sensitivity, and this can be readily ascertained by simple inspection of images of that time and images acquired now with the latest equipment.

Nonetheless, as with upper GI malignancies, the major benefit of PET in CRC seems to be in the detection of extrahepatic metastases, although the available literature is sparse. Thus, in a meta-analysis by Patel and colleagues,[38] no pooled estimates could be derived from the few data (n = 178, 3 studies), but per-patient analyses suggested that PET/CT was more sensitive than ceCT (75%–89% vs 58%–64%), albeit with comparable specificities (95%–96% vs 87%–97%). A subsequent systematic review comprising 6 studies was equivocal, however, in that half of the studies found no significant difference, whereas the other half showed superior detection rates of PET compared with ceCT in the detection of extrahepatic metastases. In 1 study, PET led to correct change in patient management in one-fourth of cases.[39]

One of the few randomized controlled trials of PET imaging was in 150 CRC patients selected for resection of liver metastases.[40] Half of the patients were randomized to conventional preoperative work-up, including ceCT of the chest and abdomen, whereas the other half had an additional PET, and the primary endpoint was futile laparotomies (ie, laparotomies not resulting in complete tumor treatment, revealing benign disease, or followed by disease-free survival <6 months). There were significantly fewer futile laparotomies in the experimental arm than in the control arm (28% vs 45% with a relative risk reduction of 38%; *P* = .042). The additional findings with PET could be disregarded by the multidisciplinary treatment team. If acceptance of PET findings had been mandatory, it would have resulted in an additional reduction in futile laparotomies (ie, a relative risk reduction of 65%). The investigators concluded that the addition of PET prevented unnecessary surgery in 1 of 6 patients. One of the few cost-effectiveness studies of PET also focused on patients with CRC and the management of metachronous liver metastases after curative resection. The investigators concluded that combined PET/CT was as effective as CT alone with regard to life expectancy but less expensive due to cost savings from avoidance of futile surgery.[41] In the setting of evaluating CRC liver metastases, postablation PET may play a role (**Fig. 2**). Several studies, albeit small ones, have shown excellent ability of early PET to rule out residual disease or recurrence with a negative predictive value of 96% to 100% of PET scans performed 2 to 3 weeks after ablation. The positive predictive values were more variable (80%–100%), probably due to abscesses or postablation inflammation.[42] Thus, the decision to institute adjuvant chemotherapy in the future could be obviated, if early PET scans are negative.

Response assessment in CRC is less well established. The studies have generally shown PET responders to have lower recurrence rates, longer PFS, and trends toward longer overall survival compared with PET nonresponders, whereas pathologic response is not necessarily correlated with these parameters. The available studies are small and heterogeneous, however, with regard to patient population, research questions, treatment regimen, scan techniques, and timing.[42–45] Furthermore, although an argument for better response assessment is the need to reduce futile treatments, at present there is no solid ground for changing the regimens based on PET response and, thus, the clinical implications for the patients may be limited and mostly of academic interest.

## GASTROINTESTINAL STROMAL TUMORS

FDG and PET were also studied early on in GISTs due to a generally high FDG avidity. As with the other GI malignancies, FDG has no established role in the initial work-up of these tumors but may have significant impact in detecting metastatic disease, which is present in more than half of patients at presentation.[46] Early stand-alone PET studies were not encouraging due to both false-positive and false-negative results, for example, 5 of 141 false-positive lesions and 25 of 141 false-negative lesions in a study by Gayed and colleagues[47] and 36 of 173 false negative lesions in a study by Choi and colleagues,[48] whereas Antoch and colleagues[49] found PET unable to diagnose smaller liver and lung lesions. False-negative findings were also encountered, however, with CT (eg, 21/137 false-negative lesions in the study by Gayed and colleagues,[47] particularly in the bones). Some of these issues have been alleviated with technologic developments, and combined FDG-PET/CT may be superior to either modality alone. In the study by Antoch and

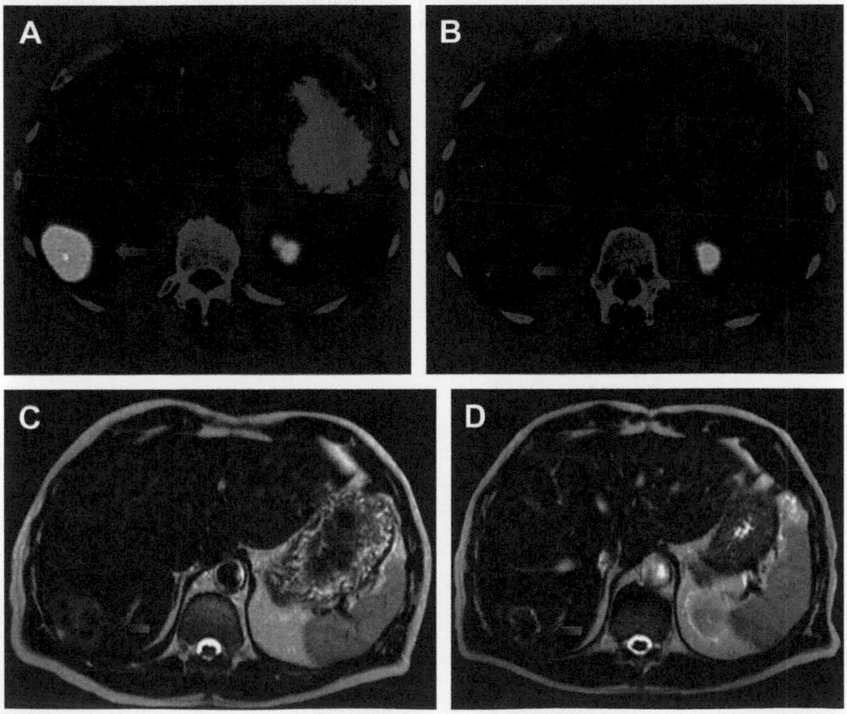


**Fig. 2.** A patient with colorectal carcinoma liver metastases treated with hepatic radioembolization. FDG-PET/CT (*A*) pretreatment and (*B*) 6 weeks post-treatment shows a marked complete metabolic response (*red arrows*), whereas MR imaging (*C*) pretreatment and (*D*) 6 weeks post-treatment shows only a partial anatomic response (*blue arrows*). (*From* Donswijk ML, Hess S, Mulders T, et al. [18F]Fluorodeoxyglucose PET/computed tomography in gastrointestinal malignancies. PET Clin 2014;9:433; with permission.)

colleagues,[49] PET/CT located 282 lesions in 20 patients, whereas CT and PET alone identified 242 and 147 lesions, respectively. Gayed and colleagues[47] found similar performance of CT and PET/CT, that is, sensitivities and positive predictive values of 93% and 100%, and 86% and 98%, respectively, the differences being nonsignificant.

Several studies have assessed the biological features of GISTs. For instance, Otomi and colleagues[50] established a relationship between FDG uptake and malignancy, that is, significantly higher values in high-risk GISTs compared with low-risk and medium-risk tumors. This apparent relationship between tumor glycolysis and malignant potential was substantiated by Kamiyama and colleagues,[51] who found significant correlation between FDG uptake and Ki67 values and mitotic index. These features may have implications for patient prognosis but may also serve as basis for early response assessment (**Fig. 3**).

In one of the first studies of early response in GISTs, Jager and colleagues[52] found FDG-PET able to differentiate metabolic responders (n = 11) from metabolic nonresponders (n = 4) after only 1 week of imatinib mesylate treatment compared with clinical and radiologic response according to RECIST. Mean SUVmax decreased significantly in the responders (64.9 ± 13.8%

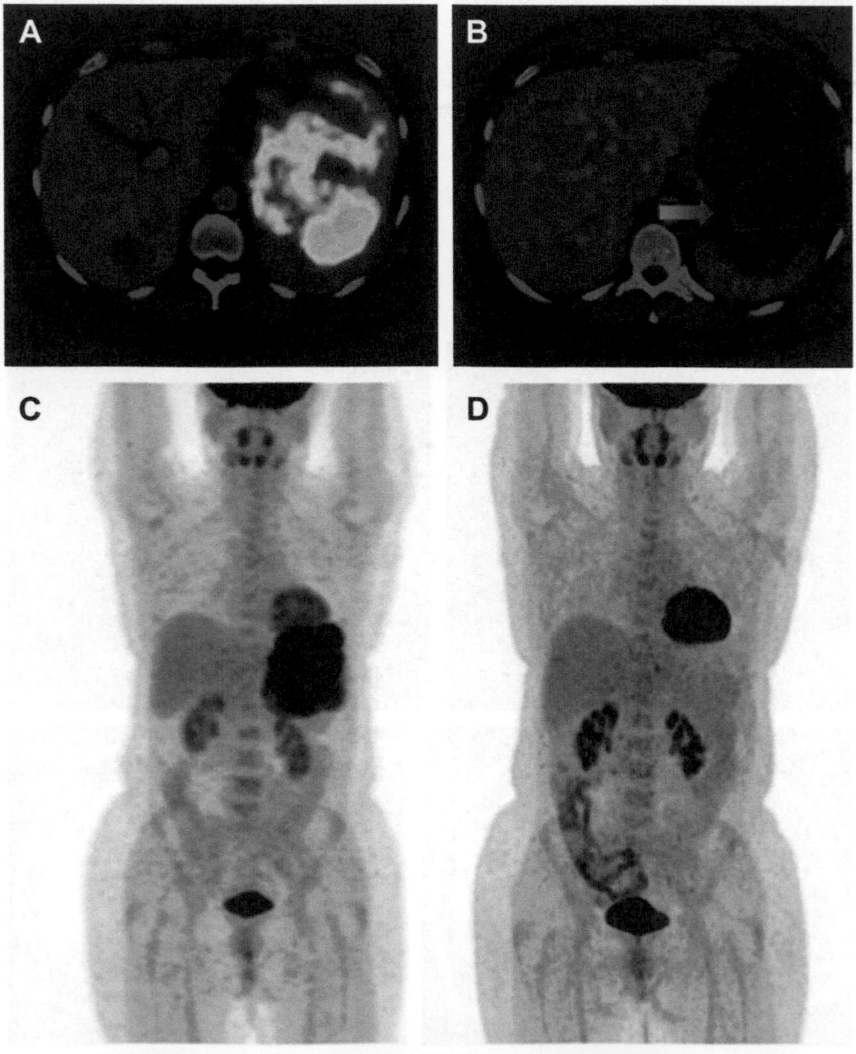


**Fig. 3.** FDG-PET/CT in a patient with GIST treated with imatinib. Transaxial slice through the stomach (*A*) and maximum intensity projection (*C*) show intense FDG uptake in a large gastric stroma cell tumor before treatment, and complete metabolic response after 3 months of treatment (*B, D*), while CT shows a residual mass (*blue arrow*). (*From* Donswijk ML, Hess S, Mulders T, et al. [18F]Fluorodeoxyglucose PET/computed tomography in gastrointestinal malignancies. PET Clin 2014;9:435; with permission.)

decrease; $P = .001$), whereas mean SUVmax actually increased in nonresponders (16.3 $\pm$ 19.1% increase; $P$ = not significant). FDG-PET also correlated with clinical disease course; PFS was significantly longer in PET responders compared with PET nonresponders, that is, after the first year, all responders were still progression free, whereas this was only the case for 1 of the nonresponders ($P = .0002$). Finally, the investigators found no significant difference in FDG uptake between scans 1 and 8 weeks after treatment initiation, which indicates that the FDG response to imatinib mesylate is genuinely an early response. This was substantiated by a case story from Shinto and colleagues,[53] who found a significant reduction in SUVmax (from 13 to 4) 24 hours after a single dose of imatinib mesylate (400 mg). These findings are underlined by the comparison with morphologic therapy assessment as presented by Heinicke and colleagues.[54] An SUVmean decrease of 60% was achieved on day 8 of imatinib mesylate treatment, whereas partial response was reached according to RECIST after in mean 23 weeks.

Progression or secondary resistance to imatinib mesylate appears as re-emergence of FDG uptake in metabolic inactive lesions. Some results suggest, however, a more complex interrelation with heterogeneous intratumoral and intertumoral clonal dedifferentiation: after cessation of imatinib mesylate therapy, flares of FDG uptake have been observed in lesions that were metabolically inactive during therapy. This suggests that some lesions may still be responsive to initial treatment, whereas only some clones progress to resistance, and this may in turn provide basis for combination therapy for different tyrosine kinase inhibitors, like imatinib mesylate and sunitinib, instead of the traditional complete switch in therapy.[55] Thus, although the optimum threshold is still under debate, the literature favors the use of FDG-PET as the primary method for treatment assessment in GISTs, with metabolic responses correlating well with PFS as well as long-term prognosis.[46,55–57]

## DISCUSSION

Currently, there seems to be no evidence to support routine application of FDG-PET/CT in the pretherapeutic evaluation of local involvement or lymph node staging in patients with GI malignancies, whereas results for distant metastatic status are more promising, especially in CRC. Some of the challenges relate to the physiologic distribution of FDG within the GI tract (discussed previously), whereas another important caveat is the differences in FDG accumulation patterns associated with different concentrations of GLUT1 glucose transporters, which is especially pronounced in gastric and pancreatic cancers.[3] Kawamura and colleagues[58] found that overall only 30% of gastric carcinomas expressed GLUT1 with the highest proportions in the rare papillary adenocarcinomas (44%) and virtually nonexistent in signet-ring cell carcinomas and mucinous adenocarcinomas (6% and 2%, respectively). Furthermore, there are certain diagnostic issues in the preoperative diagnostic work-up, especially in pancreatic cancer, for example, lesion localization, proximity to vessels, and invasion of adjacent structures. These demands are better met by EUS and special CT protocols for locoregional staging, whereas PET/CT is now primarily considered for the detection of distant metastases.[3] It seems that PET has not a sufficiently superior sensitivity compared with ceCT and MR imaging for hepatic involvement to warrant its use as first-line investigation, but it should be considered a second-line option, when ceCT or MR imaging is equivocal. In patients with solitary or oligometastatic disease, the higher sensitivity of PET for extrahepatic metastases may be of clinical significance to avoid futile surgery.

It must be pointed out that much literature information is based on older and heterogeneous studies using outdated techniques, that is, stand-alone PET, early-generation PET/CT, or PET combined with low-dose CT without contrast enhancement. These approaches can no longer be considered clinically sufficient, as illustrated by the first study to use PET/ceCT in pancreatic cancer: sensitivities of stand-alone PET and PET/low-dose CT were 100%, but specificities were only 44% and 56%, respectively, whereas the corresponding values for PET/ceCT were 96% and 82% respectively.[59] Furthermore, PET and PET/CT are often applied late in the patient course, which is a cause of selection bias. Thus, further studies on upfront PET/CT using state-of-the-art technology must be carried out to firmly evaluate the true potential of FDG-PET/CT for preoperative staging and surgical treatment decision making in GI malignancies.

Traditionally, response is evaluated using RECIST. Metabolic response seems, however, to precede morphologic changes substantially – in some cases, changes in tumor metabolism can be appreciated after few days or weeks, whereas morphologic changes are not recognizable until several weeks or months later. Also, novel targeted treatments have different modes of action. They are aimed at specific molecular or cellular pathways and cause other effects than traditional cytotoxic chemotherapy. For instance, immunotherapy can give rise to infiltratory lesions as part of their effect and this may be interpreted as novel lesions consistent with progression according to RECIST.

Overall, there seems to be a potential for using PET/CT to evaluate early response to treatment and tailor the strategy in accordance with tumor biology in gastric cancer, but to date no group has succeeded in reproducing the results of the MUNICON-trials,[16–19] and larger, preferably multicenter, studies are warranted.

In GISTs, RECIST may be especially prone to underestimate the treatment effect as judged from the simple geometric size of the primary lesions – not only is the RECIST required shrinkage not easily accomplished but also intratumoral hemorrhage, necrosis, and myxoid degeneration may actually cause morphologic augmentation. In these settings, an increasing number of reports suggest a role for FDG-PET/CT–based division of patients as PET responders or PET nonresponders, with an overall high specificity for predicting response.[45]

Due to the physiologic FDG uptake in the GI tract, other tracers have been suggested, but the experience with these is limited and results are not convincing. Thus, Staniuk and colleagues[60] evaluated the thymidine analog (proliferation marker) 3'-deoxy-3'-[18F]-fluorothymidine in preoperative staging of gastric cancer. Although the rate of detection of primary tumors was high (49/50), results for locoregional lymph node assessment was as equivocal as FDG, with a substantial fraction of false-positive and false-negative findings resulting in a mediocre overall correct delineation of lymph node involvement (73%). Another approach has been presented on molecular receptor targeting in CRC. Certain mutations, for instance in RAS genes, are associated with poor response to certain antibody treatment, for instance cetuximab. A recent in vitro study on human CRC cells imaged with $^{64}$Cu-DOTA-cetuximab suggested that cetuximab accumulated sufficiently in both RAS wild-type and RAS mutant tumor cells, and in the future pretherapeutic assessment of labeled antibody uptake may help to stratify patients eligible for such treatment.[45] Although the work on alternative tracers is interesting, often well-executed, and necessary, the challenges related to other tracers are not straightforward, and at present no tracer has emerged as a true competitor to FDG for most applications.[2] One reason may be the inherent heterogeneity of most malignancies (discussed previously), which is increasingly recognized as important because metastatic clones may be significantly different from the primary tumor.[3,61,62] Thus, a sensitive, general-purpose tracer like FDG may be the natural first-line tracer despite its potential shortcomings.

Furthermore, in the authors' opinion, evaluation of FDG is still in its infancy and with regard to several important aspects of FDG the surface has only been scratched, in particular when it comes to quantification. The most common way of evaluating response is still by (semi)quantitative assessment using SUV-based parameters as the predominant method despite the inherent technical and patient related pitfalls, for example, using SUVmax instead of SUVmean values in heterogeneous tumors, timing of the scan, and blood glucose levels. No consensus on SUV reporting has been established, for example, the use of fixed values or changes in SUV from scan to scan or the application of conceptually more attractive approaches, like measurement and monitoring of total lesion glycolysis and the like.[63,64] This lack of standardization along with a relative lack of standardization of scanner hardware impedes the conductance of multicenter studies, because comparison of quantitative variables obtained by different centers with various scanners of different ages is at present a challenging task.[65,66]

In conclusion, the use of FDG-PET/CT in GI malignancies is not as straightforward as in many other malignancies. The potential is clearly there, and some aspects are promising, but further studies using state-of-the-art approaches in multidisciplinary settings are required.

## REFERENCES

1. Jameson JL, Longo DL. Precision medicine–personalized, problematic, and promising. N Engl J Med 2015;372(23):2229–34.
2. Hess S, Blomberg BA, Zhu HJ, et al. The pivotal role of FDG-PET/CT in modern medicine. Acad Radiol 2014;21(2):232–49.
3. Donswijk ML, Hess S, Mulders T, et al. [18f]fluorodeoxyglucose PET/computed tomography in gastrointestinal malignancies. PET Clin 2014;9(4):421–41, v–vi.
4. Lordick F, Allum W, Carneiro F, et al. Unmet needs and challenges in gastric cancer: the way forward. Cancer Treat Rev 2014;40(6):692–700.
5. de Geus-Oei LF, Vriens D, Arens AI, et al. FDG-PET/CT based response-adapted treatment. Cancer Imaging 2012;12:324–35.
6. Eisenhauer EA, Therasse P, Bogaerts J, et al. New response evaluation criteria in solid tumours: revised RECIST guideline (version 1.1). Eur J Cancer 2009;45(2):228–47.
7. Podoloff DA, Ball DW, Ben-Josef E, et al. NCCN task force: clinical utility of PET in a variety of tumor types. J Natl Compr Canc Netw 2009;7(Suppl 2):S1–26.

8. Filik M, Kir KM, Aksel B, et al. The role of 18F-FDG PET/CT in the primary staging of gastric cancer. Mol Imaging Radionucl Ther 2015;24(1):15–20.
9. Park K, Jang G, Baek S, et al. Usefulness of combined PET/CT to assess regional lymph node involvement in gastric cancer. Tumori 2014;100(2):201–6.
10. Cui JX, Li T, Xi HQ, et al. Evaluation of (18)F-FDG PET/CT in preoperative staging of gastric cancer: a meta-analysis. Zhonghua Wei Chang Wai Ke Za Zhi 2013;16(5):418–24 [in Chinese].
11. Smyth E, Schoder H, Strong VE, et al. A prospective evaluation of the utility of 2-deoxy-2-[(18) F]fluoro-D-glucose positron emission tomography and computed tomography in staging locally advanced gastric cancer. Cancer 2012;118(22):5481–8.
12. Ha TK, Choi YY, Song SY, et al. F18-fluorodeoxyglucose-positron emission tomography and computed tomography is not accurate in preoperative staging of gastric cancer. J Korean Surg Soc 2011;81(2):104–10.
13. Li B, Zheng P, Zhu Q, et al. Accurate preoperative staging of gastric cancer with combined endoscopic ultrasonography and PET-CT. Tohoku J Exp Med 2012;228(1):9–16.
14. Yang QM, Bando E, Kawamura T, et al. The diagnostic value of PET-CT for peritoneal dissemination of abdominal malignancies. Gan To Kagaku Ryoho Chemother 2006;33(12):1817–21.
15. Couper GW, McAteer D, Wallis F, et al. Detection of response to chemotherapy using positron emission tomography in patients with oesophageal and gastric cancer. Br J Surg 1998;85(10):1403–6.
16. Weber WA, Ott K, Becker K, et al. Prediction of response to preoperative chemotherapy in adenocarcinomas of the esophagogastric junction by metabolic imaging. J Clin Oncol 2001;19(12):3058–65.
17. Ott K, Herrmann K, Lordick F, et al. Early metabolic response evaluation by fluorine-18 fluorodeoxyglucose positron emission tomography allows in vivo testing of chemosensitivity in gastric cancer: long-term results of a prospective study. Clin Cancer Res 2008;14(7):2012–8.
18. Lordick F. Optimizing neoadjuvant chemotherapy through the use of early response evaluation by positron emission tomography. Recent Results Cancer Res 2012;196:201–11.
19. Ott K, Herrmann K, Krause BJ, et al. The value of PET imaging in patients with localized gastroesophageal Cancer. Gastrointest Cancer Res 2008;2(6):287–94.
20. Kauhanen SP, Komar G, Seppanen MP, et al. A prospective diagnostic accuracy study of 18F-fluorodeoxyglucose positron emission tomography/computed tomography, multidetector row computed tomography, and magnetic resonance imaging in primary diagnosis and staging of pancreatic cancer. Ann Surg 2009;250(6):957–63.
21. Asagi A, Ohta K, Nasu J, et al. Utility of contrast-enhanced FDG-PET/CT in the clinical management of pancreatic cancer: impact on diagnosis, staging, evaluation of treatment response, and detection of recurrence. Pancreas 2013;42(1):11–9.
22. Heinrich S, Goerres GW, Schafer M, et al. Positron emission tomography/computed tomography influences on the management of resectable pancreatic cancer and its cost-effectiveness. Ann Surg 2005; 242(2):235–43.
23. Bang S, Chung HW, Park SW, et al. The clinical usefulness of 18-fluorodeoxyglucose positron emission tomography in the differential diagnosis, staging, and response evaluation after concurrent chemoradiotherapy for pancreatic cancer. J Clin Gastroenterol 2006;40(10):923–9.
24. Wang XY, Yang F, Jin C, et al. Utility of PET/CT in diagnosis, staging, assessment of resectability and metabolic response of pancreatic cancer. World J Gastroenterol 2014;20(42):15580–9.
25. Sahani DV, Bonaffini PA, Catalano OA, et al. State-of-the-art PET/CT of the pancreas: current role and emerging indications. Radiographics 2012;32(4):1133–58 [discussion: 1158–60].
26. Lordick F, Ott K, Krause BJ. New trends for staging and therapy for localized gastroesophageal cancer: the role of PET. Ann Oncol 2010;21(Suppl 7):vii294–9.
27. Maemura K, Takao S, Shinchi H, et al. Role of positron emission tomography in decisions on treatment strategies for pancreatic cancer. J Hepatobiliary Pancreat Surg 2006;13(5):435–41.
28. Sperti C, Pasquali C, Bissoli S, et al. Tumor relapse after pancreatic cancer resection is detected earlier by 18-FDG PET than by CT. J Gastrointest Surg 2010;14(1):131–40.
29. Kittaka H, Takahashi H, Ohigashi H, et al. Role of (18)F-fluorodeoxyglucose positron emission tomography/computed tomography in predicting the pathologic response to preoperative chemoradiation therapy in patients with resectable T3 pancreatic cancer. World J Surg 2013;37(1):169–78.
30. Mori S, Oguchi K. Application of (18)F-fluorodeoxyglucose positron emission tomography to detection of proximal lesions of obstructive colorectal cancer. Jpn J Radiol 2010;28(8):584–90.
31. Peng J, He Y, Xu J, et al. Detection of incidental colorectal tumours with 18F-labelled 2-fluoro-2-deoxyglucose positron emission tomography/computed tomography scans: results of a prospective study. Colorectal Dis 2011;13(11):e374–8.
32. Lu YY, Chen JH, Ding HJ, et al. A systematic review and meta-analysis of pretherapeutic lymph node staging of colorectal cancer by 18F-FDG PET or PET/CT. Nucl Med Commun 2012;33(11):1127–33.
33. Spolverato G, Ejaz A, Azad N, et al. Surgery for colorectal liver metastases: the evolution of determining

prognosis. World J Gastrointest Oncol 2013;5(12): 207–21.

34. Niekel MC, Bipat S, Stoker J. Diagnostic imaging of colorectal liver metastases with CT, MR imaging, FDG PET, and/or FDG PET/CT: a meta-analysis of prospective studies including patients who have not previously undergone treatment. Radiology 2010;257(3):674–84.
35. Bipat S, van Leeuwen MS, Comans EF, et al. Colorectal liver metastases: CT, MR imaging, and PET for diagnosis–meta-analysis. Radiology 2005; 237(1):123–31.
36. Floriani I, Torri V, Rulli E, et al. Performance of imaging modalities in diagnosis of liver metastases from colorectal cancer: a systematic review and meta-analysis. J Magn Reson Imaging 2010;31(1):19–31.
37. Wiering B, Ruers TJ, Krabbe PF, et al. Comparison of multiphase CT, FDG-PET and intra-operative ultrasound in patients with colorectal liver metastases selected for surgery. Ann Surg Oncol 2007;14(2): 818–26.
38. Patel S, McCall M, Ohinmaa A, et al. Positron emission tomography/computed tomographic scans compared to computed tomographic scans for detecting colorectal liver metastases: a systematic review. Ann Surg 2011;253(4):666–71.
39. Chan K, Welch S, Walker-Dilks C, et al. Evidence-based guideline recommendations on the use of positron emission tomography imaging in colorectal cancer. Clin Oncol 2012;24(4):232–49.
40. Ruers TJ, Wiering B, van der Sijp JR, et al. Improved selection of patients for hepatic surgery of colorectal liver metastases with (18)F-FDG PET: a randomized study. J Nucl Med 2009;50(7):1036–41.
41. Langer A. A systematic review of PET and PET/CT in oncology: a way to personalize cancer treatment in a cost-effective manner? BMC Health Serv Res 2010; 10:283.
42. de Geus-Oei LF, Vriens D, van Laarhoven HW, et al. Monitoring and predicting response to therapy with 18F-FDG PET in colorectal cancer: a systematic review. J Nucl Med 2009;50(Suppl 1):43S–54S.
43. de Geus-Oei LF, van Laarhoven HW, Visser EP, et al. Chemotherapy response evaluation with FDG-PET in patients with colorectal cancer. Ann Oncol 2008; 19(2):348–52.
44. Martoni AA, Di Fabio F, Pinto C, et al. Prospective study on the FDG-PET/CT predictive and prognostic values in patients treated with neoadjuvant chemoradiation therapy and radical surgery for locally advanced rectal cancer. Ann Oncol 2011;22(3): 650–6.
45. Kruse V, Belle SV, Cocquyt V. Imaging requirements for personalized medicine: the oncologists point of view. Curr Pharm Des 2014;20(14):2234–49.
46. Malle P, Sorschag M, Gallowitsch HJ, et al. FDG PET and FDG PET/CT in patients with gastrointestinal stromal tumours. Wien Med Wochenschr 2012; 162(19–20):423–9.
47. Gayed I, Vu T, Iyer R, et al. The role of 18F-FDG PET in staging and early prediction of response to therapy of recurrent gastrointestinal stromal tumors. J Nucl Med 2004;45(1):17–21.
48. Choi H, Charnsangavej C, de Castro Faria S, et al. CT evaluation of the response of gastrointestinal stromal tumors after imatinib mesylate treatment: a quantitative analysis correlated with FDG PET findings. AJR Am J Roentgenol 2004; 183(6):1619–28.
49. Antoch G, Kanja J, Bauer S, et al. Comparison of PET, CT, and dual-modality PET/CT imaging for monitoring of imatinib (STI571) therapy in patients with gastrointestinal stromal tumors. J Nucl Med 2004;45(3):357–65.
50. Otomi Y, Otsuka H, Morita N, et al. Relationship between FDG uptake and the pathological risk category in gastrointestinal stromal tumors. J Med Invest 2010;57(3–4):270–4.
51. Kamiyama Y, Aihara R, Nakabayashi T, et al. 18F-fluorodeoxyglucose positron emission tomography: useful technique for predicting malignant potential of gastrointestinal stromal tumors. World J Surg 2005;29(11):1429–35.
52. Jager PL, Gietema JA, van der Graaf WT. Imatinib mesylate for the treatment of gastrointestinal stromal tumours: best monitored with FDG PET. Nucl Med Commun 2004;25(5):433–8.
53. Shinto A, Nair N, Dutt A, et al. Early response assessment in gastrointestinal stromal tumors with FDG PET scan 24 hours after a single dose of imatinib. Clin Nucl Med 2008;33(7):486–7.
54. Heinicke T, Wardelmann E, Sauerbruch T, et al. Very early detection of response to imatinib mesylate therapy of gastrointestinal stromal tumours using 18fluoro-deoxyglucose-positron emission tomography. Anticancer Res 2005;25(6C):4591–4.
55. Van den Abbeele AD. The lessons of GIST–PET and PET/CT: a new paradigm for imaging. Oncologist 2008;13(Suppl 2):8–13.
56. Holdsworth CH, Badawi RD, Manola JB, et al. CT and PET: early prognostic indicators of response to imatinib mesylate in patients with gastrointestinal stromal tumor. AJR Am J Roentgenol 2007;189(6): W324–30.
57. Goerres GW, Stupp R, Barghouth G, et al. The value of PET, CT and in-line PET/CT in patients with gastrointestinal stromal tumours: long-term outcome of treatment with imatinib mesylate. Eur J Nucl Med Mol Imaging 2005;32(2):153–62.
58. Kawamura T, Kusakabe T, Sugino T, et al. Expression of glucose transporter-1 in human gastric carcinoma: association with tumor aggressiveness, metastasis, and patient survival. Cancer 2001; 92(3):634–41.

59. Strobel K, Heinrich S, Bhure U, et al. Contrast-enhanced 18F-FDG PET/CT: 1-stop-shop imaging for assessing the resectability of pancreatic cancer. J Nucl Med 2008;49(9):1408–13.
60. Staniuk T, Zegarski W, Malkowski B, et al. Evaluation of FLT-PET/CT usefulness in diagnosis and qualification for surgical treatment of gastric cancer. Contemp Oncol (Pozn) 2013;17(2):165–70.
61. Kuukasjarvi T, Karhu R, Tanner M, et al. Genetic heterogeneity and clonal evolution underlying development of asynchronous metastasis in human breast cancer. Cancer Res 1997;57(8):1597–604.
62. Kroigard AB, Larsen MJ, Laenkholm AV, et al. Clonal expansion and linear genome evolution through breast cancer progression from pre-invasive stages to asynchronous metastasis. Oncotarget 2015;6(8):5634–49.
63. Basu S, Zaidi H, Salavati A, et al. FDG PET/CT methodology for evaluation of treatment response in lymphoma: from "graded visual analysis" and "semiquantitative SUVmax" to global disease burden assessment. Eur J Nucl Med Mol Imaging 2014;41(11):2158–60.
64. Hess S, Blomberg BA, Rakheja R, et al. A brief overview of novel approaches to FDG PET imaging and quantification. Clin Transl Imaging 2014;2:11.
65. Boellaard R, Delgado-Bolton R, Oyen WJ, et al. FDG PET/CT: EANM procedure guidelines for tumour imaging: version 2.0. Eur J Nucl Med Mol Imaging 2015;42(2):328–54.
66. Tahari AK, Wahl RL. Quantitative FDG PET/CT in the community: experience from interpretation of outside oncologic PET/CT exams in referred cancer patients. J Med Imaging Radiat Oncol 2014;58(2):183–8.

# The Possible Role of PET Imaging Toward Individualized Management of Bone and Soft Tissue Malignancies

Elena Tabacchi, MD, Stefano Fanti, MD,
Cristina Nanni, MD*

**KEYWORDS**

• Sarcoma • Musculoskeletal • Bone • Soft tissue • Cancer

**KEY POINTS**

- PET/computed tomography (CT) for sarcoma detection and grading: Usually higher-grade tumors are more metabolically active than lower-grade tumors, but this is not always true so that PET/CT does not provide excellent performance in this field.
- PET/CT has a significant impact on staging and restaging sarcomas especially for lymph nodal metastases, distant metastases and local relapse; sensitivity is lower for lung metastases, so that a thorax diagnostic CT is suggested.
- There is a significant association between tumor standardized uptake value (SUV) and several pathologic markers correlated to prognosis. The amount of necrosis (easily detected by PET/CT) is a predictor of good therapy response.
- Tumor SUV changes provides additional information to assess the treatment response.
- The routine use of PET-guided biopsy is not well established yet, but in some cases benefits may come from a biopsy targeted on the hottest area within a suspect sarcoma.

## INTRODUCTION

Bone and soft tissue sarcomas represent a heterogeneous group of malignancies including more than 50 histologic subtypes.[1,2]

Soft tissue sarcomas (mesodermal origin) represent approximately 1% of adult malignancies and 7% of pediatric malignancies and are generally sporadic with no specific etiologic agent. In some cases, exposure to alkylating chemotherapeutic agents, Paget disease, areas of bone infarction, irradiated bones, neurofibromatosis, tuberous sclerosis, Gardner syndrome, and Li Fraumeni syndrome could be considered as predisposing factors.

Bone sarcomas represent only 0.2% of all new cancer diagnoses and have a peak of presentation in adolescence (primary sarcomas) and a peak in the elderly (secondary sarcomas associated with Paget disease and irradiated bones).

Soft tissue sarcomas arise predominantly in the abdomen and in the extremities, instead bone sarcomas may arise in any bone and within any region of a given bone. However, osteosarcoma arises most frequently in the long bones of the lower extremities, whereas Ewing sarcoma arises in the long tubular bones, the flat bones of the pelvis, and the ribs.

Disclosure Statement: The authors have nothing to disclose.
Nuclear Medicine, AOU di Bologna Policlinico S. Orsola-Malpighi, Via Massarenti 9, Bologna 40138, Italy
* Corresponding author.
*E-mail address:* cristina.nanni@aosp.bo.it

PET Clin 11 (2016) 285–296
http://dx.doi.org/10.1016/j.cpet.2016.02.011

The typical clinical presentation of patients with soft tissue sarcoma is an enlarging mass: the size greater than 5 cm, location deep to fascia, and rapid tumor growth are worrisome characteristics. Important elements are duration of mass, rate of growth, pain, weakness, history of trauma, exposure to radiation or other carcinogenic toxins, personal or family history of cancer, and smoking history. Other important considerations are the consistency of the mass, presence of pain with palpation, its anatomic location (relative to the fascia and neurovascular structures), evaluation of regional lymph nodes, and neurovascular examination of the affected extremity.[3,4] Unlike bone sarcomas, soft tissue sarcomas are generally not associated with pain; for this reason, lack of pain does not make a mass more likely to be benign.[5]

Up to 60% of patients who initially receive treatment with curative intent present local recurrence or distant metastases and prognosis is strongly related to several factors, like the extent of the disease at diagnosis, the grade of the tumor, the age of the patient, the presence of microscopically positive margins after resection, and the presence of metastasis at diagnosis.[6–9]

Surgery is the standard treatment for sarcomas in a curative setting. On the basis of the histologic subtype, tumor grade, and tumor site, patients receive radiotherapy and/or chemotherapy (adjuvant or neoadjuvant) so as to facilitate surgical excision of large tumors or to consolidate local treatment after surgical resection.[10–12]

Follow-up of patients treated for soft tissue or bone sarcoma is related to the risk of recurrence and the amount of time elapsed after treatment. Long-term follow-up studies demonstrate that approximately 80% of patients had a relapse in the first 3 years after therapy, and that patients who are alive without recurrence at 5 and 10 years after therapy apparently still have a risk for a subsequent late recurrence. Surveillance strategies include physical examination, appropriate imaging of the primary site of the tumor, and chest imaging for the risk of lung metastasis.[6]

In this patient population, the accurate and early detection of local or metastatic recurrent lesions is highly warranted, because early treatment can prolong survival.[13]

## NORMAL ANATOMY AND IMAGING TECHNIQUE

Anatomically based imaging modalities like computed tomography (CT) and magnetic resonance (MR) imaging represent the primary diagnostic modalities for evaluating sarcomas.[14–17]

Regarding soft tissue sarcoma, radiographs of the affected extremity should be obtained and analyzed for the presence and size of a soft tissue shadow, bony destruction, and intratumoral calcifications. Radiographs can help identify a primary bone tumor associated with a large soft tissue mass such as happens in Ewing sarcoma. In particular, if a bone lesion is considered an "indeterminate lesion" by radiography, namely not clearly consistent with a single diagnosis, typically the doubt is clarified by MR imaging, which is the primary imaging method for evaluating bone lesions, their exact location, and their proximity to neurovascular structures.[18]

The amount and type of bony destruction can provide evidence of the biologic activity of tumor: slow growing masses may present a pressure effect with cortical remodeling marked by a well-defined reactive rim; rapidly growing masses may produce a more irregular cortical destruction. Phleboliths are generally found in benign hemangiomas, whereas amorphous calcification is typical of synovial sarcoma and some liposarcomas.[19]

MR imaging, which should be performed with and without intravenous gadolinium enhancement,[3] is the best modality for evaluation of a potential soft tissue sarcoma in particular for diagnostic characterization and staging and to plan effective management. If MR imaging is not feasible (incompatible medical device or high-risk metallic foreign body), a CT scan with and without intravenous contrast is recommended with 3-dimensional (3D) reconstruction to assess local extent of disease. Soft tissue sarcomas typically exhibit heterogeneous high signal intensity on T2-weighted images, whereas T1-weighted images best demonstrate normal anatomy and its relation to the tumor. As the sequence is not fluid sensitive, it will help differentiate tumor from the edema seen on T2 sequences. Often the delineation between tumor tissue and uninvolved tissue is further defined by T1 postgadolinium images. Sometimes the tumor extent can be overestimated on T2 sequences, as the fluid-sensitive nature of the sequence cannot easily define edema as opposed to actual tumor extent.

Dynamic contrast-enhanced MR imaging (DCE-MR imaging) is a method of physiologic imaging that uses bolus administration of water-soluble and paramagnetic contrast, rapidly obtained sequences, and software to measure perfusion and diffusion characteristics of the imaged tissue.[20]

DCE–MR imaging relies on the contrast agent first passing through the capillaries of the tumor and then rapidly diffusing into the interstitial compartment evaluating increased vascular density, high perfusion, and increased permeability associated with soft tissue sarcomas. Viable tumor enhances rapidly, whereas areas of necrosis, degeneration, hemorrhage, and fibrosis enhance much more slowly. The major advantage of DCE–MR imaging is the ability to potentially reflect tumor biology defining the most aggressive part of a tumor for biopsy, determine response to chemotherapy, and differentiate recurrence from inflammatory tissue.[20]

In addition to cross-sectional imaging, a CT scan of the chest should be performed on initial presentation of sarcoma and after any neoadjuvant therapy, as the finding of metastatic disease (often pulmonary metastases) may alter the goals of the surgical treatment plan. Bone scans could be used for staging purposes even if the incidence of bone metastasis is extremely low.[21]

PET with the glucose analog $^{18}$F-fluorodeoxyglucose ($^{18}$F-FDG) is used increasingly to provide complementary information in sarcoma diagnosis and treatment planning. The acquisition of PET data is not affected by metal implants (frequently present when patients have undergone limb-sparing bone resection and prosthetic bone reconstruction); PET/CT enables fast and accurate full-body evaluation that potentially may add relevant diagnostic information to whole-body CT or MR imaging studies.[14–17]

PET/CT is very sensitive and specific for detection of high-grade bone and soft tissue sarcoma but has a low positive predictive value for evaluation of nodal metastases.[22]

PET/CT has been studied in sarcoma detection and grading,[23] initial staging,[24] assessing response to neoadjuvant therapy,[25] determining prognosis,[25,26] investigating potential local recurrence,[27] and biopsy guidance.[28,29]

## *PET/Computed Tomography for Sarcoma Detection and Grading*

This is the most researched area for PET scanning in sarcoma. The standardized uptake value (SUV) is a measure of radioactivity in a specific area of interest, and a higher SUV value means that this area is more metabolically active. Usually higher-grade tumors are more metabolically active than lower grade tumors[23]; however, high-grade tumors may have a low metabolic activity and not every highly metabolically active area is necessarily a malignant entity.[30]

Folpe and colleagues[31] used an SUV value greater than 7.5 as a cutoff to determine if SUV can predict grade and found that 93% of tumors in this group were high-grade sarcomas (7% of benign tumors were also in this group) and 52% of high-grade malignancies had an SUV value less than 7.5. They found a correlation between higher SUV value and histologic findings of increased mitosis rate and cellularity.[31]

Charest and colleagues[32] found that all lesions in their study (212 bone and soft tissue sarcomas) with an SUV value greater than 6.5 were high grade although many high-grade sarcomas had an SUV less than 6.5.

Bastiaannet and colleagues[23] performed a meta-analysis in 2004 regarding the detection of sarcomas using PET scan and found an overall sensitivity, specificity, and accuracy, respectively, of 91%, 85%, and 88%.

SUV can thus give an estimation of tumor grade before biopsy but PET/CT does not replace biopsy of the lesion and histologic examination by a pathologist to determine the grade.

## *PET/Computed Tomography for Initial Staging and Restaging*

Metastasis in soft tissue and bone sarcoma is predominantly (75%) to the lung (**Fig. 1**).[33] Mixoid/round cell liposarcomas have predilection for retroperitoneal involvement and may benefit, in the initial staging, from abdominal imaging in association with chest.[34] Synovial sarcoma, rhabdomyosarcoma, clear cell sarcoma, and epithelioid sarcoma have a predilection to lymph node involvement.[35,36]

Many studies underline the impact of 18F-FDG PET/CT on the management of pediatric sarcomas compared with conventional imaging (MR, CT, bone scintigraphy, ultrasound, and chest radiography). For example, Völker and colleagues[16] evaluated, in a multicenter study, 46 pediatric patients affected by Ewing, osteo/rhabdomyosarcoma who underwent FDG-PET for staging. The results of the study showed that FDG-PET and conventional imaging were equally accurate for detecting the primary tumor (100% accuracy), PET was superior in assessing lymph node involvement and bone localizations, and CT turned out to be more accurate for the detection of pulmonary metastasis.

Similarly, Tateishi and colleagues[37] evaluated 117 patients and found a very high accuracy in defining the exact TNM when FDG-PET/CT was combined with conventional imaging results.

FDG-PET/CT is important even in detecting sarcoma recurrence in pediatric patients. This was demonstrated by Arush and colleagues[38] on 19 patients who presented an FDG-PET scan that was useful for the correct interpretation of conventional imaging findings and was able to detect otherwise unknown metastasis in 2 patients.

Fuglo and colleagues[22] retrospectively evaluated 89 patients with bone and soft tissue

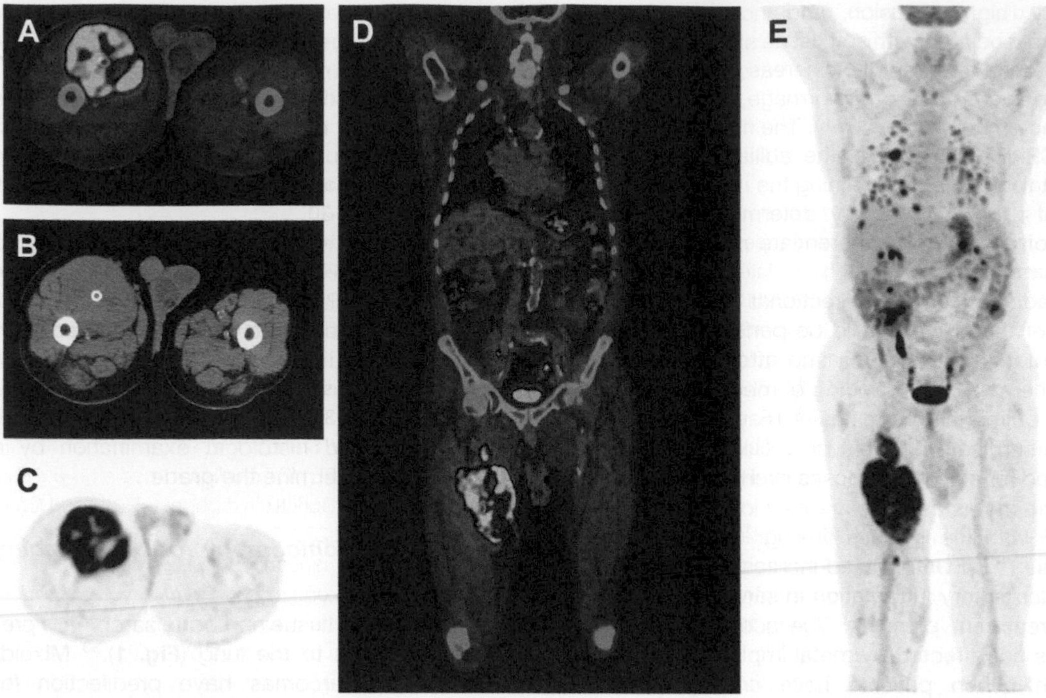


**Fig. 1.** Soft tissue sarcoma of the right thigh in an 85-year-old man, stadiation. (*A*) PET/CT, transaxial view. (*B*) CT, transaxial view. (*C*) PET, transaxial view. (*D*) PET/CT coronal view. (*E*) Maximum intensity projection (MIP) shows intense focal uptake (SUVmax = 22) at the middle third anteromedial of the right thigh with 2 additional small hypermetabolic foci above and below the main lesion (T). Faint uptake against some bilateral inguinal lymph nodes (N). Numerous bilateral pulmonary nodules hypermetabolic (M).

sarcomas: the positive predictive value for lymph node involvement was only 27%, whereas sensitivity, specificity, positive predictive value, and negative predictive value for distant metastasis was 95%, 95%, 87%, and 98%, respectively.

The use of PET/CT for staging may be useful as an adjunct, especially in certain histologies that are more likely to have nonpulmonary metastasis.

### *PET/Computed Tomography and Prediction of Prognosis*

In patients with sarcoma, it is very important to detect the major number of prognostic factors so as to define the best therapeutic approach and schedule follow-up examinations. Tumor type and site are associated with a risk for poor outcome[39]; in particular, patients with bone sarcoma generally have a better outcome than patients with high-grade soft tissue sarcoma, and extremity tumors present less risk for a poor outcome compared with those in truncal sites. Even tumor size is recognized as a significant prognostic factor in the planning of treatment for soft tissue sarcoma tumors[39] and histologically intermediate-grade soft tissue sarcomas that are larger than 5 cm in diameter are considered in the same high-risk category for reduced survival as histologically high-grade tumors.

Many investigators analyzed the possible role of FDG-PET in predicting the prognosis both when performed at diagnosis and after the presurgical chemotherapy.

A study of Folpe and colleagues[31] that includes a large number of well-characterized soft tissue and bone tumors, has shown a significant association between the tumor SUV and several pathologic markers, including histopathological grade, tumor cellularity, proliferative activity as measured by mitotic figure counts, and overexpression of p53.

Eary and colleagues[40] evaluated 238 patients affected by different kinds of sarcomas who underwent FDG-PET before chemotherapy or surgical resection and compared the PET result with the overall survival and the disease-free survival. PET images were analyzed in terms of maximum SUV (SUVmax) and heterogeneity of FDG distribution within the primary mass: biologic heterogeneity (including proliferation, necrosis, noncellular accumulations like fibrous tissue, differences in blood flow, oxygenation, receptorial expression, cellular metabolism) is a very important feature of malignant tumors. The investigators found that both SUVmax and FDG heterogeneous distribution can distinguish between higher-risk patients and lower-risk patients.

Even Lisle and colleagues,[41] analyzing 44 patients affected by synovial sarcoma, found a correlation between pretherapy SUVmax and overall survival and progression-free survival. Patients with SUVmax greater than 4.35 at diagnosis had a decreased disease-free survival and thus a higher risk for recurrences and metastatic disease.

Sato and colleagues[42] evaluated 13 patients by measuring the sarcoma SUVmax before and after the neoadjuvant chemotherapy and correlated them with the expression of metastasis-related glycolytic enzyme and autocrine motility factor/phosphoglucose isomerase in surgically excised tumors. They considered a follow-up of 4 years and found that mean SUV before therapy was similar in patients with and without metastasis, whereas mean SUV after therapy was significantly lower in those without metastasis. Therefore, SUV was significantly correlated with the presence of glycolytic enzyme and autocrine motility factor/phosphoglucose isomerase.

Many published reports focused on the association between tumor FDG uptake and tumor necrosis: the presence of a high level of tumor necrosis in sarcomas is thought to be a strong predictor of long-term treatment response.[43–46]

## PET/Computed Tomography and Evaluation of Response to Therapy

Assessment of tumor response on the basis of criteria involving changes in tumor size is not particularly helpful in sarcomas (**Fig. 2**).[47]

A study by Bredella and colleagues[48] demonstrated that tumor FDG SUV changes contributed additional information to assessment of the treatment response with MR imaging and a study of Evilevitch and colleagues[47] showed that the difference between the SUV pre- and post-therapy (SUVdiff) value was more accurate for assessing the response than either the presence of substantial tumor necrosis or the RECIST (Response Evaluation Criteria in Solid Tumors) when these were applied to the same group of soft tissue sarcomas. They evaluated 42 patients with resectable biopsy-proven soft tissue sarcomas who underwent an FDG-PET before and after therapy, and found that the reduction of FDG uptake in histopathological responders was significantly greater than in nonresponders. Considering a 60% decrease in tumor FDG uptake as a

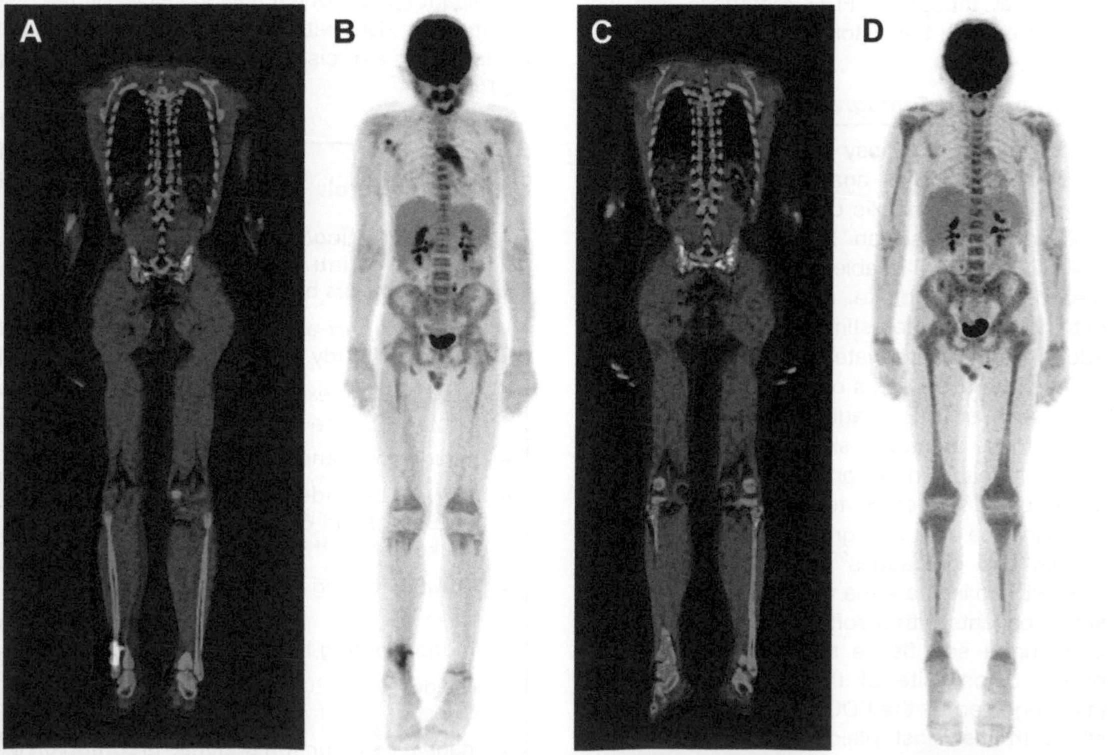


**Fig. 2.** Sarcoma of the distal third of the right leg in a 12-year-old boy. (*A, C*) PET/CT coronal view. (*B, D*) MIP. (*A, B*) Stadiation: focal uptake (SUVmax = 3.4) at the distal third of the right leg. (*B, C*) After neoadjuvant chemotherapy: persistence of small area of uptake at the distal third of the right tibia.

threshold, they found a sensitivity of 100% and a specificity of 71% for assessment of histopathological response.

Ye and colleagues[45] evaluated 15 patients with osteosarcoma and found that it was possible to discriminate between responders and nonresponders on the basis of PET results. In particular, they used the measurement of tumour-to-background ratio (TBR) considered significantly better than SUV.

Despite these results, Benz and colleagues[49] found that the most effective method in measuring the response to therapy on PET images were SUVmax and SUVpeak and not TBR, as the interobserver variability of TBR seems to be very high.

Benz and colleagues[50] reported that a reduction in tumor FDG uptake of greater than 35% from the pretherapy value was predictive of histologically assessed treatment response. These results established specific criteria for posttherapy treatment response assessment In clinical practice.

Regarding bone sarcomas, Cheon and colleagues[51] found that the MR-based volume change, used in combination with pretherapy and posttherapy tumor FDG SUV data, was associated with the histologic response of the tumor. Dimitrakopoulou-Strauss and colleagues[52] used multiparameter FDG kinetic analysis to demonstrate that the tumor FDG metabolic rate was associated with the histologic response.

### *PET/Computed Tomography in Biopsy*

PET/CT-guided biopsy combines the well-established value of anatomic information from CT with PET metabolic characterization.[53] Large malignant lesions can be heterogeneous and 18F-FDG PET/CT is able to guide biopsy to the area of highest uptake, reducing the probability of tumor grade underestimation and consequential adoption of inappropriate approach.[54,55]

Often there are areas of necrosis or inhomogeneity seen on MR imaging in a sarcoma mass and if these areas are sampled the diagnosis is subject to sampling error. To avoid this situation, it has been suggested to use PET scanning for sampling the area with greatest SUV.

Hain and colleagues[29] evaluated the use of FDG-PET to indicate the most appropriate biopsy site in patients with a soft tissue mass suspected of being a soft tissue sarcoma. The histology of the biopsy site of the 8 malignant lesions (as suggested by the FDG-PET scan) showed the site with the most pleiomorphism and highest mitotic index within the sarcoma. The ability of FDG-PET to predict soft tissue tumor grade, as a complement to biopsy to deepen the biological behavior of these tumors, was also reviewed by Israel-Mardirosian and Adler.[56]

PET-guided biopsy enables further evaluation of lesions with exclusively FDG uptake without corresponding anatomic findings on CT.[57]

The routine use of PET-guided biopsy is not yet well established, but, especially when biopsy results are inconclusive or not consistent with the overall clinical and radiologic images, the patient may benefit from a target second biopsy with the use of PET scan to find the best area of a large tumor that needs to be sampled.

## IMAGING PROTOCOLS

The procedure for PET/CT image acquisition is standard and includes several steps, from appropriate preparation of patients to image acquisition and reconstruction (**Box 1**).

A contraindication to perform PET/CT scan is the state of pregnancy. It is always required to exclude pregnancy at the start of the examination for each woman of childbearing age.

Patients are required to fast (for at least 6 hours before the start of the PET study), and interrupt parenteral nutrition/intravenous fluid with glucose (at least 4 hours before PET scan) and antidiabetic therapy (from the day before the PET scan) due a significant impact of circulating insulin on the distribution of FDG within the body. Patients must avoid strong exercise at least 6 hours before the PET study.

**Box 1**
**Imaging protocols**

- 6 hours fasting/interruption of parenteral nutrition or intravenous fluid with glucose at least 4 hours before PET study
- Interruption of antidiabetic therapy the day before PET study
- Avoid strong exercise 6 hours before PET study
- Exclude pregnancy
- Intravenous fludeoxyglucose (FDG) injection (3 MBq/Kg) and 60 minutes ($\pm$10 minutes) of uptake before the scan
- Hydration during the 60 minutes ($\pm$10 minutes) of uptake
- Bladder voiding before the scan (2 min/bed)
- Low-dose CT (120 kV, 80 mA) for attenuation correction and for image interpretation
- Image reconstruction and interpretation on a dedicated workstation providing image fusion and multiplanar cuts

It would be preferable to test the blood glucose level before FDG administration and to avoid FDG injection if glucose levels are higher than 120 mg/dL for a possible reduction in sensitivity.

The injected dose depends on patient weight, system sensitivity, and acquisition time. Injection should be fully intravenous and an optimal uptake time before the scan is 60 minutes (±10 minutes). Meanwhile, patients need to stand still and to hydrate to increase the renal excretion of unbound tracer and reduce background activity. Renal insufficiency and impossibility to hydrate are not contraindications to the examination. Bladder voiding is required before image acquisition to reduce the dose in the pelvis.

A supine decubitus is preferred under the scanner for image acquisition even if any other antalgic position is acceptable.

The standard field of view includes acquisition from the skull (from a line passing through the eyes) to half femurs, but further acquisitions depend on primary tumor location.

Acquisition time depends on the system and injected dose, but generally, for a 3D system and 3 MBq/Kg of FDG, 2 minuted per bed position is enough, leading to an average overall acquisition time of 14 minutes.

Low-dose CT (120 kV, 80 mA) is necessary both for attenuation correction and for image interpretation and allows evaluation of anatomic structure and recognition of, for example, bone aspecific uptake related to degeneration or fractures.

Bone metallic implants are not a contraindication, even if they can determine some artifacts both on CT and PET images, reducing accuracy.

After reconstruction, images must be interpreted on a dedicated workstation, providing image fusion and multiplanar cuts.

SUVmax (based on body weight) is the standard semiquantitative index and it is very useful especially in the evaluation of response to therapy.

## DIFFERENTIAL DIAGNOSIS

Sometimes avid FDG uptake may occur in benign conditions that could be falsely interpreted as malignancy (**Box 2**).

Among benign skeletal lesions with intense FDG uptake are fibro-osseus defects (common in childhood),[58] osteochondromas, giant cell tumors, chondroblastomas, Langerhans cells histiocytosis, fibro-xanthomas, desmoid tumors, and fibrous dysplasia.

For all such situations, the qualitative or quantitative analysis of SUV has not a great value[58,59] and remains essential in the evaluation of the tomographic characteristics of the lesions.

**Box 2**
**Differential diagnosis**

*Benign skeletal lesions*

Fibro-osseus defects

Osteochondromas

Giant cell tumors

Chondroblastomas

Langerhans cell histiocytosis

Fibro-xanthomas

Desmoid tumors

Fibrous dysplasia

*Infectious/inflammatory diseases*

Abscess

Osteomyelitis

Postsurgical status

Postradiotherapy status

Granulocyte colony-stimulating factors

Traumatic alterations

Granulomas

Another source of misinterpretation is represented by infectious/inflammatory diseases (eg, tuberculosis, pneumonia, abscess, osteomyelitis), postsurgical and postradiotherapy status, and the use of granulocyte colony-stimulating factors that promote expansion with consequential uptake by the bone marrow. Inflammatory alterations after surgery, traumatic event, or radiotherapy procedures may demonstrate glycolytic activity even 3 months after the event. This is important especially in the evaluation of patients with sarcoma after treatment.

Even granulomas, resulting from injection or foreign bodies, can occasionally mimic neoplasms on physical examination and imaging.[60]

Granulomas due to a parasite infection (less common), also can be mistaken for soft tissue tumors.[61]

Therefore correlation with clinical history, such as underlying diseases, age, trauma history, surgery, or procedures, is mandatory for an accurate diagnosis.

## PITFALLS, PEARLS, VARIANTS

PET has some disadvantages as compared with anatomic imaging methods: CT, for example, is capable of detecting small lung lesions, as it allows for the performance of metastasectomy or radiotherapy with increase of patient survival (**Box 3**).[16,54,62,63]

**Box 3**
**Pitfalls, pearls, variants**

- Low sensitivity for pulmonary lesions
- Skip lesions
- Different physiologic FDG uptake in children

Indeed, the sensitivity of PET in detecting pulmonary metastases has been reported to be as low as 24% for lesions smaller than 1 cm.[16] Fused PET/CT improves detection of pulmonary metastases above PET alone,[64] but, seeing that PET/CT is generally undertaken with a reduced-dose CT protocol, image quality may still not be sufficient to detect small pulmonary metastases. A diagnostic-quality CT of the chest, therefore, remains an essential part of the staging and follow-up of sarcoma.[65]

This reduced sensitivity is multifactorial and can be due to other technical limitations and not only to the finite spatial resolution of the scanner (a lesion smaller than 3–4 mm may not be identified), but even to the partial volume effect (PVE) and respiratory movement during emission acquisition.

PVE can result in significant qualitative/quantitative changes to PET studies and it results in the signals of small avid lesions being spread over larger volumes. It generally occurs whenever the avid lesion is smaller than 3 times the full width at half maximum, and is exacerbated when surrounding tissue uptake is particularly low (as happens in lung tissue). PVE results in small lesions appearing larger in size but less avid.[66]

In addition, respiratory movements affect PET images due to the long acquisition times involved,[67] and the movement of lung lesions during respiration results in overestimated tracer avid volumes and reduced apparent tracer uptake,[68] especially in lung tissue closest to the diaphragm. Respiratory gating is a technique whereby the respiratory cycle is divided into multiple phases and the acquired events sorted into temporal bins to improve the spatial resolution of thoracic PET images at the expense of increased image noise. Respiratory gating allows more accurate SUV and volume measurements of pulmonary nodules.[69]

Despite those technical limitations that affect small pulmonary metastases, PET sensitivity is reduced compared with conventional imaging even for pulmonary metastases larger than 1 cm. This may be due to reduced perfusion of lesions, downregulation of glucose receptors, or altered glucose metabolism.[70]

Seeing that sarcomas often involve young patients, it is important to know variant patterns of physiologic FDG uptake that differ in children as compared with adults to avoid pitfalls in their interpretation. Some of this sites include brown adipose tissue,[71,72] thymus,[73] brain,[74] epiphyseal plates,[58] pharyngeal lymphatic tissue of Waldeyer ring, salivary glands, and hematopoietic bone marrow.[75] Additionally, pediatric patients suffer from a multitude of community-acquired infections that may prompt intense reactive nodal avidity and thus mimic malignancy.

Skeletally immature pediatric patients present physiologic linear uptake in physes and apophyses (see **Fig. 2**).[58]

Such uptake could hide small skeletal lesions, or may be exchanged for pathologic activity. In addition, loss of the normal sharp demarcation of uptake in the physes may reflect bone marrow infiltration or activation and should be recognized.

An advantage of PET/CT, compared with other imaging modalities, is the possibility to detect skip lesions. In addition, PET/CT may be especially indicated for detecting skip lesions whose differentiation from physiologic medullary hematopoiesis is difficult in MR imaging, in particular in childhood, as the physiologic hematopoietic medulla may be quite extensive.[63]

## DIAGNOSTIC CRITERIA

FDG PET/CT relies on the quantitative analysis of SUV as well as on visual qualitative analysis to evaluate the degree of FDG uptake by the lesion (**Box 4**).[48]

Based on the intensity of FDG uptake, PET/CT allows the detection of tumor regression/progression even before the identification of morphologic alterations by anatomic imaging methods such as CT and MR imaging.[48,76]

Indeed, it is important to remember that the metabolic response precedes the volumetric decrease of the tumors and PET/CT findings can aid in important decision making about maintaining or modifying therapy, besides providing prognostic data.

**Box 4**
**Diagnostic criteria**

- Visual qualitative analysis
- Quantitative analysis (standardized uptake value)
- Metabolic response/progression before morphological alterations
- FDG avidity related to individuals pathology

Neoplastic tissues with 30% decrease in SUV (quantitative analysis), as compared with the baseline scan performed before chemotherapy, are classified as good responders to the instituted treatment.[48]

On the other hand, a 30% increase of SUV characterizes disease progression. Some investigators declare that an SUV reduction less than 2.5 after chemotherapy is associated with an increase in disease-free survival, with 79% positive predictive value for favorable response (less than 10% of viable neoplastic tissue in the lesion).[77]

It should be noticed that the degree of FDG avidity in sarcoma mainly depends on individual pathology and can range from low grade to markedly avid. This is particularly the case for soft tissue sarcomas including rhabdomyosarcoma, and needs to be appreciated when FDG is used for this indication.[78]

## WHAT THE REFERRING PHYSICIAN NEEDS TO KNOW

1. PET/CT provides metabolic information about the primary tumor (T) but its main advantage is the evaluation of lymph node involvement (N), identification of distant metastasis (M), and local relapse.
2. PET/CT does not provide anatomic details, so cannot be used to evaluate local infiltration.
3. SUVmax before therapy is prognostic and is fundamental if the therapy assessment is needed as compared with posttherapy SUVmax.
4. After radiotherapy, some false positives may occur because of radiotherapy-related inflammation. The likelihood of this event reduces proportionally to the time after therapy.
5. A diagnostic-quality chest CT without contrast media must be performed beside each PET/CT evaluation due to the low sensitivity of PET in detecting lung metastases. A diagnostic chest CT can be acquired also on conventional PET/CT tomographs.
6. Some benign diseases arising especially in the bone can be intensely hypermetabolic so that PET/CT can result in a false positive.

## SUMMARY

PET seems to be useful for evaluating patients with soft tissue and bone sarcomas in particular for tumor detection and grading, determining patient prognosis, assessing the response to neoadjuvant chemotherapy, staging/restaging the disease, and for guiding biopsies.

## REFERENCES

1. Engellau J, Bendahl PO, Persson A, et al. Improved prognostication in soft tissue sarcoma: independent information from vascular invasion, necrosis, growth pattern, and immunostaining using whole tumor sections and tissue microarrays. Hum Pathol 2005;36: 994–1002.
2. International Agency for Research on Cancer. WHO Classification of soft tissue tumours. Available at: http://www.iarc.fr/en/publications/pdfs-online/pat-gen/bb5/bb5-classifsofttissue.pdf. Accessed August 26, 2012.
3. Martin CT, Morcuende J, Buckwalter JA, et al. Prereferral MRI use in patients with musculoskeletal tumors is not excessive. Clin Orthop Relat Res 2012; 470(11):3240–5.
4. Styring E, Billing V, Hartman L, et al. Simple guidelines for efficient referral of soft-tissue sarcomas: a population-based evaluation of adherence to guidelines and referral patterns. J Bone Joint Surg Am 2012;14:1291–6.
5. Peabody TD, Simon MA. Principles of staging of soft-tissue sarcomas. Clin Orthop Relat Res 1993; 289:19–31.
6. Skubitz KM, D'Adamo DR. Sarcoma. Mayo Clin Proc 2007;82(11):1409–32.
7. Johnson GR, Zhuang H, Khan J, et al. Roles of positron emission tomography with fluorine-18-deoxyglucose in the detection of local recurrent and distant metastatic sarcoma. Clin Nucl Med 2003;28: 815–20.
8. Pisters PW, Leung DH, Woodruff J, et al. Analysis of prognostic factors in 1041 patients with localized soft tissue sarcomas of the extremities. J Clin Oncol 1996;14:1679–89.
9. Eilber FC, Rosen G, Nelson SD, et al. High-grade extremity soft tissue sarcomas: factors predictive of local recurrence and its effect on morbidity and mortality. Ann Surg 2003;237:218–26.
10. Ballo MT, Zagars GK. Radiation therapy for soft tissue sarcoma. Surg Oncol Clin N Am 2003;12:449–67.
11. Bacci G, Lari S. Current treatment of high grade osteosarcoma of the extremity: review. J Chemother 2001;13:235–43.
12. Phan A, Patel S. Advances in neoadjuvant chemotherapy in soft tissue sarcomas. Curr Treat Options Oncol 2003;4:433–9.
13. Cormier JN, Pollock RE. Soft tissue sarcomas. CA Cancer J Clin 2004;54:94–109.
14. Ceyssens S, Stroobants S. Sarcoma. Methods Mol Biol 2011;727:191–203.
15. Eary JF, Conrad EU. Imaging in sarcoma. J Nucl Med 2011;52:1903–13.
16. Volker T, Denecke T, Steffen I, et al. Positron emission tomography for staging of pediatric sarcoma patients: results of a prospective multicenter trial. J Clin Oncol 2007;25:5435–41.

17. Hicks RJ. Functional imaging techniques for evaluation of sarcomas. Cancer Imaging 2005;5:58–65.
18. Lietman SA, Joyce MJ. Bone sarcomas: overview of management, with a focus on surgical treatment considerations. Cleve Clin J Med 2010;77(Suppl 1): S8–12.
19. Aboulafia AJ, Levine AM, Schmidt DP. Musculoskeletal tumors 2. Rosemont (IL): American Academy of Orthopaedic Surgeons; 2007.
20. Shapeero LG, Vanel D, Verstraete KL, et al. Fast magnetic resonance imaging with contrast for soft tissue sarcoma viability. Clin Orthop Relat Res 2002;397:212–27.
21. Lukas M, Reimer NB, Reith JD, et al. Multidisciplinary management of soft tissue sarcoma. ScientificWorldJournal 2013;2013:852462.
22. Fuglo HM, Jorgensen SM, Loft A, et al. The diagnostic and prognostic value of 18F-FDG PET/CT in the initial assessment of high-grade bone and soft tissue sarcoma. A retrospective study of 89 patients. Eur J Nucl Med Mol Imaging 2012;39(9):1416–24.
23. Bastiaannet E, Groen H, Jager PL, et al. The value of FDG-PET in the detection, grading and response to therapy and soft tissue and bone sarcomas: a systematic review and meta-analysis. Cancer Treat Rev 2004;30(1):83–101.
24. Roberge D, Vakilian S, Alabed YZ, et al. FDG PET/CT in initial staging of adult soft-tissue sarcoma. Sarcoma 2012;2012:960194.
25. Schuetze SM, Rubin BP, Vernon C, et al. Use of positron emission tomography in localized extremity soft tissue sarcoma treated with neoadjuvant chemotherapy. Cancer 2005;103(2):339–48.
26. Schwarzbach MHM, Hinz U, Dimitrakopoulou-Strauss A, et al. Prognostic significance of preoperative [18-F] fluorodeoxyglucose (FDG) positron emission tomography (PET) imaging in patients with resectable soft tissue sarcomas. Ann Surg 2005;241(2):286–94.
27. Al-Ibraheem A, Buck AK, Benz MR, et al. (18) F-Fluorodeoxyglucose positron emission tomography/computed tomography for the detection of recurrent bone and soft tissue sarcoma. Cancer 2013;119(6):1227–34.
28. Park JH, Park EK, Kang CH, et al. Intense accumulation of 18F-FDG, not enhancement on MRI, helps to guide the surgical biopsy accurately in soft tissue tumors. Ann Nucl Med 2009;23(10):887–9.
29. Hain SF, O'Doherty MJ, Bingham J, et al. Can FDG PET be used to successfully direct preoperative biopsy of soft tissue tumors? Nucl Med Commun 2003;24(11):1139–43.
30. Ioannidis JP, Lau J. 18F-FDG PET for the diagnosis and grading of soft-tissue sarcoma: a meta-analysis. J Nucl Med 2003;44(5):717–24.
31. Folpe AL, Lyles RH, Sprouse JT, et al. (F-18) fluorodeoxyglucose positron emission tomography as a predictor of pathologic grade and other prognostic variables in bone and soft tissue sarcoma. Clin Cancer Res 2000;6:1279–87.
32. Charest M, Hickeson M, Lisbona R, et al. FDG PET/CT imaging in primary osseous and soft tissue sarcomas: a retrospective review of 212 cases. Eur J Nucl Med Mol Imaging 2009;36(12):1944–51.
33. Billingsley KG, Lewis JJ, Leung DH, et al. Multifactorial analysis of the survival of patients with distant metastasis arising from primary extremity sarcoma. Cancer 1999;85(2):389–95.
34. Moreau LC, Turcotte R, Ferguson P, et al. Myxoid/round cell liposarcoma (MRCLS) revisited: an analysis of 418 primarily managed cases. Ann Surg Oncol 2012;19(4):1081–8.
35. Fong Y, Coit DG, Woodruff JM, et al. Lymph node metastasis from soft tissue sarcoma in adults. Analysis of data from a prospective database of 1772 sarcoma patients. Ann Surg 1993;217(1):72–7.
36. Riad S, Griffin AM, Liberman B, et al. Lymph node metastasis in soft tissue sarcoma in an extremity. Clin Orthop Relat Res 2004;426:129–34.
37. Tateishi U, Yamaguchi U, Seki K, et al. Bone and soft-tissue sarcoma: preoperative staging with fluorine 18 fluorodeoxyglucose PET/CT and conventional imaging. Radiology 2007;245(3):839–47.
38. Arush MW, Israel O, Postovsky S, et al. Positron emission tomography/computed tomography with 18fluoro-deoxyglucose in the detection of local recurrence and distant metastases of pediatric sarcoma. Pediatr Blood Cancer 2007;49(7):901–5.
39. Coindre JM. Grading of soft tissue sarcomas: review and update. Arch Pathol Lab Med 2006;130(10): 1448–53.
40. Eary JF, O'Sullivan F, O'Sullivan J, et al. Spatial heterogeneity in sarcoma 18F-FDG uptake as a predictor of patient outcome. J Nucl Med 2008;49(12):1973–9.
41. Lisle JW, Eary JF, O'Sullivan J, et al. Risk assessment based on FDG-PET imaging in patients with synovial sarcoma. Clin Orthop Relat Res 2009;467(6):1605–11.
42. Sato J, Yanagawa T, Dobashi Y, et al. Prognostic significance of 18F-FDG uptake in primary osteosarcoma after but not before chemotherapy: a possible association with autocrine motility factor/phosphoglucose isomerase expression. Clin Exp Metastasis 2008;25(4):427–35.
43. Jones DN, McCowage GB, Sostman HD, et al. Monitoring of neoadjuvant therapy response of soft-tissue and musculoskeletal sarcoma using fluorine-18-FDG PET. J Nucl Med 1996;37(9):1438–44.
44. Iagaru A, Masamed R, Chawla SP, et al. F-18 FDG PET and PET/CT evaluation of response to chemotherapy in bone and soft tissue sarcomas. Clin Nucl Med 2008;33(1):8–13.
45. Ye Z, Zhu J, Tian M, et al. Response of osteogenic sarcoma to neoadjuvant therapy: evaluated by 18F-FDG-PET. Ann Nucl Med 2008;22(6):475–80.

46. Hamada K, Tomita Y, Inoue A, et al. Evaluation of chemotherapy response in osteosarcoma with FDG-PET. Ann Nucl Med 2009;23(1):89–95.
47. Evilevitch V, Weber WA, Tap WD, et al. Reduction of glucose metabolic activity is more accurate than change in size at predicting histopathologic response to neoadjuvant therapy in high-grade soft-tissue sarcomas. Clin Cancer Res 2008;14(3):715–20.
48. Bredella MA, Caputo GR. Steinbach LS.Value of FDG positron emission tomography in conjunction with MR imaging for evaluating therapy response in patients with musculoskeletal sarcomas. AJR Am J Roentgenol 2002;179(5):1145–50.
49. Benz MR, Evilevitch V, Allen-Auerbach MS, et al. Treatment monitoring by 18F-FDG PET/CT in patients with sarcomas: interobserver variability of quantitative parameters in treatment-induced changes in histopathologically responding and non responding tumors. J Nucl Med 2008;49(7): 1038–46.
50. Benz MR, Czernin J, Allen-Auerbach MS, et al. FDG-PET/CT imaging predicts histopathologic treatment responses after the initial cycle of neoadjuvant chemotherapy in high-grade soft-tissue sarcomas. Clin Cancer Res 2009;15(8):2856–63.
51. Cheon GJ, Kim MS, Lee JA, et al. Prediction model of chemotherapy response in osteosarcoma by 18F-FDG PET and MRI. J Nucl Med 2009;50(9): 1435–40.
52. Dimitrakopoulou-Strauss A, Strauss LG, Egerer G, et al. Impact of dynamic 18F-FDG PET on the early prediction of therapy outcome in patients with high-risk soft-tissue sarcomas after neoadjuvant chemotherapy: a feasibility study. J Nucl Med 2010;51(4):551–8.
53. Kobayashi K, Bhargava P, Raja S, et al. Image-guided biopsy: what the interventional radiologist needs to know about PET/CT. Radiographics 2012; 32(5):1483–501.
54. Eary JF, Conrad EU, Bruckner JD, et al. Quantitative [F-18]fluoro- deoxyglucose positron emission tomography in pretreatment and grading of sarcoma. Clin Cancer Res 1998;4:1215–20.
55. Klaeser B, Mueller MD, Schmid RA, et al. PET-CT-guided interventions in the management of FDG-positive lesions in patients suffering from solid malignancies: initial experiences. Eur Radiol 2009;19(7):1780–5.
56. Israel-Mardirosian N, Adler LP. Positron emission tomography of soft tissue sarcomas. Curr Opin Oncol 2003;15:327–30.
57. Klaeser B, Wiskirchen J, Wartenberg J, et al. PET/CT-guided biopsies of metabolically active bone lesions: applications and clinical impact. Eur J Nucl Med Mol Imaging 2010;37(11):2027–36.
58. Goodin GS, Shulkin BL, Kaufman RA, et al. PET/CT characterization of fibroosseous defects in children: 18F-FDG uptake can mimic metastatic disease. AJR Am J Roentgenol 2006;187:1124–8.
59. Franzius C, Daldrup-Link HE, Wagner-Bohn A, et al. FDG-PET for detection of recurrences from malignant primary bone tumors: comparison with conventional imaging. Ann Oncol 2002;13:157–60.
60. Schwartzfarb EM, Hametti JM, Romanelli P, et al. Foreign body granuloma formation secondary to silicone injection. Dermatol Online J 2008;14:20.
61. Useche JN, de Castro AM, Galvis GE, et al. Use of US in the evaluation of patients with symptoms of deep venous thrombosis of the lower extremities. Radiographics 2008;28:1785–97.
62. Franzius C, Daldrup-Link HE, Sciuk J, et al. FDG-PET for detection of pulmonary metastases from malignant primary bone tumors: comparison with spiral CT. Ann Oncol 2001;12:479–86.
63. Brenner W, Bohuslavizki KH, Eary JF. PET imaging of osteosarcoma. J Nucl Med 2003;44:930–42.
64. Gerth HU, Juergens KU, Dirksen U, et al. Significant benefit of multimodal imaging: PET/CT compared with PET alone in staging and follow-up of patients with Ewing tumors. J Nucl Med 2007;48:1932–9.
65. McCarville MB. PET-CT imaging in pediatric oncology. Cancer Imaging 2009;9:35–43.
66. Soret M, Bacharach SL, Buvat I. Partial-volume effect in PET tumor imaging. J Nucl Med 2007;48: 932–45.
67. Allen-Auerbach M, Yeom K, Park J, et al. Standard PET/CT of the chest during shallow breathing is inadequate for comprehensive staging of lung cancer. J Nucl Med 2006;47:298–301.
68. Erdi YE, Nehmeh SA, Pan T, et al. The CT motion quantitation of lung lesions and its impact on PET-measured SUVs. J Nucl Med 2004;45: 1287–92.
69. Werner MK, Parker JA, Kolodny GM, et al. Respiratory gating enhances imaging of pulmonary nodules and measurement of tracer uptake in FDG PET/CT. AJR Am J Roentgenol 2009;193:1640–5.
70. Iagaru A, Chawla S, Menendez L, et al. 18F-FDG PET and PET/CT for detection of pulmonary metastases from musculoskeletal sarcomas. Nucl Med Commun 2006;27:795–802.
71. Hany TF, Gharehpapagh E, Kamel EM, et al. Brown adipose tissue: a factor to consider in symmetrical tracer uptake in the neck and upper chest region. Eur J Nucl Med Mol Imaging 2002;29:1393–8.
72. Yeung HW, Grewal RK, Gonen M, et al. Patterns of (18)F-FDG uptake in adipose tissue and muscle: a potential source of false-positives for PET. J Nucl Med 2003;44:1789–96.
73. Brink I, Reinhardt MJ, Hoegerle S, et al. Increased metabolic activity in the thymus gland studied with 18F-FDG PET: age dependency and frequency after chemotherapy. J Nucl Med 2001;42:591–5.

74. London K, Howman-Giles R. Normal cerebral FDG uptake during childhood. Eur J Nucl Med Mol Imaging 2014;41:723–35.
75. Shammas A, Lim R, Charron M. Pediatric FDG PET/CT: physiologic uptake, normal variants, and benign conditions. Radiographics 2009;29:1467–86.
76. Franzius C, Sciuk J, Brinkschmidt C, et al. Evaluation of chemotherapy response in primary bone tumors with F-18 FDG positron emission tomography compared with histologically assessed tumor necrosis. Clin Nucl Med 2000;25:874–81.
77. Hawkins DS, Schuetze SM, Butrynski JE, et al. [18F] Fluorodeoxyglucose positron emission tomography predicts outcome for Ewing sarcoma family of tumors. J Clin Oncol 2005;23:8828–34.
78. Portwine C, Marriott C, Barr RD. PET imaging for pediatric oncology: an assessment of the evidence. Pediatr Blood Cancer 2010;55:1048–106.

# PET/Computed Tomography in Breast Cancer

## Can It Aid in Developing a Personalized Treatment Design?

Sumeet Suresh Malapure, MD[a], Kalpa Jyoti Das, MD[b], Rakesh Kumar, MD, PhD[b,*]

**KEYWORDS**

• Breast cancer • Receptor imaging • $^{18}$F-FDG PET/CT • $^{18}$F-16α-17β-Fluoroestradiol PET/CT

**KEY POINTS**

- In an estimated two-thirds of receptor positive (especially ER+) breast cancer patients adjuvant endocrine therapy had led to increased survival rates and better outcome.
- Characterization of such tumors and metastatic lesions and categorizing the patients accordingly can aid in predicting response and planning treatment strategies in a personalized manner.
- In vivo characterization and predictive tests using PET/computed tomography with various radiopharmaceuticals may reduce both undertreatment and overtreatment and play a significant role in future management of breast cancer that will be personalized and tailored to fit a particular subset of patient.

## INTRODUCTION

Worldwide, breast cancer is the most frequently diagnosed life-threatening cancer. It is the leading cause of cancer death among women in developing countries and stands second in developed countries accounting for 29% of all cancers in the United States.[1,2] Increased public awareness and improved screening have led to earlier diagnosis, at stages amenable to complete surgical resection and curative therapies. Along with improvements in therapy, these factors have led to improved survival rates for women diagnosed with breast cancer. Over the past 3 decades, extensive breast cancer research has led to extraordinary progress in the understanding of the disease. This has resulted in the development of more targeted and less toxic treatments and with changing health economics, personalized treatment is rapidly gaining importance. Personalized medicine according to the US National Institutes of Health (NIH) has been defined as "an emerging practice of medicine that uses an individual's genetic profile to guide decisions made in regard to the prevention, diagnosis, and treatment of disease."[3] With personalized health regimens, physicians can make optimal choices to maximize the likelihood of effective treatment and simultaneously avoid the risks of adverse drug reactions that are seen in approximately

The authors have nothing to disclose.

[a] Department of Nuclear Medicine, Kasturba Medical College, Manipal University, SH 65, Manipal 576104, Karnataka, India; [b] Diagnostic Nuclear Medicine Division, Department of Nuclear Medicine, All India Institute of Medical Sciences, Sri Aurobindo Marg, New Delhi 110029, India
* Corresponding author.
*E-mail address:* rkphulia@yahoo.com

PET Clin 11 (2016) 297–303
http://dx.doi.org/10.1016/j.cpet.2016.02.006

6.7% of the hospitalized cases, amounting to more than 100,000 deaths annually.

## PATHOPHYSIOLOGY

Latest research has demonstrated that different sets of molecular alterations lead to pathogenesis of different subtypes of breast cancer and each of these subtypes are distinctly different from each other in terms of their natural history and clinical behavior.[4] These alterations generally express themselves in terms of presence or absence of hormonal receptor status. This knowledge of different pathogenetic pathways along with their subtypes and type-specific risk factors have significantly altered the management of breast cancer. According to the Cancer Genome Atlas Network (TCGA) there are 4 main breast tumor subtypes with distinct genetic aberrations:

- Luminal A
- Luminal B
- Basal-like
- HER2-positive

Along with this, numerous prognostic and predictive factors have been identified by the College of American Pathologists (CAP) to guide the clinical management of women with breast cancer. These include the following:

1. Axillary lymph node status
2. Tumor size
3. Lymphatic/vascular invasion
4. Patient age
5. Histologic grade
6. Histologic subtypes (eg, tubular, mucinous [colloid], or papillary)
7. Response to neoadjuvant therapy
8. Estrogen receptor (ER)/progesterone receptor (PR) status
9. HER2 gene amplification or overexpression.

In addition to TNM factors, expression of hormonal receptors by tumor cells play an important role in breast cancer prognostication and treatment. ER and PR status predict both long-term survival and response to therapy.[5] Hormone receptor–positive tumors generally have a more indolent course and are responsive to hormone therapy. The presence of the ER/PR is the most important determinant of response, and response is unlikely in the absence of sufficient tumor ER expression.[6] Expression is routinely measured in clinical practice by in vitro assay of biopsy material. For ER-expressing metastatic breast cancer, hormonal therapy is often first-line treatment.[7] Thus, it is critically important to know the receptor status for the treatment of metastatic breast cancer. This information, however, is difficult to obtain, particularly when there is widespread metastases and to places from which a biopsy is difficult to obtain. Also, the receptor status of metastatic disease can vary from that of the primary tumor.[8] Histopathological receptor expression determination from every metastatic lesion is impractical. In this setting, receptor-based in vivo quantitative studies using receptor-specific imaging can give valuable information and lead to optimal treatment.

HER2 overexpression is associated with a more aggressive tumor phenotype and a worse prognosis (higher recurrence rate and increased mortality), independent of other clinical features (eg, age, stage, and tumor grade). Prognosis has improved with the routine use of HER2-targeted therapies like trastuzumab, pertuzumab, lapatinib (oral TKI), trastuzumab-emtansine (an antibody-drug conjugate) and combination therapies. HER2 status has also been shown to predict response to certain chemotherapeutic agents like doxorubicin, anthracycline-based regimens, and paclitaxels.[9]

Molecular classification of breast cancer provides a link between the molecular biology of breast cancer and the behavior of cancer cells in the corresponding subtypes.[10] It also provides more accurate information about the molecular profile of the tumor than the clinical or phenotypic classification.[10–12] However, true molecular profiling has not yet reached clinical implementation as a routine aspect of patient management.

In the past decade, significant advances in molecular biology technologies, such as microarrays, next-generation sequencing, and whole-exome sequencing, have allowed researchers to better understand tumor cell biology to identify complex genomic abnormalities (ie, gene mutation, copy number aberrations, methylation, and translocations), and to identify biomarkers involved in multiple signaling pathways that can improve general clinical practice contributing to a personalized prognostic and predictive approach to management.[13]

## ROLE OF PET WITH FLUDEOXYGLUCOSE F 18/ COMPUTED TOMOGRAPHY

The goal of molecular imaging in personalized medicine is to be a biomarker that can be predictive as well as a prognostic factor. A prognostic biomarker is one that is related to a patient's clinical outcome and can be used to select patients for an adjuvant systemic treatment irrespective of the patient response to treatment, whereas a predictive biomarker is related to the patient's response to a particular intervention. In several studies done in breast cancer, PET with fludeoxyglucose F 18 (18F-FDG PET)/computed tomography (CT) has shown good results in this direction (**Fig. 1**). Degree of FDG uptake correlates well with prognosis (**Fig. 2**). Management of breast cancer consists of locoregional and systemic therapy, which is largely based on the T, N, and M staging. Locoregional surgical treatment can be given with curative intent in early stages, whereas in advanced stages, in which tumor has spread outside the axillary basin, surgery is rarely curable. Therefore, detection of metastases and proper staging is critical in breast cancer treatment (**Fig. 3**). Osseous metastases are present in 8% of breast cancer patients overall and in 65% to 75% of patients with stage IV disease.[14] PET/CT has demonstrated its superiority in detecting skeletal metastases in comparison with radiography, MR imaging, and bone scans.[15–17]

Lin and colleagues[18] evaluated the role of FDG PET/CT in predicting response to combination therapy in HER2-positive tumors with lapatinib and trastuzumab. HER 2/erbB2 belongs to the erbB family, which has a kinase unit except erbB-3. The combination therapy has thus shown synergistic action in previously conducted trials.[19–21] This along with the fact that HER2 activates PI3K/AKT pathway, which regulates glucose uptake, and effective HER2 blockade will decrease glucose uptake, they hypothesized that decreased FDG uptake would reflect effective treatment. A total of 87 patients were divided into cohort 1 and 2. Cohort 1 had no prior trastuzumab for metastatic breast cancer (MBC) or greater than 1 year from adjuvant trastuzumab if given and in cohort 2, 1 to 2 lines of chemotherapy including trastuzumab for MBC and/or recurrence less than 1 year from adjuvant trastuzumab. The confirmed objective response rate was 50.0% (95% confidence interval [CI] 33.8%–66.2%) in cohort 1 and 22.2% (95% CI 11.3%–37.3%) in cohort 2. Clinical benefit rate, which was defined as complete/partial response plus stable disease $\geq$24 weeks, was 57.5% (95% CI 40.9%–73.0%) in cohort 1 and 40.0% (95% CI 25.7%–55.7%) in cohort 2. Median progression-free survival was 7.4 and 5.3 months, respectively. Lack of metabolic response in FDG PET/CT done at week 1 was associated with failure to achieve an objective response by RECIST (negative predictive value, 91% [95% CI 74%–100%] for cohort 1 and 91% [95% CI 79%–100%] for cohort 2).

Kitajima and coworkers[22] retrospectively analyzed pretherapeutic FDG PET/CT of 306 patients with breast cancer to determine whether there is any association between FDG uptake and the molecular subtype of breast cancer. Mean maximum standardized uptake values (SUVmax) were 3.41 $\pm$ 2.07 (range 1.18–14.30), 5.17 $\pm$ 3.52 (range 1.35–19.01), 6.57 $\pm$ 3.84 (range 1.42–15.58), 7.55 $\pm$ 3.63 (range 2.30–13.60), and

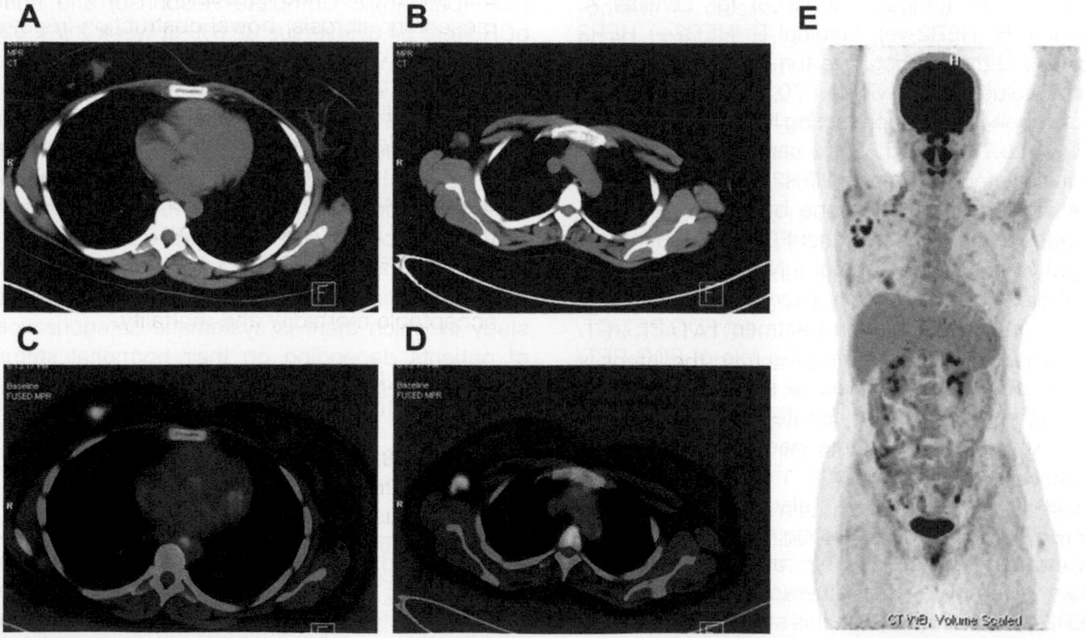


**Fig. 1.** A 27-year-old woman with known case of right breast cancer underwent a whole-body F18 FDG PET/CT scan for staging, which revealed a nodular lesion in the right breast (*A*) and axillary lymph nodes (*B*) with abnormal FDG uptake in breast (*C*) and right axillary lymph nodes (*D*). The same findings are also seen in maximum intensity projection image (MIP) (*E*).

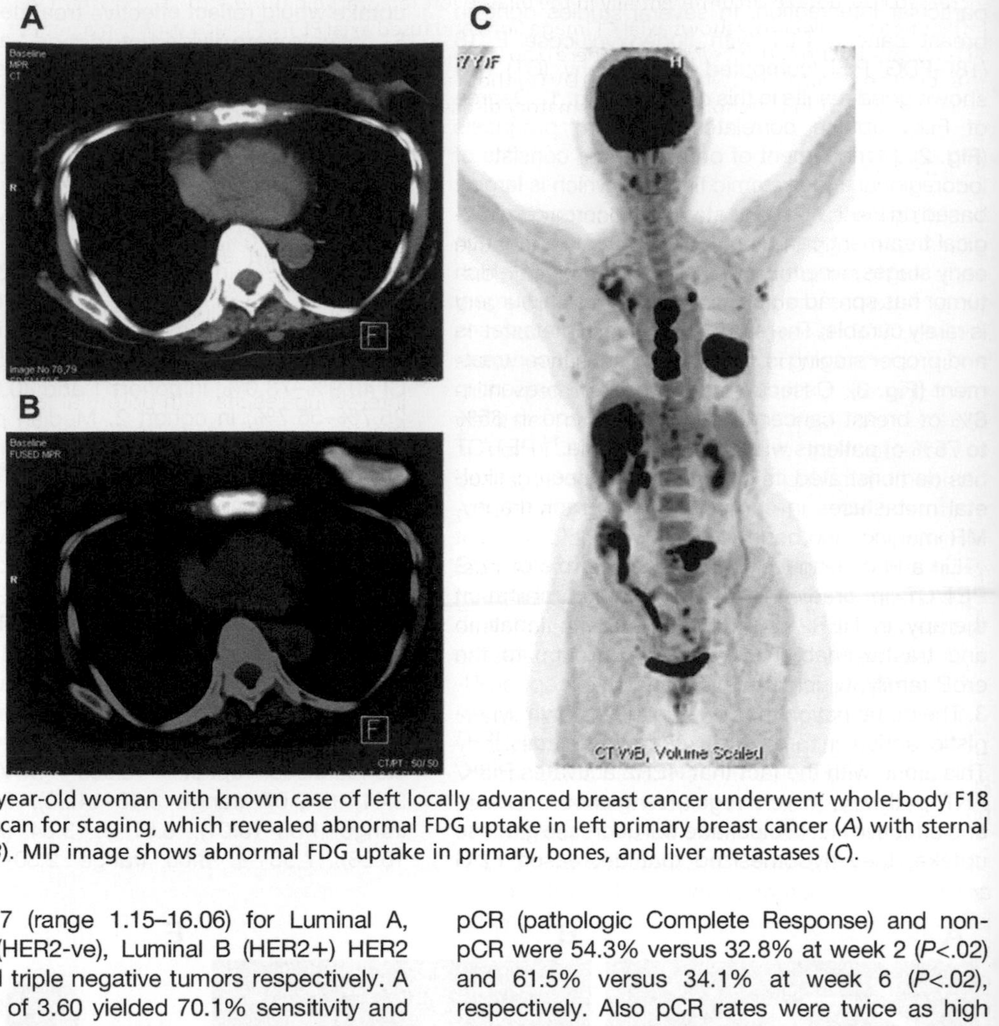


**Fig. 2.** A 67-year-old woman with known case of left locally advanced breast cancer underwent whole-body F18 FDG PET/CT scan for staging, which revealed abnormal FDG uptake in left primary breast cancer (*A*) with sternal metastasis (*B*). MIP image shows abnormal FDG uptake in primary, bones, and liver metastases (*C*).

6.97 ± 4.17 (range 1.15–16.06) for Luminal A, Luminal B (HER2-ve), Luminal B (HER2+) HER2 positive and triple negative tumors respectively. A cutoff value of 3.60 yielded 70.1% sensitivity and 66.1% specificity for predicting luminal A and cutoff value of 6.75 yielded 65.4% sensitivity and 75.2% specificity for predicting a HER2-positive subtype.

A similar study was done by Koolen and colleagues[23] and showed higher FDG uptake for triple negative and grade 3 tumors. No single molecular subtype showed uniformly decreased FDG uptake to warrant exclusion of pretreatment FDG PET/CT.

In other study correlating the role of FDG PET/CT in differentiating molecular subtypes, Koo and colleagues[24] also demonstrated that SUVmax of FDG was higher in triple negative and HER2-positive tumors.

Gebhart and colleagues[25] also tested the utility of early FDG PET/CT in predicting response to neoadjuvant trastuzumab, lapatinib, or their combination when given with chemotherapy (Neo-ALTTO) in HER2-positive patients. In this study, a 6-week biologic window with only anti-HER2 therapy was given and serial FDG PET/CT scans were done at baseline, week 2, and week 6. Of 66 evaluable FDG PET/CT scans, mean SUVmax reductions for pCR (pathologic Complete Response) and non-pCR were 54.3% versus 32.8% at week 2 ($P<.02$) and 61.5% versus 34.1% at week 6 ($P<.02$), respectively. Also pCR rates were twice as high for 18F-FDG PET/CT responders than nonresponders (week 2: 42% vs 21%, $P = .12$; week 6: 44% vs 19%, $P = .05$). In this study, hormone receptor (HR)-positive tumors showed lower rates of pCR as compared with HR-negative tumors. However, hormonal therapy was not administered in these patients and the investigators suggested a study in which there is systematic categorization of patients depending on their hormonal status and evaluating with proper hormonal therapy.

## RECEPTOR-BASED PET/COMPUTED TOMOGRAPHY

### *18F-16α-17β-Fluoroestradiol*

As mentioned earlier, noninvasive characterization of metastatic disease can be very useful particularly in metastatic breast cancer in which hormonal therapy is the first line of treatment if found to be receptor positive. Many studies have been done in this area among these18F-16α-17β-Fluoroestradiol (FES), with a target to background tissue

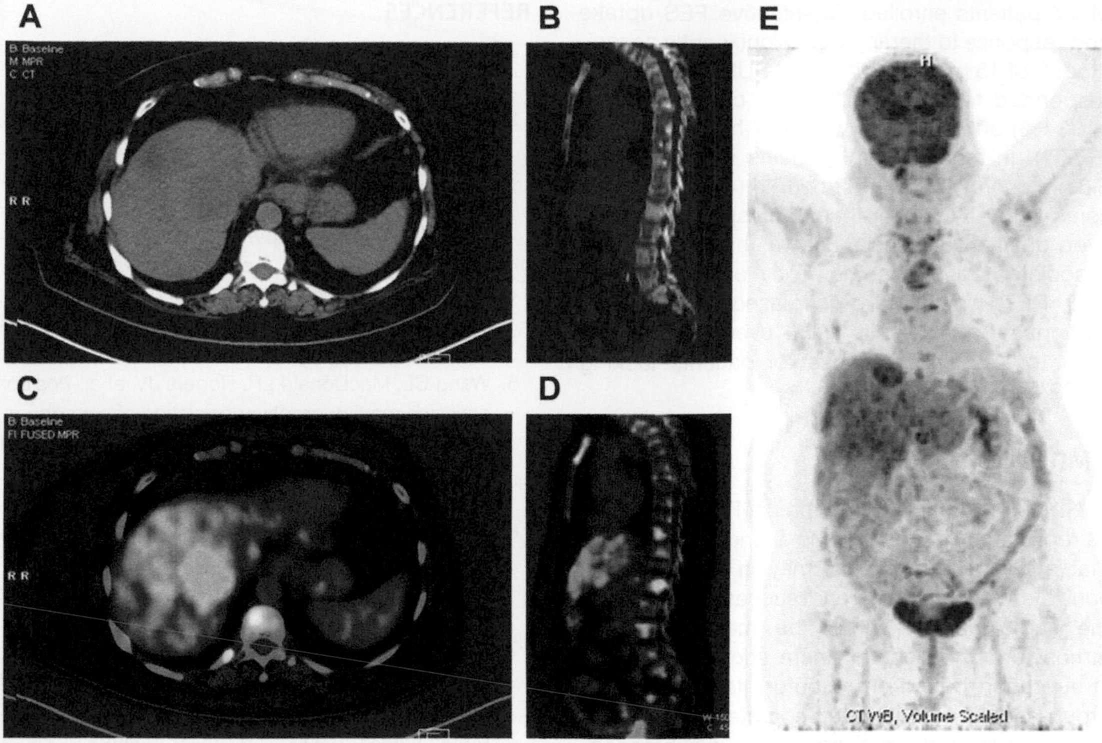


**Fig. 3.** A 67-year-old woman with known case of recurrent left breast cancer underwent whole-body F18 FDG PET/CT scan for restaging that revealed multiple hypodense lesion in liver and sclerotic lesions in multiple vertebrae (*A, B*) with FDG uptake (*C, D*). The same findings are also seen in the MIP image (*E*).

activity ratios exceeding 80:1,[26] has shown promising results. Excellent correlation between FES uptake in the primary tumor and the tumor ER concentration measured in vitro by radioligand binding on primary tumors were found by Mintun and colleagues.[27] Preliminary comparison of FES uptake in the primary and also metastatic tumor showed good correlation with the immunohistochemistry assay of the biopsied material.

In a study done by Mortimer and coworkers,[28] the baseline FES uptake and percentage change in uptake after tamoxifen therapy showed correlation with the effectives of the therapy. A baseline arbitrary cutoff SUV value of 2 had a positive predictive value (PPV) and negative predictive value (NPV) of 79% and 88%, respectively. None of patients with SUV less than 1.5 showed response to treatment. The percentage change in FES (55% in responders vs 19% in nonresponders) and change in absolute SUV value (2.5 in responders vs 0.5 in nonresponders) predicted response to tamoxifen therapy.

Interestingly apart from antiestrogen therapy, estrogen therapy can also induce tumor regression. Diethylstilbestrol (DES) showed equal efficacy with a response rate of 41% as compared with 33% in those treated with tamoxifen,[29] and in a recent study, DES showed a better 5-year survival rate than tamoxifen (35% vs 16%).[30] Patients who progressively acquire resistance to antiestrogen therapy despite being receptor positive, tend to gain by estrogen therapy.[31] However, response to additive estrogen therapy is not uniform and patient selection holds the key to successful treatment. Van Kruchten and colleagues[32] conducted a study to demonstrate the utility of FES PET in such cases hypothesizing that long-term antiestrogen therapy would have upregulated ER expression and prior evidence of estrogen hypersensitivity might help to select patients for agonist treatment. FES PET showed varied uptake between the 19 patients (median 2.5; range 1.1–15.5) and 255 lesions (median 2.8; range 0.6–24.3) analyzed. With an SUVmax cutoff of 1.5, the PPV/NPV of 18F-FES-PET for response to treatment was 60% (95% CI 31%–83%) and 80% (95% CI 38%–96%), respectively. Explorative analysis done in the same study in 3 patients who had FES PET done before antiestrogen therapy, the PPV and NPV increased to 64% and 100%, respectively. They concluded that FES PET/CT can aid in selection of refractory patients who would benefit from estrogen therapy.

Linden and colleagues[33] studied the utility of FES PET in determining response to tamoxifen therapy. They observed objective response in 11 of 47 patients enrolled. Quantitative FES uptake and response to therapy were significantly associated; 0 of 15 patients with initial SUV less than 1.5 responded to hormonal therapy, compared with 11 (34%) of 32 patients with SUV higher than 1.5 (*P*<.01). In the subset of patients whose tumors did not overexpress HER2/neu, 11 (46%) of 24 patients with SUV higher than 1.5 responded. However, qualitative assessment was not significantly associated with outcome. They concluded that FES PET would have increased the rate of response from 23% to 34% overall, and from 29% to 46% in the subset of patients lacking HER2/neu overexpression.

## LIMITATIONS

The major limitation of SUVmax of FDG PET/CT is its reproducibility. As there is a long list of factors that affect SUVmax, uniformity in scan acquisitions between patients and successive scans in the same patient should be maintained with utmost priority. Second, there should be proper stratification based on receptor status and each group should be analyzed separately with proper treatment for individual groups. Larger prospective randomized controlled trials are required to accurately determine the role of early FDG PET/CT scans in clinical management of breast cancer.

## SUMMARY

More than 70% of the breast tumors are ER+ and adjuvant endocrine therapy in such patients had led to increased survival rates and better outcome. However, most of the metastatic disease varies in nature and initial responders later become refractory to hormonal therapy, decreasing the response rate to less than 20%. In vivo characterization of such tumors and metastatic lesions and categorizing the patients accordingly can aid in predicting response and planning treatment strategies in a personalized manner.

Because the number of treatment options and their cost for patients with HER2-positive breast cancer continues to increase, a key question is how best to tailor therapies to individual patients. In the metastatic setting, predictive tests for clinical benefit could spare patients unnecessary toxicity and cost from ineffective therapies and maximize the likelihood of response to treatment. In vivo characterization and predictive tests may reduce both undertreatment and overtreatment and play a significant role in future management of breast cancer that will be personalized and tailored to fit a particular subset of patients in whom response to treatment will be uniform.

## REFERENCES

1. Torre LA, Bray F, Siegel RL, et al. Global cancer statistics, 2012. CA Cancer J Clin 2015;65(2):87–108.
2. Siegel RL, Miller KD, Jemal A. Cancer statistics, 2015. CA Cancer J Clin 2015;65(1):5–29.
3. Genetics home reference: Glossary. U.S. National Institutes of Health U.S. National Library of Medicine. Available at: http://ghr.nlm.nih.gov/glossary=personalizedmedicine. Accessed July 1, 2012.
4. The Cancer Genome Atlas Network. Comprehensive molecular portraits of human breast tumours. Nature 2012;490(7418):61–70.
5. Wang CL, MacDonald LR, Rogers JV, et al. Positron emission mammography: correlation of estrogen receptor, progesterone receptor, and human epidermal growth factor receptor 2 status and 18F-FDG. Am J Roentgenol 2011;197(2):W247–55.
6. Osborne CK, Yochmowitz MG, Knight WA 3rd, et al. The value of estrogen and progesterone receptors in the treatment of breast cancer. Cancer 1980;46:2884–8.
7. Mouridsen H, Gershanovich M, Sun Y, et al. Superior efficacy of letrozole versus tamoxifen as first-line therapy for postmenopausal women with advanced breast cancer: results of a phase III study of the International Letrozole Breast Cancer Group. J Clin Oncol 2001;19:2596–606.
8. Kuukasjarvi T, Kononen J, Helin H, et al. Loss of estrogen receptor in recurrent breast cancer is associated with poor response to endocrine therapy. J Clin Oncol 1996;14:2584–9.
9. Baselga J, Seidman AD, Rosen PP, et al. HER2 overexpression and paclitaxel sensitivity in breast cancer: therapeutic implications. Oncology (Williston Park) 1997;11(3 Suppl 2):43–8.
10. Rivenbark AG, O'Connor SM, Coleman WB. Molecular and cellular heterogeneity in breast cancer: challenges for personalized medicine. Am J Pathol 2013;183:1113–24.
11. Pusztai L, Mazouni C, Anderson K, et al. Molecular classification of breast cancer: limitations and potential. Oncologist 2006;11:868–77.
12. Eroles P, Bosch A, Pérez-Fidalgo JA, et al. Molecular biology in breast cancer: intrinsic subtypes and signaling pathways. Cancer Treat Rev 2012;38:698–707.
13. Allison KH. Molecular pathology of breast cancer: what a pathologist needs to know. Am J Clin Pathol 2012;138:770–80.
14. Grankvist J, Fisker R, Iyer V, et al. MRI and PET/CT of patients with bone metastases from breast carcinoma. Eur J Radiol 2012;81(1):e13–8.
15. Niikura N, Costelloe CM, Madewell JE, et al. FDGPET/CT compared with conventional imaging in the detection of distant metastases of primary breast cancer. Oncologist 2011;16(8):1111–9.

16. Koolen BB, VranckenPeeters MJ, Aukema TS, et al. 18F-FDG PET/CT as a staging procedure in primary stage II and III breast cancer: comparison with conventional imaging techniques. Breast Cancer Res Treat 2012;131(1):117–26.
17. Hahn S, Heusner T, Kümmel S, et al. Comparison of FDG-PET/CT and bone scintigraphy for detection of bone metastases in breast cancer. Acta Radiol 2011;52(9):1009–14.
18. Lin NU, Guo H, Yap JT, et al. Phase II study of lapatinib in combination with trastuzumab in patients with human epidermal growth factor receptor 2-positive metastatic breast cancer: clinical outcomes and predictive value of early [18F]fluorodeoxyglucose positron emission tomography imaging (TBCRC 003). J Clin Oncol 2015;33(24):2623–31.
19. Storniolo AM, Pegram MD, Overmoyer B, et al. Phase I dose escalation and pharmacokinetic study of lapatinib in combination with trastuzumab in patients with advanced ErbB2-positive breast cancer. J Clin Oncol 2008;26:3317–23.
20. Blackwell KL, Burstein HJ, Storniolo AM, et al. Randomized study of lapatinib alone or in combination with trastuzumab in women with ErbB2-positive, trastuzumab-refractory metastatic breast cancer. J Clin Oncol 2010;28:1124–30.
21. Baselga J, Bradbury I, Eidtmann H, et al, NeoALTTO Study Team. Lapatinib with trastuzumab for HER2-positive early breast cancer (NeoALTTO): a randomised, open-label, multicentre, phase 3 trial. Lancet 2012;379(9816):633–40.
22. Kitajima K, Fukushima K, Miyoshi Y, et al. Association between $^{18}$F-FDG uptake and molecular subtype of breast cancer. Eur J Nucl Med Mol Imaging 2015; 42(9):1371–7.
23. Koolen BB, VranckenPeeters MJ, Wesseling J, et al. Association of primary tumour FDG uptake with clinical, histopathological and molecular characteristics in breast cancer patients scheduled for neoadjuvant chemotherapy. Eur J Nucl Med Mol Imaging 2012; 39(12):1830–8.
24. Koo HR, Park JS, Kang KW, et al. 18F-FDG uptake in breast cancer correlates with immunohistochemically defined subtypes. Eur Radiol 2014;24(3):610–8.
25. Gebhart G, Gámez C, Holmes E, et al. 18F-FDG PET/CT for early prediction of response to neoadjuvant lapatinib, trastuzumab, and their combination in HER2-positive breast cancer: results from Neo-ALTTO. J Nucl Med 2013;54(11):1862–8.
26. Kiesewetter DO, Kilbourn MR, Landvatter SW, et al. Preparation of four fluorine-18-labeled estrogens and their selective uptakes in target tissues of immature rats. J Nucl Med 1984;25:1212–21.
27. Mintun MA, Welch MJ, Siegel BA, et al. Breast cancer: PET imaging of estrogen receptors. Radiology 1988;169:45–8.
28. Mortimer JE, Dehdashti F, Siegel BA, et al. Metabolic flare: indicator of hormone responsiveness in advanced breast cancer. J Clin Oncol 2001;19: 2797–803.
29. Ingle JN, Ahmann DL, Green SJ, et al. Randomized clinical trial of diethylstilbestrol versus tamoxifen in postmenopausal women with advanced breast cancer. N Engl J Med 1981;304:16–21.
30. Peethambaram PP, Ingle JN, Suman VJ, et al. Randomized trial of diethylstilbestrol vs. tamoxifen in postmenopausal women with metastatic breast cancer. An updated analysis. Breast Cancer Res Treat 1999;54:117–22.
31. Ellis MJ, Gao F, Dehdashti F, et al. Lower-dose vs high-dose oral estradiol therapy of hormone receptor-positive, aromatase inhibitor-resistant advanced breast cancer: a phase 2 randomized study. JAMA 2009;302:774–80.
32. van Kruchten M, Glaudemans AW, de Vries EF, et al. Positron emission tomography of tumour [(18)F]fluoroestradiol uptake in patients with acquired hormone-resistant metastatic breast cancer prior to oestradiol therapy. Eur J Nucl Med Mol Imaging 2015;42(11):1674–81.
33. Linden HM, Stekhova SA, Link JM, et al. Quantitative fluoroestradiol positron emission tomography imaging predicts response to endocrine treatment in breast cancer. J Clin Oncol 2006;24(18):2793–9.

# PET Imaging of Skeletal Metastases and Its Role in Personalizing Further Management

Abhishek Mahajan, MBBS, MD, MRes[a], Gurdip Kaur Azad, MBBS, MRCP, FRCR[b], Gary J. Cook, MBBS, MSc, MD, FRCR, FRCP[b,c,*]

**KEYWORDS**

• Neoplasms/Carcinoma • Bone • Skeletal metastasis • Tumor biology • Functional imaging • Radionuclide imaging • Translational medicine • Evidence based medicine

**KEY POINTS**

- It is crucial to accurately detect, quantify, and evaluate treatment response in skeletal metastatic disease so that the patient is appropriately staged and optimally managed.
- Multimodal PET/computed tomography imaging is not only accurate but superior for the assessment of skeletal metastatic disease.
- Multiparametric hybrid PET/MR imaging is emerging as an innovative and potential multimodality imaging tool for detecting and delineating metastatic skeletal disease.
- PET-based bone-specific and tumor-specific methods for noninvasively imaging bone metastases have the ability to contribute to individual patient management decisions at all stages of diagnosis and treatment.

## INTRODUCTION

The skeleton is one of the most common sites for metastatic disease and the related complications pose a major management challenge, significantly affecting the quality of life of these patients.[1] These complications have been described as skeletal-related events (SREs) and include a range of clinical presentations, including bone pain, pathologic fractures, hypercalcemia, nerve root compression, myelosuppression, and cord compression.[2–4] Bone is the most frequent and may be the first and only involved metastatic site in patients with solid tumors. Therapeutic options have improved. For example, in prostate cancer, skeletal metastases are associated with overall survival (OS) ranging from 12 to 53 months.[5] Other solid tumors that are frequently associated with skeletal metastases are breast, lung, thyroid, kidney, and urinary bladder and the incidence of bone metastases at the time of diagnosis in such patients is as high as 40%.[6,7] The overall survival of patients with cancer has significantly improved over the past 2 decades, and this has led to increase in the incidence of metastatic disease. It has been found that approximately 70% of the patients with advanced breast or prostate cancer

The authors have nothing to disclose.

[a] Department of Radiodiagnosis, Tata Memorial Hospital, Parel, Mumbai 400012, India; [b] Division of Imaging Sciences and Biomedical Engineering, Cancer Imaging Department, King's College London, St Thomas' Hospital, Westminster Bridge Road, London SE1 7EH, UK; [c] Clinical PET Centre, St Thomas' Hospital, Westminster Bridge Road, London SE1 7EH, UK
* Corresponding author. Clinical PET Centre, St Thomas' Hospital, Westminster Bridge Road, London SE1 7EH, UK.
*E-mail address:* gary.cook@kcl.ac.uk

PET Clin 11 (2016) 305–318
http://dx.doi.org/10.1016/j.cpet.2016.02.003
1556-8598/16/$ – see front matter 

have bone metastases.[7,8] Thus, it is crucial to accurately detect, quantify, and evaluate treatment response in skeletal metastatic disease so that the patient is appropriately staged and optimally managed.[9,10] A wide range of imaging modalities are available for diagnosing bone metastases.[11] The main recommended anatomic modalities are computed tomography (CT) and magnetic resonance (MR) imaging, and the main functional modalities widely accepted and recommended for diagnosing bone metastases are bone scintigraphy and PET imaging with tumor-specific or bone-specific tracers.[12,13] In this review, we summarize the current state of PET imaging of the skeleton as an established tool for diagnosing bone metastases and monitoring response to treatment.

## PATHOPHYSIOLOGY OF SKELETAL METASTASES

Breast and prostate cancers have a high predisposition for skeletal metastases and are also known as osteotropic malignancies, whereas other cancers, including cervix, endometrium, and gastrointestinal tract, have a very low incidence of skeletal metastases.[14] The "seed and soil" hypothesis of the tumor biology first described by Stephen Paget explains the selective affinity of circulating malignant cells for deposition and further proliferation of some cancer cells in the bone environment.[15] Metastatic spread to bones can occur by direct extension but more commonly by hematogenous dissemination.[7] Adhesion molecules play an important role in homing of the circulating tumor cells, where chemotactic and growth factors secreted by the normal bone remodeling process provide the required nutritive support for their growth.[16] Some tumors release factors, such as parathyroid hormone–related protein, tumor necrosis factor $\alpha$ or $\beta$, and interleukin (IL)-1 and IL-6, that upregulate osteoclastic activity leading to osteolysis. There are certain tumors in which factors such as insulinlike growth factors, epidermal growth factors and transforming growth factors $\alpha$ and $\beta$ cause upregulation of osteoblastic activity leading to predominant osteosclerosis.[17] These form the basis of bone forming, that is, osteoblastic (eg, prostate cancer) or bone destructive, that is, osteolytic metastases (eg, kidney, thyroid, and lung). However, many tumors present with a spectrum of blastic and lytic bone lesions with abnormal osteoblast and osteoclast activity whatever the dominant morphology. Compared with osteoblastic metastases, osteolytic metastases generally have a more aggressive course with early clinical presentation and progression.[18] Also noteworthy is that bone marrow involvement usually predates bone destruction, and metastases at this stage may be more easily detected with tumor-specific rather than bone-specific imaging techniques, a process that may contribute to false negatives on conventional nuclear bone scintigraphic imaging.[19]

## IMAGING OF SKELETAL METASTASES: AN OVERVIEW

In the emerging era of "personalized medicine" in oncology, imaging acts as both a predictive and prognostic biomarker that in turn permits clinicians to individualize treatment for patients by identifying those who may or may not benefit from a particular treatment plan.[20]

With skeletal metastases, the main questions that will affect an individual patient's management include the following:

1. Are there any bone metastases? If skeletal metastases are diagnosed, then treatment for the patient will generally become palliative rather than curative and so a sensitive diagnostic test is required to ensure correct prognostication and treatment strategy.
2. Is there a single, multiple, or (oligo) metastasis, and are metastases confined to the skeleton? Patients with a solitary bone metastasis or metastases confined to the skeleton generally have a better prognosis than those with multiple skeletal metastases or a combination of skeletal and visceral disease. A solitary metastasis may be eligible for attempted curative therapy, for example, stereotactic radiotherapy or surgery.[21,22] As well as a sensitive and specific test, this management will require an imaging method that can also detect or exclude nodal and visceral disease with high accuracy.
3. Are there any metastases that may lead to an SRE, for example, spinal cord compression? For this complication there is generally a requirement for good morphologic characterization of a bone lesion to assess the amount of bone destruction and risk of fracture, as well as the relation to adjacent structures at risk, such as the spinal cord. Systemic treatments, as well as being palliative can reduce future SREs and local radiotherapy or kyphoplasty may be required for symptomatic lesions or where there is risk of an SRE.
4. Should treatment be systemic, local, or both? Systemic treatment is generally palliative but may reduce SREs and prolong progression-free survival (PFS) and OS. As well as cytotoxic chemotherapy, for example, docetaxel in

prostate cancer, bone-specific drugs with antiosteoclastic properties, such as bisphosphonates and denosumab, are also used.
5. Is the patient suitable for targeted radionuclide therapy for bone metastases? The principle of radionuclide therapy is to confirm specific uptake in target lesions by imaging analogs before therapy with alpha-emitting or beta-emitting radionuclides, for example, 89Strontium, 153Samarium, or 223Radium.[23]
6. Is the patient responding to treatment? It may be impossible to predict which patients will respond to different types of treatment aimed at skeletal metastases. Response rates are generally less than 50%, and it is therefore imperative to assess response as soon as possible so that nonresponding patients can be changed to more effective treatment and avoid unnecessary toxicity from futile treatment regimes. This remains a challenge for oncology in general and imaging specifically. RECIST 1.1 criteria do not generally cater for bone assessment and conventional assessment with bone scan or CT may take many months before an accurate assessment can be made with the risk of false progressive disease (PD) assessments from bone-specific methods that may show a flare during an initial healing phase.[24–26]

The diagnostic strategy depends on the availability of an imaging modality and its diagnostic performance. The most common routinely used investigation for diagnosing bone metastases is bone scintigraphy (BS), using 99mTc-labeled diphosphonates.[27] However, it has limited sensitivity in the early stages of the disease when tumor is confined to the marrow, and lesions without an osteoblastic response remain invisible. Due to the nonspecific nature of bone accumulation of bone scan radiopharmaceuticals, a few conditions may lead to false-positive results, including trauma, healing factures, degenerative changes, and benign bone neoplasms.[28] Despite advantages over standard imaging methods such as radiographs or CT, BS has limited sensitivity and poor specificity for identifying bone metastases.[29] This is overcome to some extent by the addition of single-photon emission computed tomography (SPECT), which has the advantage of providing anatomic localization of abnormal tracer uptake with better contrast resolution. It allows approximately 20% to 50% greater lesion detection than planar scintigraphy imaging.[30] Furthermore, it has been found that SPECT/CT significantly outperforms SPECT alone and when available SPECT/CT should be performed in patients in whom correct classification of equivocal lesions is expected to alter the patient's management.[31] A recently published prospective study in 308 patients (211 with breast cancer, 97 with prostate cancer) imaged with whole-body scintigraphy (WBS), SPECT, and SPECT/CT for staging and restaging reported that SPECT/CT significantly improved the specificity and positive predictive value of BS. SPECT/CT helped in downstaging of metastatic disease in the total, breast cancer, and prostate cancer groups (32.1%, 33.8%, and 29.5% of patients, respectively). Three patients (2.1%) with breast cancer who were previously negative were upstaged by additional SPECT/CT and the study concluded that SPECT/CT has a significant effect on clinical management and reduces further diagnostic investigations.[32]

An alternative strategy is PET-based radionuclide imaging. The commonly used radiopharmaceuticals are 18F-fluoro-2-D-glucose (FDG) and 18F/11C-choline as tumor-specific agents or sodium fluoride as a bone-specific tracer (NaF).[33] The main advantages of PET imaging are its higher resolution and inherent quantitative nature that enable absolute determination of activity per unit volume of tissue.[34]

## PET

Morphologic bone imaging, such as radiographs, CT, and MR imaging delineate the structure of lesions within bone whereas functional bone imaging such as SPECT and PET assess the abnormal functional or metabolic aspects of bone or tumor cells.[35] 99mTc-labeled-diphosphonate is the most commonly used osteotropic tracer for SPECT and 18F-NaF for PET. Other oncotropic tracers being used are Carbon-11 (11C) and 18F-radiolabeled acetate and choline, particularly for prostate cancer. These agents identify tumor cells based on upregulated lipid synthesis and choline kinase activity, respectively.[13,27] Oncotropic radiopharmaceuticals can be classified as either specific or nonspecific. Specific oncotropic agents target specific biological abnormalities in tumors and those that can also give information on bone metastases include metaiodobenzylguanidine analogs, 111Indium-pentetreotide (OctreoScan), and 68Gallium-labeled somatostatin. The most commonly used nonspecific oncotropic radioisotope is the glucose analog 18F-labeled -FDG.[13,27]

### *18F Sodium Fluoride PET*

18F-NaF was first described in 1962 as a radionuclide bone scan tracer for $\gamma$-camera imaging and in 1972 the Food and Drug Administration approved 18F-NaF imaging.[36,37] However, the introduction of 99mTc-diphosphonates in 1975 led to its withdrawal from the market and it was listed as a discontinued drug in 1984. It remained underutilized for bone imaging until recent developments in PET/CT hardware lead to a resurgence of the clinical use of 18F-NaF for bone imaging.[38] The skeletal clearance of 18F-NaF is very similar to 99mTc-labeled diphosphonates and is dependent on local bone metabolism and blood flow. At physiologic blood flow rates, the first pass extraction of 18F-NaF approaches 100% and allows estimation of bone blood flow. Uptake is not specific to bone metastases and as with 99mTc-diphosphonates there may be false-positive results with 18F-NaF. However, with the morphologic information available from modern PET/CT (and more recently PET/MR imaging) scanners, the specificity for differentiating these lesions into benign and malignant has significantly improved.[35] The extracted 18F-NaF is subsequently chemisorbed into the bone crystals to form fluoroapatite and fluorohydroxyapatite. The selective accumulation is mainly seen in actively mineralizing bone and bone formation. Contrary to 99mTc-labeled diphosphonates, 18F-NaF is not bound to protein and has a rapid skeletal uptake as early as 1 hour after injection. Higher lesion-to-background ratios for both osteoblastic and osteolytic metastases makes it an important imaging tool for detecting skeletal metastases.[39] This provides high-quality images within short scan times and a low patient radiation dose (approximately 4.3 mSv for a 250-MBq injection). An important limiting factor to wide clinical use of 18F-NaF is the requirement of a cyclotron for its production.[40] Overall, 18F-NaF-PET has the advantages of improved sensitivity with superior image quality, higher bone uptake with reasonable patient radiation dose, and better pharmacokinetics with faster clearance from blood with a short time from time of injection to imaging (**Fig. 1**).

The Centers for Medicare and Medicaid Services (CMS) initiated the approval of reimbursement for 18F-NaF-PET at the beginning of April 2009 and in February 2011 CMS culminated the decision with approval of its use for imaging skeletal metastatic disease in sites participating in the National Oncology PET Registry.[41]

Compared with 99mTechnetium-methylene diphosphonate (MDP) planar or SPECT BS, 18F-NaF-PET has higher sensitivity and specificity for detecting bone metastases in various primary malignancies, including breast, lung, and prostate cancer.[42] One of the earliest studies reported in 2001, in 44 patients with primary malignancies of the lung, prostate, and thyroid, that 18F-NaF-PET correctly detected 96 metastatic lesions in 15 patients and was found to have better accuracy than that of 99mTc-MDP BS, which could identify only 46 metastases in 13 patients. 18F-NaF-PET was shown to have better diagnostic accuracy than planar BS with the area under the receiver operating curve being 0.99 versus 0.64 on a lesion-by-lesion basis and 1.0 versus 0.82 on a patient-by-patient basis, respectively.[43] Another study in 34 patients with breast or prostate cancer compared 18F-NaF-PET/CT and 99mTc-MDP SPECT BS and concluded that for detecting pelvic

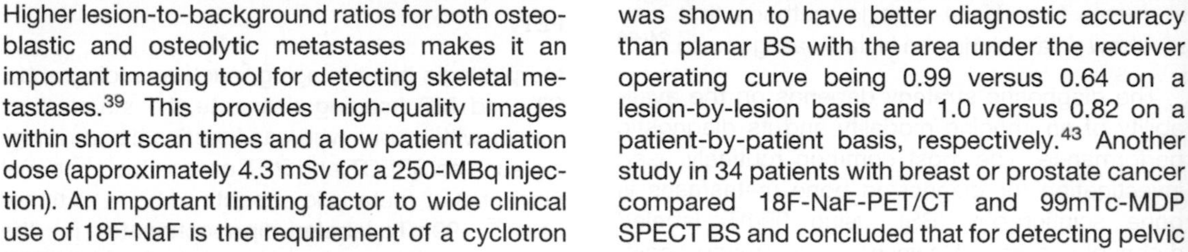

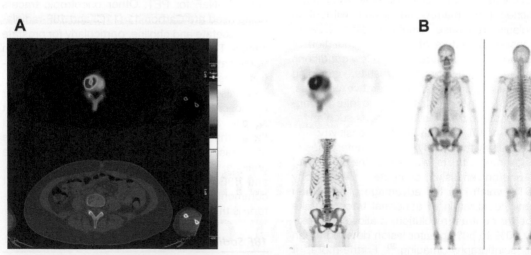


**Fig. 1.** A patient with metastatic breast cancer. (*A*) 18F-NaF PET/CT showing axial fused, CT and PET slices through the lower lumbar spine as well as the maximum intensity projection (MIP) image. The axial images clearly show that the lower lumbar spine abnormality is caused by a lytic metastasis in the vertebral body and is not due to benign degenerative disease. (*B*) A 99mTc-MDP bone scan in the same patient. The spatial and contrast resolution of the bone scan is inferior to that of the 18F-NaF PET/CT scan.

and lumbar lesions, 18F-NaF-PET/CT has a significantly higher accuracy than that for 99mTc-MDP BS. Compared with 99mTc-MDP BS with SPECT, which could correctly diagnose only 28 of 33 patients, 18F-NaF-PET/CT diagnosed 32 of 33 patients.[44] Compared with 18F-FDG-PET/CT and BS, the reported sensitivity and negative predicted values of 18F-NaF-PET/CT in breast, prostate, and lung cancers was 100%.[45] Studies have shown that using a maximum standardized uptake value (SUVmax) threshold of 10 can exclude nearly all normal bone activity from volumetric calculations for determination of skeletal tumor burden and a cutoff of SUVmax over 50 almost always represents bone metastases, whereas an SUVmax less than 12 always represents degenerative joint disease (*P*<.001).[46,47]

Recently published literature supports the fact that 18F-NaF-PET/CT is a potential alternative biomarker for assessment of treatment response of bone metastases. A pilot study evaluated the change in SUVmax on follow-up 18-F-NaF-PET/CT to assess response to (223)Ra dichloride (Alpharadin) therapy in castrate-resistant prostate cancer (CRPC) and found it to be consistent with prostate-specific antigen (PSA) response and alkaline phosphatase activity at 12 weeks after starting treatment.[48] Similar results were reported in ACRIN 6687, another study in which patients with prostate cancer treated with dasatinib were imaged with 18F-NaF-PET/CT. Changes in 18F-NaF incorporation in tumor and normal bone that occurred in response to dasatinib were correlated with PFS, PSA, and serum markers. The study concluded that 18F-NaF PET is capable of identifying dasatinib treatment response in CRPC bone metastases with a significant differential 18F-NaF PET response between tumor and normal bone.[49] 18F-NaF-PET/CT–based skeletal tumor burden indices of total fluoride skeletal metastatic lesion uptake and total volume of fluoride avid bone metastases in hormone-refractory prostate cancer treated with (223)Ra dichloride therapy has been found to be a predictive biomarker of OS and SREs related to Ra-223 chloride therapy.[50] Similar results were reported in a feasibility study in breast cancer; 18F-NaF-PET-CT was shown to be useful for evaluating changes in bone turnover in response to treatment.[51]

Finally, Hillner and colleagues[42] reported a study that evaluated the role of 18F-NaF-PET for monitoring response to treatment during systemic therapy in a large set of cancers from the National Oncologic PET Registry and found that 18F-NaF-PET imaging has a significant clinical impact on management, especially in those who had progressive osseous disease. The same group also reported that for imaging skeletal metastatic disease, 18F-NaF-PET can potentially replace the intended use of other advanced imaging (body CT, MR imaging, or FDG-PET) for restaging or suspected recurrence in prostate and other cancer types.[52]

In summary, F18-NaF-PET may help detect early disease progression in the bones, giving patients the opportunity to be treated with more effective treatments early and thus avoiding potentially toxic side effects from ineffective treatments.

### 18F Fluorodeoxyglucose PET/Computed Tomography

18F-FDG-PET/CT provides a unique combination of functional information about the metabolic activity of tumor and associated anatomic information, which makes it an apt modality for staging and monitoring of patients with cancer. Similar to the activity in the primary lesion, the abnormal uptake in the bone infiltrated by tumor cells is in proportion to levels of glucose metabolism.[53] This makes 18F-FDG-PET/CT a nonspecific oncotropic radionuclide tracer that detects bone or bone marrow metastases often before bone destruction on a CT or osteoblastic activity on a bone scan becomes detectable.[54,55] 18F-FDG-PET/CT can potentially differentiate between metabolically active disease in blastic metastases versus the inactive tumor in treated sclerotic bone lesions (**Fig. 2**). However, it is more likely to be positive and show higher avidity for osteolytic metastases than for untreated sclerotic metastases and the sensitivity to detect residual microscopic elements is limited.[56,57]

18F-FDG-PET and BS have been compared and studies have reported mixed results. A lesion-based analysis in 17 patients with metastatic prostate cancer found 18F-FDG-PET to be superior in characterizing active and dormant bone lesions and also reported that it recognizes new lesions earlier than BS.[58] Subsequently, 2 other studies found 18F-FDG-PET sensitivity to be lower than for BS in prostate cancer.[59,60] Another study found that the SUVmax correlates strongly with prognosis in patients with progressive prostate cancer and is associated with poor prognosis. The study concluded that FDG-SUVmax is an independent prognostic factor and provides complementary prognostic information in CRPC. However, 18F-FDG-PET was reported to be of limited value in assessing treatment response in patients with hormone-responsive nonprogressive metastatic prostate cancer, as these lesions were found to have low glycolytic activity.[61]

A small study in 9 patients with CRPC treated with abiraterone and cabozantinib imaged with

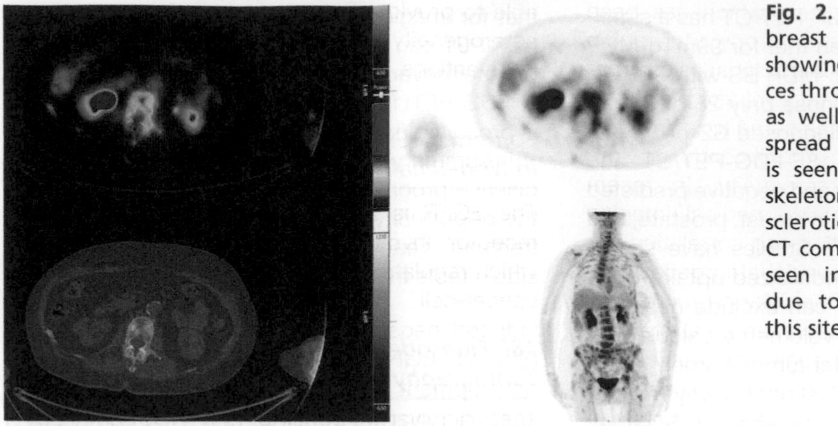

Fig. 2. A patient with metastatic breast cancer. 18F-FDG PET/CT showing axial fused, CT and PET slices through the upper lumbar spine as well as the MIP image. Widespread abnormal 18F-FDG activity is seen throughout much of the skeleton corresponding to active sclerotic metastases as seen on the CT component. Reduced uptake is seen in the lower thoracic spine due to previous radiotherapy at this site.

18F-FDG-PET/CT and 18F-NaF-PET/CT for response assessment found 18F-FDG-PET/CT to be superior to 18F-NaF-PET-CT and conventional imaging.[62] Notably, compared with 11C-acetate PET, the reported sensitivity for detection of osseous metastases is higher for 18F-FDG-PET but the sensitivity for accurately measuring disease response is higher with 11C-acetate-PET.[63] Another retrospective study analyzed 38 patients with prostate cancer bone metastases targeting the androgen receptor signaling pathway and assessed the changes in morphologic patterns of prostate cancer bone metastases on CT, their associated glycolytic activity based on FDG uptake and relative androgen receptor expression based on uptake of 18F-16β-fluoro-5-dihydrotestosterone (FDHT). Numbers of bone lesions detected on 18F-FDG-PET and 18F-FDHT-PET scans were significantly associated with OS and higher FDHT uptake was found to be associated with shorter OS. However, 18F-FDG uptake did not show any association with OS.[64] This indicates that 18F-FDHT, an analog of the primary ligand of the androgen receptor, provides clinically relevant prognostic information in patients with bone metastases in CRPC.

Much of the reported literature describing PET and bone metastases compares BS with 18F-FDG-PET in patients with breast cancer and it has better diagnostic accuracy than BS. Sensitivity for lytic metastases is higher than for osteoblastic metastases, which are less FDG avid.[65] For detecting bone metastases in patients with breast cancer on a per-lesion–based analysis, 18F-FDG-PET is reported to be more sensitive than BS (96% vs 76%) with similar specificity (92% vs 95%).[66] A meta-analysis reported that 18F-FDG-PET has higher diagnostic performance for detection of breast cancer recurrence and metastases, and in a per-patient analysis the reported pooled sensitivity was 90% with a false-positive rate of 12%, false-negative rate of 10%, and overall diagnostic accuracy of 86%.[67] Another meta-analysis of 7 studies evaluated the diagnostic performance of 18F-FDG-PET/CT for detection of bone metastases in breast cancer and found it to be more accurate with a higher sensitivity than planar BS (93% vs 81%).[68]

Most of the studies that have evaluated the changes in SUVmax and the role in predicting osseous response to therapy are retrospective and have reported 18F-FDG-PET to be an independent biomarker for monitoring therapy and predicting response.[69,70] A study in 32 patients with breast cancer with bone metastases being evaluated with 18F-FDG-PET/CT and 18F-NaF-PET/CT with respect to disease prognostication and outcome reported that baseline 18F-FDG-PET/CT predicts the prognosis of these patients more accurately than the conventional and biological prognostic factors, and was independently associated with OS. The investigators also concluded that when compared with 18F-FDG-PET/CT, 18F-NaF-PET/CT had a higher diagnostic sensitivity but was not independently associated with OS.[71] To summarize, in breast cancer, not only is F18-FDG-PET accurate at detecting bone metastases, but there is increasing evidence to support its use in the assessment of treatment response of bone disease.

A meta-analysis in lung cancer evaluated and compared the capability of 18F-FDG-PET/CT, 18F-FDG-PET, MR imaging, and BS imaging for assessment of bone metastases. 18F-FDG-PET/CT and 18F-FDG-PET showed better performance than the other imaging modalities. The pooled sensitivity and specificity for the detection of bone metastases in lung cancer with 18F-FDG-PET/CT was 92% and 98%, for 18F-FDG-PET was 87% and 94%, for MR imaging was 77%

and 92%, and for BS was 86% and 88%, respectively.[72] A recently published study in a mixed cohort of primary malignancies was evaluated with 18F-FDG-PET/CT before and after treatment and a statistically significant correlation was found between regression in the metabolic activity and increase in the attenuation of the target bone lesions. It was concluded that lesion metabolic activity is a more reliable parameter for response assessment than the changes in their radiographic patterns.[73]

Overall, F18-FDG-PET provides valuable information in the initial diagnosis of bone metastases, especially if the patient has oligo-metastatic disease in which the intent of treatment may well change from palliative to curative and from systemic to local, thus avoiding unnecessary treatment-related toxicities.

## *Choline PET/Computed Tomography*

Although 18F-FDG-PET showed promising results in hormone-resistant poorly differentiated prostate cancer, it was found to have limited value in well-differentiated types, and 11C-choline or 18F-Fluorocholine (FCH)-PET/CT add valuable information in both primary and recurrent prostate cancer, especially in cases with equivocal lesions on BS (**Fig. 3**). One such study showed that when imaged with 11C-choline-PET/CT detected multiple sites of unknown relapses in 44% (11/25) of patients and of these, 2 had a single bone lesion with associated extraosseous metastases; 6 with multiple bone lesions and 3 with multiple bone lesions and associated extraosseous disease lesions.[74] On a per-patient basis, the reported sensitivity and specificity of 11C-choline-PET/CT was 86% (19/22) and 100% (19/19). The detection rate of previously undetected disease in patients with biochemical recurrence and negative bone scans is reported to be 14.6%.[75] Another study that compared the value of BS and 11C-choline-PET/CT in 78 patients with prostate cancer showed that 11C-choline-PET/CT could correctly detect bone metastases with high specificity of 98% (98% vs 75%, respectively) with a lower sensitivity (89% vs 100%).[76] Beauregard and colleagues[77] reported that compared with BS, 18F-choline-PET/CT and 18F-FDG-PET/CT were 100% sensitive for detecting lymph node and distant metastases in prostate cancer compared with a sensitivity of 67% for BS. Another prospective study reported a 20% (17/83) change in the management of patients with high-risk prostate cancer and 15% of all patients (19/130) based on metastatic disease detected on preoperative 18F-choline-PET. Of the 132 patients, 13 had 43 bone metastases.[78] The investigator suggested this modality will be helpful in the triage of prostate cancers that are at high risk for extracapsular disease. A meta-analysis compared choline-PET/CT, MR imaging, SPECT, and BS in the diagnosis of bone metastases in patients with prostate cancer. On a per-patient basis, the pooled sensitivities of choline-PET/CT, MR imaging, and BS for detection of metastases were found to be 91%, 97%, and 79%, respectively, and pooled specificities were 99%, 95%, and 82%, respectively. On a per-lesion basis, the pooled sensitivity of choline-PET/CT, SPECT, and BS were 84%, 90%, and 59%, and the pooled specificities were 93%, 85%, and 75%, respectively. The study concluded that for detecting bone metastases in prostate cancer, on a per-patient basis, MR imaging is better than choline-PET/CT and BS. On a per-lesion basis compared with bone SPECT and BS, choline-PET/CT showed a higher diagnostic odds ratio (78.16, 6.21, and 99.78, respectively) and better Q* values (proportion of false positives incurred when the test was called significant, ie, false discovery rate), which were 0.8751, 0.7132, and 0.8896, respectively.[79]

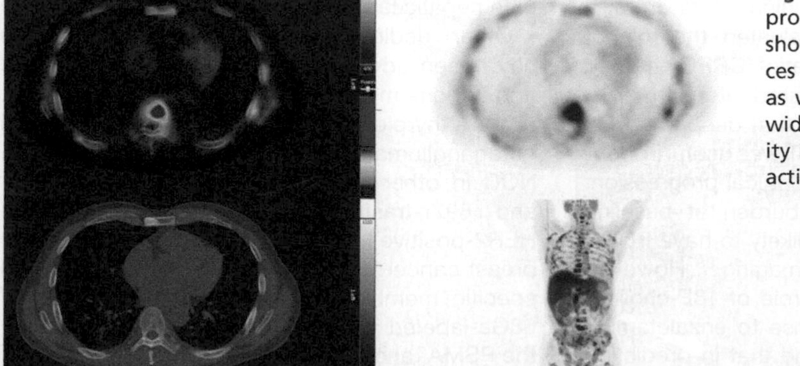

**Fig. 3.** A patient with metastatic prostate cancer. 11C-choline-PET/CT showing axial fused, CT and PET slices through the mid-thoracic spine as well as the MIP image. There is widespread abnormal choline activity in the skeleton in keeping with active metastatic disease.

It is important to note that compared with sclerotic lesions, lytic metastases show a higher uptake of choline and an inverse relationship is found between the intensity of 18F-choline uptake and the degree of lesion sclerosis. Beheshti and colleagues[80] reported normal 18F-choline uptake in sclerotic lesions on CT >825 HU and such lesions were commonly seen in patients who were on androgen deprivation therapy, suggesting these were successfully treated inactive lesions with osteoblastic response leading to sclerosis and a reduction in choline activity within the tumor cells. Overall sensitivity, specificity, positive predictive value, and negative predictive value for lesion detection in CRPC using 18F-choline-PET has been reported to be 96%, 96%, 99%, and 81%, respectively.[81] Another study compared the diagnostic accuracy of MR imaging: BS, 18F-NaF-PET/CT, and 18F-choline-PET/CT for spinal metastases in prostate cancer with MR imaging as the reference and found that 18F-choline-PET/CT and 18F-NaF-PET/CT were superior to BS, and questioned the present use of BS as the method of choice in patients with hormone-naïve prostate cancer.[82] A study correlated choline metabolism and proliferation assessed by 11C-choline-PET in estrogen receptor (ER)-positive breast cancer and compared it with 18F-fluorothymidine (FLT) PET and found that higher choline uptake was a measure of cellular activity and was found to be related to cytoplasmic choline kinase-alpha expression.[83] It has been shown that 18F-choline-PET/CT is significantly more accurate than BS for detecting bone metastases from breast and prostate cancers.[84]

Studies have reported that both 18F and 11C-choline-PET–positive imaging findings in patients with prostate cancer with biochemical recurrence are predictive markers of a shorter PFS and have a major impact on the clinical management of these patients.[85,86] Data from a preclinical study showed that 11C-choline-PET has potential for monitoring early response to docetaxel in metastatic prostate cancer.[87] Clinical data from a recently published study evaluated the role of 11C-choline-PET in metastatic CRPC treated with docetaxel and compared it with PSA response. The study showed that despite a PSA response, 11C-choline-PET/CT was useful in identifying patients who had radiological progression. Patients with higher tumor burden at baseline 11C-choline-PET were more likely to have PD on follow-up 11C- choline-PET imaging.[88] However, another study evaluated the role of 18F-choline-PET/CT for predicting response to enzalutamide in metastatic CRPC and found that in predicting OS, 18F-choline-PET/CT did not add any further information beyond that obtained from PSA.[89] Serial measurements of choline uptake measured on 11C-choline-PET have also been found to correlate with clinical response to trastuzumab in patients with breast cancer.[90]

In patients with high-risk prostate cancer treated with curative intent, F18-choline can help detect previously undetected metastatic disease, thereby warranting systemic treatment instead. However, clinical trials are currently ongoing, looking at the role of C11-choline/F18-choline-PET scans in the diagnosis and monitoring of treatment response.

## *Specific PET Tracers*

Specific tracers have been found to be useful for detecting skeletal metastatic disease for particular tumor types; such examples are 124Iodine for differentiated thyroid cancer and 18F-fluoroestradiol (FES) for breast cancer, and studies have suggested that these may replace or complement 18F-FDG-PET imaging.[91,92] There have been significant advances in development of these targeted agents that have enabled accurate characterization in various primary tumor types that have not only improved the specificity of early detection and monitoring of such osteotropic metastases, but have potential significant impact on personalized patient management.[93] In one such study that evaluated the role of 18F-FES-PET in patients with breast cancer presenting with a clinical dilemma despite complete standard workup (when imaging methods were inconclusive and performing biopsy was not feasible), it was found that 18F-FES-PET is more sensitive for detecting bone lesions and detected 341 bone lesions, compared with 246 by conventional imaging in 33 patients.[93] 18F-FES-PET is shown to be a noninvasive method of obtaining molecular information about ER expression and can be used as a diagnostic tool when conventional workup is ambiguous and biopsies are not feasible or inconclusive; however, it is not recommended to evaluate hepatic lesions.[93]

Other dedicated radiopharmaceuticals that have been advocated for tumor-specific detection of bone metastases are 18F-FDOPA in medullary thyroid cancer, pheochromocytoma, paraganglioma, and 68Ga-DOTATOC or DOTANOC in other types of neuroendocrine tumors and 89Zr-trastuzumab in PET imaging for HER2-positive lesions in patients with metastatic breast cancer.[94,95] Another example is prostate-specific membrane antigen (PSMA) PET using 68Ga-labeled small molecule antagonist against the PSMA, and is found to have higher tracer uptake in dedifferentiated malignancies with high detection rates in patients with low PSA levels.[96,97]

The clinical applications of these tracers have been extended to "theranostics" and are being investigated for identifying patients who may benefit from therapeutic tumor-targeted drug derivatives of such tracer compounds; for example, ER imaging before anti-estrogen therapy or increased osteoblastic activity before radionuclide-targeted therapy, such as 186Rhenium, 183Samarium, or 223Radium.[98,99] Targeted PET imaging of HER2 with radiolabeled trastuzumab (89Zr-trastuzumab PET) has been found to be a noninvasive method for characterizing HER2 expression in primary and distant lesions.[100] Preclinical studies of 66 and 68Ga-DOTA-E-(c[RGDfK])$_2$ PET in a nude mouse model have shown promising results for imaging of $\alpha v\beta 3$ and $\alpha v\beta 5$ integrins that are overexpressed in bone metastases and are proposed to be novel companion diagnostics for detection and follow-up of osseous metastases.[101]

## PET/MR IMAGING

Hybrid multimodal PET/MR has emerged as a novel imaging modality that may impact on management of patients with bone metastases. It has improved spatial and contrast resolution from MR imaging and is expected to decrease the imaging false-positive rate and improve cancer staging and monitoring sensitivity.[102] A recent feasibility study comparing PET/MR imaging with PET/CT found that PET/MR imaging led to higher reader confidence and improved conspicuity. It was proposed that the highest clinical impact will be in patients with limited and early metastatic skeletal disease.[103] Another study reported that compared with 18F-FDG-PET/MR imaging, hypersclerotic benign bone lesions showed significantly higher ($P$<.05) conspicuity and diagnostic confidence on 18F-FDG-PET/CT, and 18F-FDG-PET/CT still sets the reference.[104] A recently published study reported that 18F-FDG-PET/MR with diagnostic T1-weighted turbo spin echo (TSE) sequences is superior to 18F-FDG-PET/CT and 18F-FDG-PET/MR with T1-weighted Dixon in-phase images. The investigators found that there was no correlation between the degree of sclerosis and the mean underestimation for 18F-FDG-PET/MR compared with 18F-FDG-PET/CT.[105] In terms of overall performance, 18F-FDG-PET/MR imaging was shown to be comparable to 18F-FDG-PET/CT but had a higher diagnostic accuracy for early bone marrow infiltration and for bone tumors with low 18F-FDG uptake. They recommended the use of a diagnostic T1-weighted TSE sequence for the PET/MR imaging protocol.[105] The use of T1-weighted spin-echo sequences for attenuation correction in PET/MR is found to have superior quantitative analysis of tracer uptake and thus superior analysis of PET tracer distribution for detecting and assessing response to therapy in bone metastases. The Food and Drug Administration has approved 2-point Dixon-based MR sequence for attenuation correction in a commercially available integrated PET/MR system. Two-point Dixon sequence delivers water-weighted and fat-weighted images and the contribution from bone signal is neglected by this approach; however, the technical challenge is most evident in the separation of cortical bone and air interface, where it can potentially lead to inaccuracies in quantifying PET signal from cortical bone or areas adjacent to bone.[106,107]

A recent study in 109 patients with breast cancer found that contrast-enhanced 18F-FDG-PET/MR detected a higher number of osseous metastases than did same-day contrast-enhanced 18F-FDG-PET/CT with sensitivities of 85% and 96% for contrast-enhanced PET/CT and contras-enhanced PET/MR, respectively, with an estimated specificity of 98% for 18F-FDG-PET/MR. The reported false-positive rate for contrast-enhanced PET/CT was 12%.[108] A further study quantitatively analyzed 18F-choline-PET/MR imaging for bone metastases from prostate cancer and reported that the SUVs from hybrid 18F-choline-PET had an inverse correlation with apparent diffusion coefficient values in diffusion-weighted (DW) MR imaging,[109] supporting the relationship in prostate cancer of high cellularity expressed by low ADC and the metabolic activity of phospholipid turnover expressed by high SUV. The study concluded that the advantage of combining high-resolution anatomic imaging with functional studies and metabolic/molecular imaging adds to diagnostic confidence and characterization of different aspects of tumor biology. At the same time combined simultaneous PET/MR imaging (DW MR imaging and choline-PET) is proposed to have potential for monitoring hormonal deprivation therapies as well as radiation therapy in prostate cancer.

Recently published literature has shown promising results in the implementation of choline-PET/MR imaging and multiparametric-MR imaging in assessing recurrent prostate cancer after external beam radiotherapy (EBRT) and found it to be a feasible and effective diagnostic tool for detecting prostate cancer recurrence in patients showing biochemical relapses after first-line treatment with EBRT.[110] With regard to patient-based analysis for detection of relapses, 18F-choline-PET/MR imaging had an overall detection rate of 86%

(18/21), which was higher in comparison with 18F-choline-PET/CT, contrast-enhanced CT, and multiparametric-MR imaging (76%, 43%, and 81%, respectively) and 18F-choline-PET/MR imaging performed significantly better than contrast-enhanced CT for detection of skeletal metastases in pelvic bones. On a patient-based analysis for bone lesions, 18F-PET/MR imaging provided the highest detection rate of 100% (9/9), which was higher than 18F-choline-PET/CT (89%; 8/9) and contrast-enhanced CT (44%; 4/9).

Another study evaluated the reproducibility of combined hybrid PET/MR imaging and 68Ga-PSMA-tracer for depiction of nodal and skeletal bone metastases in prostate cancer and compared it with 68Ga-PSMA PET/CT reporting 68Ga-PSMA PET/MR imaging to be accurate and reliable with very low discordance when compared with 68Ga-PSMA PET/CT.[111]

Overall PET/MR imaging is an evolving and promising imaging technique for detection of skeletal metastases and assessment of response to therapy in skeletal metastatic disease. The highest potential clinical impact of PET/MR imaging appears to be in bone-marrow metastases, early bone metastatic disease, and extraosseous tumor extension assessment. Finally, when it comes to providing personalized patient care, simultaneous combined PET and MR imaging is justified to be "state-of-the-art imaging" and offers the potential of a "one-stop shop" imaging modality.

## SUMMARY

Ongoing developments and improvements in the personalized management of cancer have led to better symptom control, reduced SREs, and better survival. In accordance with the highest standards of cancer management, substantial advancement in the field of imaging is required for reliable detection and characterization of bone metastases and treatment response assessment. Due to the complex morphology, slow metabolism, tumor biology, and heterogeneity on the molecular level; the evaluation of the osseous lesions still remains a challenge. To overcome this, optimized multimodal imaging using PET/CT that fuses morphologic and functional data is found not only to be accurate but superior for the assessment of skeletal metastatic disease across most tumor types and clinical scenarios. Multiparametric hybrid PET/MR imaging has emerged as an innovative and potential multimodality imaging tool that combines the advantage of 2 important imaging modalities and is expected to lead to further improvements over PET/CT in detecting and delineating metastatic skeletal disease. The future of imaging skeletal metastases is an evolving process and potential remains for exploring further tumor-specific radiotracers that will not only increase diagnostic accuracy but when used as theranostics, will have a significant impact on personalized cancer management. PET-based bone-specific and tumor-specific methods for noninvasively imaging bone metastases have the ability to contribute to individual patient management decisions at all stages of diagnosis and treatment.

## ACKNOWLEDGMENTS

The authors acknowledge financial support from the Department of Health via the National Institute for Health Research (NIHR) Biomedical Research Center award to Guy's & St Thomas' NHS Foundation Trust in partnership with King's College London and the King's College London/University College London Comprehensive Cancer Imaging Centre funded by the CRUK and EPSRC in association with the MRC and DoH (England) (16463) and research grants from Prostate Cancer UK (PA12-04) and Breast Cancer Now (2012NovPR013).

## REFERENCES

1. Brown JE, Cook RJ, Major P, et al. Bone turnover markers as predictors of skeletal complications in prostate cancer, lung cancer, and other solid tumors. J Natl Cancer Inst 2005;97(1):59–69.
2. Coleman RE, Rubens RD. Bone metastases. In: Abeloff MD, Armitage JO, Niederhuber JE, et al, editors. Clinical oncology. 3rd edition. New York: Churchill Livingstone; 2004. p. 1091–128.
3. Weinfurt KP, Li Y, Castel LD, et al. The impact of skeletal-related events on health-related quality of life of patients with metastatic prostate cancer [abstract]. Ann Oncol 2002;13(Suppl 5):180.
4. Pelger RC, Soerdjbalie-Maikoe V, Hamdy NA. Strategies for management of prostate cancer-related bone pain. Drugs Aging 2001;18:899–911.
5. Coleman RE. Metastatic bone disease: clinical features, pathophysiology and treatment strategies. Cancer Treat Rev 2001;27:165–76.
6. Mundy GR. Metastasis to bone: causes, consequences and therapeutic opportunities. Nat Rev Cancer 2002;2:584–93.
7. Bussard KM, Gay CV, Mastro AM. The bone microenvironment in metastasis; what is special about bone? Cancer Metastasis Rev 2008;27:41–55.
8. Yu HH, Tsai YY, Hoffe SE. Overview of diagnosis and management of metastatic disease to bone. Cancer Control 2012;19:84–91.
9. Ulmert D, Solnes L, Thorek DL. Contemporary approaches for imaging skeletal metastasis. Bone Res 2015;3:15024.

10. Choi J, Raghavan M. Diagnostic imaging and image-guided therapy of skeletal metastases. Cancer Control 2012;19:102–12.
11. Talbot JN, Paycha F, Balogova S. Diagnosis of bone metastasis: recent comparative studies of imaging modalities. Q J Nucl Med Mol Imaging 2011; 55(4):374–410.
12. Chua S, Gnanasegaran G, Cook GJ. Miscellaneous cancers (lung, thyroid, renal cancer, myeloma, and neuroendocrine tumors): role of SPECT and PET in imaging bone metastases. Semin Nucl Med 2009; 39(6):416–30.
13. Cuccurullo V, Cascini GL, Tamburrini O, et al. Bone metastases radiopharmaceuticals: an overview. Curr Radiopharm 2013;6(1):41–7.
14. Talmadge JE, Fidler IJ. AACR centennial series: the biology of cancer metastasis: historical perspective. Cancer Res 2010;70(14):5649–69.
15. Langley RR, Fidler IJ. The seed and soil hypothesis revisited—the role of tumor-stroma interactions in metastasis to different organs. Int J Cancer 2011; 128(11):2527–35.
16. Kang Y, Siegel PM, Shu W, et al. A multigenic program mediating breast cancer metastasis to bone. Cancer Cell 2003;3:537–49.
17. Weilbaecher KN, Guise TA, McCauley LK. Cancer to bone: a fatal attraction. Nat Rev Cancer 2011; 11(6):411–25.
18. Morrissey C, Lai JS, Brown LG, et al. The expression of osteoclastogenesis-associated factors and osteoblast response to osteolytic prostate cancer cells. Prostate 2010;70(4):412–24.
19. Bäuerle T, Semmler W. Imaging response to systemic therapy for bone metastases. Eur Radiol 2009;19:2495–507.
20. Mahajan A, Goh V, Basu S, et al. Bench to bedside molecular functional imaging in translational cancer medicine: to image or to imagine? Clin Radiol 2015;70(10):1060–82.
21. De Ruysscher D, Wanders R, van Baardwijk A, et al. Radical treatment of non-small-cell lung cancer patients with synchronous oligometastases: long-term results of a prospective phase II trial (Nct01282450). J Thorac Oncol 2012;7(10): 1547–55.
22. Bhattacharya IS, Woolf DK, Hughes RJ, et al. Stereotactic body radiotherapy (SBRT) in the management of extracranial oligometastatic (OM) disease. Br J Radiol 2015;88(1048):20140712.
23. Rubini G, Nicoletti A, Rubini D, et al. Radiometabolic treatment of bone-metastasizing cancer: from 186rhenium to 223radium. Cancer Biother Radiopharm 2014;29(1):1–11.
24. Pollen JJ, Witztum KF, Ashburn WL. The flare phenomenon on radionuclide bone scan in metastatic prostate cancer. AJR Am J Roentgenol 1984; 142(4):773–6.
25. Wade AA, Scott JA, Kuter I, et al. Flare response in 18F-fluoride ion PET bone scanning. AJR Am J Roentgenol 2006;186(6):1783–6.
26. Messiou C, Cook G, Reid AH, et al. The CT flare response of metastatic bone disease in prostate cancer. Acta Radiol 2011;52(5):557–61.
27. O'Sullivan GJ, Carty FL, Cronin CG. Imaging of bone metastasis: an update. World J Radiol 2015; 7(8):202–11.
28. Schmidt GP, Reiser MF, Baur-Melnyk A. Whole-body MRI for the staging and follow-up of patients with metastasis. Eur J Radiol 2009;70(3): 393–400.
29. Gnanasegaran G, Cook G, Adamson K, et al. Patterns, variants, artifacts, and pitfalls in conventional radionuclide bone imaging and SPECT/CT. Semin Nucl Med 2009;39:380–95.
30. Apostolova I, Gölcük E, Bohuslavizki KH, et al. Impact of additional SPECT in bone scanning in tumor patients with suspected metastatic bone disease. Ann Nucl Med 2009;23(10):869–75.
31. Ndlovu X, George R, Ellmann A, et al. Should SPECT-CT replace SPECT for the evaluation of equivocal bone scan lesions in patients with underlying malignancies? Nucl Med Commun 2010; 31(7):659–65.
32. Palmedo H, Marx C, Ebert A, et al. Whole-body SPECT/CT for bone scintigraphy: diagnostic value and effect on patient management in oncological patients. Eur J Nucl Med Mol Imaging 2014;41(1): 59–67.
33. Ota N, Kato K, Iwano S. Comparison of (1)(8)F-fluoride PET/CT, (1)(8)F-FDG PET/CT and bone scintigraphy (planar and SPECT) in detection of bone metastases of differentiated thyroid cancer: a pilot study. Br J Radiol 2014;87:20130444.
34. Cheng X, Li Y, Xu Z, et al. Comparison of 18F-FDG PET/CT with bone scintigraphy for detection of bone metastasis: a meta-analysis. Acta Radiol 2011;52(7):779–87.
35. Bombardieri E, Setti L, Kirienko M, et al. Which metabolic imaging, besides bone scan with 99mTc-phosphonates, for detecting and evaluating bone metastases in prostatic cancer patients? An open discussion. Q J Nucl Med Mol Imaging 2015;59(4):381–99.
36. Blau M, Nagler W, Bender MA. Fluorine-18: a new isotope for bone scanning. J Nucl Med 1962;3: 332–4.
37. Vallabhajosula S, Solnes L, Vallabhajosula B. A broad overview of positron emission tomography radiopharmaceuticals and clinical applications: what is new? Semin Nucl Med 2011;41: 246–64.
38. Grant FD, Fahey FH, Packard AB, et al. Skeletal PET with 18F-fluo-ride: applying new technology to an old tracer. J Nucl Med 2008;49:68–78.

39. Petren-Mallmin M, Andreasson I, Liunggren O, et al. Skeletal metastases from breast cancer: uptake of18F-fluoride measured with PET in correlation with CT. Skeletal Radiol 1998;27:72–6.
40. Love C, Din AS, Tomas MB, et al. Radionuclide bone imaging: an illustrative review. Radiographics 2003;23:341–58.
41. Li Y, Schiepers C, Lake R, et al. Clinical utility of 18F-fluoride PET/CT in benign and malignant bone diseases. Bone 2012;50:128–39.
42. Hillner BE, Siegel BA, Hanna L, et al. 18F-fluoride PET used for treatment monitoring of systemic cancer therapy: results from the National Oncologic PET Registry. J Nucl Med 2015;56(2):222–8.
43. Schirrmeister H, Guhlmann A, Elsner K, et al. Sensitivity in detecting osseous lesions depends on anatomic localization: planar bone scintigraphy versus 18F PET. J Nucl Med 1999;40:1623–9.
44. Iagaru A, Young P, Mittra E, et al. Pilot prospective evaluation of 99mTc-MDP scintigraphy, 18F NaF PET/CT, 18F FDG PET/CT and whole-body MRI for detection of skeletal metastases. Clin Nucl Med 2013;38:e290–6.
45. Damle N, Bal C, Bandopadhyaya GP, et al. The role of 18F-fluoride PET-CT in the detection of bone metastases in patients with breast, lung and prostate carcinoma: a comparison with FDG PET/CT and 99mTc-MDP bone scan. Jpn J Radiol 2013;31:262–9.
46. Muzahir S, Jeraj R, Liu G, et al. Differentiation of metastatic vs degenerative joint disease using semi-quantitative analysis with (18)F-NaF PET/CT in castrate resistant prostate cancer patients. Am J Nucl Med Mol Imaging 2015;5(2):162–8.
47. Rohren EM, Etchebehere EC, Araujo JC, et al. Determination of skeletal tumor burden on 18F-fluoride PET/CT. J Nucl Med 2015;56(10):1507–12.
48. Cook G Jr, Parker C, Chua S, et al. 18F-fluoride PET: changes in uptake as a method to assess response in bone metastases from castrate-resistant prostate cancer patients treated with 223Ra-chloride (Alpharadin). EJNMMI Res 2011;1:4.
49. Yu EY, Duan F, Muzi M, et al. Castration-resistant prostate cancer bone metastasis response measured by 18F-fluoride PET after treatment with dasatinib and correlation with progression-free survival: results from American College of Radiology Imaging Network 6687. J Nucl Med 2015;56(3): 354–60.
50. Etchebehere EC, Araujo JC, Fox PS, et al. Prognostic factors in patients treated with 223Ra: the role of skeletal tumor burden on baseline 18F-Fluoride PET/CT in predicting overall survival. J Nucl Med 2015;56(8):1177–84.
51. Doot RK, Muzi M, Peterson LM, et al. Kinetic analysis of 18F-fluoride PET images of breast cancer bone metastases. J Nucl Med 2010;51(4):521–7.
52. Hillner BE, Siegel BA, Hanna L, et al. Impact of 18F-fluoride PET in patients with known prostate cancer: initial results from the National Oncologic PET Registry. J Nucl Med 2014;55(4):574–81.
53. Ozulker T, KucukozUzun A, Ozulker F, et al. Comparison of 18F-FDG-PET/CT with 99mTc-MDP bone scintigraphy for the detection of bone metastases in cancer patients. Nucl Med Commun 2010; 31:597–603.
54. Yang HL, Liu T, Wang XM, et al. Diagnosis of bone metastases: a meta-analysis comparing18FDG PET, CT, MRI and bone scintigraphy. Eur Radiol 2011;21:2604–17.
55. Evangelista L, Panunzio A, Polverosi R, et al. Early bone marrow metastasis detection: the additional value of FDG-PET/CT vs. CT imaging. Biomed Pharmacother 2012;66:448–53.
56. Cook GJ, Houston S, Rubens R, et al. Detection of bone metastases in breast cancer by 18FDG PET: differing metabolic activity in osteoblastic and osteolytic lesions. J Clin Oncol 1998;16:3375–9.
57. Escalona S, Blasco JA, Reza MM, et al. A systematic review of FDG-PET in breast cancer. Med Oncol 2010;27:114–29.
58. Morris MJ, Akhurst T, Osman I, et al. Fluorinated deoxyglucose positron emission tomography imaging in progressive metastatic prostate cancer. Urology 2002;59:913–8.
59. Shreve PD, Grossman HB, Gross MD, et al. Metastatic prostate cancer: initial findings of PET with 2-deoxy-2-[F-18]fluoro-D-glucose. Radiology 1996;199:751–6.
60. Yeh SDJ, Imbriaco M, Larson SM, et al. Detection of bony metastases of androgen-independent prostate cancer by PET-FDG. Nucl Med Biol 1996;23:693–7.
61. Meirelles GS, Schoder H, Ravizzini GC, et al. Prognostic value of baseline [18F] fluorodeoxyglucose positron emission tomography and 99mTc-MDP bone scan in progressing metastatic prostate cancer. Clin Cancer Res 2010;16:6093–9.
62. Zukotynski KA, Kim CK, Gerbaudo VH, et al. (18)F-FDG-PET/CT and (18)F-NaF-PET/CT in men with castrate-resistant prostate cancer. Am J Nucl Med Mol Imaging 2015;5:72–82.
63. Yu EY, Muzi M, Hackenbracht JA, et al. C11-acetate and F-18 FDG PET for men with prostate cancer bone metastases: relative findings and response to therapy. Clin Nucl Med 2011;36:192–8.
64. Vargas HA, Wassberg C, Fox JJ, et al. Bone metastases in castration-resistant prostate cancer: associations between morphologic CT patterns, glycolytic activity, and androgen receptor expression on PET and overall survival. Radiology 2014; 271(1):220–9.
65. Nakai T, Okuyama C, Kubota T, et al. Pitfalls of FDG-PET for the diagnosis of osteoblastic bone

metastases in patients with breast cancer. Eur J Nucl Med Mol Imaging 2005;32:1253–8.
66. Hahn S, Heusner T, Kümmel S, et al. Comparison of FDG-PET/CT and bone scintigraphy for detection of bone metastases in breast cancer. Acta Radiol 2011;52:1009–14.
67. Isasi CR, Moadel RM, Blaufox MD, et al. A meta-analysis of FDG-PET for the evaluation of breast cancer recurrence and metastases. Breast Cancer Res Treat 2005;90:105–12.
68. Rong J, Wang S, Ding Q, et al. Comparison of 18FDG PET-CT and bone scintigraphy for detection of bone metastases in breast cancer patients. A meta-analysis. Surg Oncol 2013;22:86–91.
69. De Giorgi U, Mego M, Rohren EM, et al. 18F-FDG PET/CT findings and circulating tumor cell counts in the monitoring of systemic therapies for bone metastases from breast cancer. J Nucl Med 2010; 51:1213–8.
70. Specht J, Tam S, Kurland B, et al. Serial 2-[18F] fluoro-2-deoxy-d-glucose positron emission tomography (FDG-PET) to monitor treatment of bone-dominant metastatic breast cancer predicts time to progression (TTP). Breast Cancer Res Treat 2007;105:87–94.
71. Piccardo A, Puntoni M, Morbelli S, et al. 18F-FDG PET/CT is a prognostic biomarker in patients affected by bone metastases from breast cancer in comparison with 18F-NaF PET/CT. Nuklearmedizin 2015;54(4):163–72.
72. Qu X, Huang X, Yan W, et al. A meta-analysis of $^{18}$FDG-PET-CT, $^{18}$FDG-PET, MRI and bone scintigraphy for diagnosis of bone metastases in patients with lung cancer. Eur J Radiol 2012;81(5): 1007–15.
73. Gunalp B, Oner AO, Ince S, et al. Evaluation of radiographic and metabolic changes in bone metastases in response to systemic therapy with 18FDG-PET/CT. Radiol Oncol 2015;49(2):115–20.
74. Fuccio C, Castellucci P, Schiavina R, et al. Role of 11C-choline PET/CT in the restaging of prostate cancer patients showing a single lesion on bone scintigraphy. Ann Nucl Med 2010;24:485–92.
75. Fuccio C, Castellucci P, Schiavina R, et al. Role of 11C-choline PET/CT in the re-staging of prostate cancer patients with biochemical relapse and negative results at bone scintigraphy. Eur J Radiol 2012;81:e893–6.
76. Picchio M, Spinapolice E, Fallanca F, et al. [11C] Choline PET/CT detection of bone metastases in patients with PSA progression after primary treatment for prostate cancer: comparison with bone scintigraphy. Eur J Nucl Med Mol Imaging 2012; 39:13–26.
77. Beauregard JM, Williams SG, DeGrado TR, et al. Pilot comparison of 18F-fluorocholine and 18F-fluorodeoxyglucose PET/CT with conventional imaging in prostate cancer. J Med Imaging Radiat Oncol 2010;54:325–32.
78. Beheshti M, Imamovic L, Broinger G, et al. 18F choline PET/CT in the preoperative staging of prostate cancer in patients with intermediate or high risk of extracapsular disease: a prospective study of 130 patients. Radiology 2010;254:925–33.
79. Shen G, Deng H, Hu S, et al. Comparison of choline-PET/CT, MRI, SPECT, and bone scintigraphy in the diagnosis of bone metastases in patients with prostate cancer: a meta-analysis. Skeletal Radiol 2014;43(11):1503–13.
80. Beheshti M, Vali R, Waldenberger P, et al. Detection of bone metastases in patients with prostate cancer by 18F fluorocholine and 18F fluoride PET-CT: a comparative study. Eur J Nucl Med Mol Imaging 2008;35:1766–74.
81. McCarthy M, Siew T, Campbell A, et al. (1)(8)F-Fluoromethylcholine (FCH) PET imaging in patients with castration-resistant prostate cancer: prospective comparison with standard imaging. Eur J Nucl Med Mol Imaging 2011;38:14–22.
82. Oulsen MH, Petersen H, Høilund-Carlsen PF, et al. Spine metastases in prostate cancer: comparison of technetium-99m-MDP whole-body bone scintigraphy, [(18) F]choline positron emission tomography(PET)/computed tomography (CT) and [(18) F]NaF PET/CT. BJU Int 2014;114(6):818–23.
83. Contractor KB, Kenny LM, Stebbing J, et al. Biological basis of [$^{11}$C]choline-positron emission tomography in patients with breast cancer: comparison with [$^{18}$F]fluorothymidine positron emission tomography. Nucl Med Commun 2011; 32(11):997–1004.
84. Withofs N, Grayet B, Tancredi T, et al. $^{18}$F-fluoride PET/CT for assessing bone involvement in prostate and breast cancers. Nucl Med Commun 2011; 32(3):168–76.
85. Colombié M, Campion L, Bailly C, et al. Prognostic value of metabolic parameters and clinical impact of (18)F-fluorocholine PET/CT in biochemical recurrent prostate cancer. Eur J Nucl Med Mol Imaging 2015;42(12):1784–93.
86. Garcia Garzon JR, Bassa P, Soler M, et al. Therapeutic algorithm guided by sequential 11C-choline PET/CT in a patient with metastatic castration-resistant prostate cancer. Clin Nucl Med 2015; 40(7):600–1.
87. Krause B, Souvatzoglou M, Herrmann K, et al. [11C]Choline as pharmacodynamic marker for therapy response assessment in a prostate cancer xenograft model. Eur J Nucl Med Mol Imaging 2010;37:1861–8.
88. Ceci F, Castellucci P, Graziani T, et al. (11)C-Choline PET/CT in castration-resistant prostate cancer patients treated with docetaxel. Eur J Nucl Med Mol Imaging 2015;43(1):84–91.

89. De Giorgi U, Caroli P, Scarpi E, et al. (18)F-Fluorocholine PET/CT for early response assessment in patients with metastatic castration-resistant prostate cancer treated with enzalutamide. Eur J Nucl Med Mol Imaging 2015;42(8):1276–83 [Erratum appears in Eur J Nucl Med Mol Imaging 2015; 42(8):1337–8].
90. Kenny LM, Contractor KB, Hinz R, et al. Reproducibility of [11C]choline-positron emission tomography and effect of trastuzumab. Clin Cancer Res 2010;16:4236–45.
91. Ellmann S, Beck M, Kuwert T, et al. Multimodal imaging of bone metastases: from preclinical to clinical applications. J Orthop Translat 2015. http://dx.doi.org/10.1016/j.jot.2015.07.004.
92. Van Kruchten M, Glaudemans AW, de Vries EF, et al. PET imaging of estrogen receptors as a diagnostic tool for breast cancer patients presenting with a clinical dilemma. J Nucl Med 2012;53:182–90.
93. Lecouvet FE, Talbot JN, Messiou C, et al, EORTC Imaging Group. Monitoring the response of bone metastases to treatment with magnetic resonance imaging and nuclear medicine techniques: a review and position statement by the European Organisation for Research and Treatment of Cancer imaging group. Eur J Cancer 2014;50(15): 2519–31.
94. Balogova S, Talbot JN, Nataf V, et al. 18F-fluorodihydroxyphenylalanine vs other radiopharmaceuticals for imaging neuroendocrine tumours according to their type. Eur J Nucl Med Molimag 2013;40:943–66.
95. Dijkers EC, Oude Munnink TH, Kosterink JG, et al. Biodistribution of 89Zr-trastuzumab and PET imaging of HER2-positive lesions in patients with metastatic breast cancer. Clin Pharmacol Ther 2010; 87(5):586–92.
96. Eder M, Eisenhut M, Babich J, et al. PSMA as a target for radiolabelled small molecules. Eur J Nucl Med Mol Imaging 2013;40:819–23.
97. Afshar-Oromieh A, Zechmann CM, Malcher A, et al. Comparison of PET imaging with a (68)Ga-labelled PSMA ligand and (18)F-choline-based PET/CT for the diagnosis of recurrent prostate cancer. Eur J Nucl Med Mol Imaging 2014;41:11–20.
98. Gemignani ML, Patil S, Seshan VE, et al. Feasibility and predictability of perioperative PET and estrogen receptor ligand in patients with invasive breast cancer. J Nucl Med 2013;54(10):1697–702.
99. Kratochwil C, Giesel FL. Radionuclide therapy of endocrine-related cancer. Radiologe 2014;54(10): 1007–15.
100. Chang AJ, DeSilva R, Jain S, et al. 89zr-radiolabeled trastuzumab imaging in orthotopic and metastatic breast tumors. Pharmaceuticals (Basel) 2012;5(1):79–93.
101. Lopez-Rodriguez V, Gaspar-Carcamo RE, Pedraza-Lopez M, et al. Preparation and preclinical evaluation of (66)Ga-DOTA-E(c(RGDfK))2 as a potential theranostic radiopharmaceutical. Nucl Med Biol 2015;42(2):109–14.
102. Rosenkrantz AB, Friedman K, Chandarana H, et al. Current status of hybrid PET/MRI in oncologic imaging. AJR Am J Roentgenol 2015; 206(1):162–72.
103. Samarin A, Hüllner M, Queiroz MA, et al. 18F-FDG-PET/MR increases diagnostic confidence in detection of bone metastases compared with 18F-FDG-PET/CT. Nucl Med Commun 2015; 36(12):1165–73.
104. Beiderwellen K, Huebner M, Heusch P, et al. Whole-body [$^{18}$F]FDG PET/MRI vs. PET/CT in the assessment of bone lesions in oncological patients: initial results. Eur Radiol 2014;24(8):2023–30.
105. Eiber M, Takei T, Souvatzoglou M, et al. Performance of whole-body integrated 18F-FDG PET/MR in comparison to PET/CT for evaluation of malignant bone lesions. J Nucl Med 2014;55:191–7.
106. Gaertner FC, Furst S, Schwaiger M. PET/MR: a paradigm shift. Cancer Imaging 2013;13:36–52.
107. Azad GK, Taylor B, Rubello D, et al. Molecular and functional imaging of bone metastases in breast and prostate cancers: an overview. Clin Nucl Med 2016;41:e44–50.
108. Catalano OA, Nicolai E, Rosen BR, et al. Comparison of CE-FDG-PET/CT with CE-FDG-PET/MR in the evaluation of osseous metastases in breast cancer patients. Br J Cancer 2015;112(9):1452–60.
109. Wetter A, Lipponer C, Nensa F, et al. Quantitative evaluation of bone metastases from prostate cancer with simultaneous [18F] choline PET/MRI: combined SUV and ADC analysis. Ann Nucl Med 2014; 28:405–10.
110. Piccardo A, Paparo F, Picazzo R, et al. Value of fused 18F-Choline-PET/MRI to evaluate prostate cancer relapse in patients showing biochemical recurrence after EBRT: preliminary results. Biomed Res Int 2014;2014:103718.
111. Freitag MT, Radtke JP, Hadaschik BA, et al. Comparison of hybrid (68)Ga-PSMA PET/MRI and (68) Ga-PSMA PET/CT in the evaluation of lymph node and bone metastases of prostate cancer. Eur J Nucl Med Mol Imaging 2016;43(1):70–83.

# PET-Based Thoracic Radiation Oncology

Charles B. Simone II, MD[a,*], Sina Houshmand, MD[b], Anusha Kalbasi, MD[a], Ali Salavati, MD, MPH[b,c], Abass Alavi, MD[b]

**KEYWORDS**

• PET/CT • Radiation oncology • Lung cancer • Target delineation • Proton therapy
• Adaptive planning • Personalized • Stereotactic body radiation therapy

**KEY POINTS**

- PET plays a critical role in the initial identification and staging of thoracic malignancies, and pretreatment PET scans can help guide treatment decisions.
- PET scans are particularly useful for thoracic malignancies, such as lung cancer, to aid in radiation therapy contouring and target volume delineation and also to monitor treatment response, evaluate for posttreatment recurrence, and assess for prognosis.
- PET is currently being evaluated to assess for radiation-induced toxicities and potentially even to verify radiation dose delivery.

## INTRODUCTION

Thoracic malignancies are among the most common cancers diagnosed both in the United States and worldwide. The most prominent thoracic malignancy, lung cancer, is the second most common cancer diagnosed in the United States, with an estimated 224,390 cases expected to occur in 2016; it is also the leading cause of death from cancer, with 158,080 expected deaths from lung cancer this year alone.[1] Similarly, lung cancer remains the greatest cause of mortality from cancer worldwide, with approximately 1.6 million deaths expected globally each year.[2]

Radiation therapy plays an important role in the treatment of thoracic malignancies. Depending on the primary disease site and tumor stage, radiation therapy can be used as monotherapy for curative intent, as part of multimodality therapy with chemotherapy and/or surgery for curative intent, or for palliation of symptomatic advanced disease.[3,4] In fact, more than half of all patients with thoracic malignancies will receive radiation therapy as part of their multidisciplinary care.[5]

Over the past decade, PET, especially fluorodeoxyglucose (FDG)-PET, has become integrated into multiple aspects of oncology. PET imaging has been particularly transformative in the diagnosis and staging of tumors. PET imaging, and particularly integrated PET/computed tomography (PET/CT), has been especially important in radiation oncology.[6–10] As advanced techniques like intensity-modulated radiation therapy (IMRT) and proton therapy have increased in utilization, PET/CT scans have played increasingly critical roles in the target delineation of tumors for radiation oncologists delivering conformal treatment

Disclosure Statement: The authors have nothing to disclose.
[a] Department of Radiation Oncology, Hospital of the University of Pennsylvania, University of Pennsylvania, 3400 Civic Center Boulevard, TRC 2 West, Philadelphia, PA 19104, USA; [b] Department of Radiology, Hospital of the University of Pennsylvania, University of Pennsylvania, 3400 Spruce Street, Philadelphia, PA 19104, USA; [c] Department of Radiology, University of Minnesota, 420 Delaware Street Southeast, Minneapolis, MN 55455, USA
* Corresponding author. Department of Radiation Oncology, Hospital of the University of Pennsylvania, Perelman Center for Advanced Medicine, Perelman School of Medicine, University of Pennsylvania, 3400 Civic Center Boulevard, TRC 2 West, Philadelphia, PA 19104.
*E-mail address:* charles.simone@uphs.upenn.edu

PET Clin 11 (2016) 319–332
http://dx.doi.org/10.1016/j.cpet.2016.03.001

techniques, especially when treating thoracic malignancies. This article details the current uses of PET/CT in thoracic radiation oncology (**Box 1**) with a focus on lung cancer and describes future roles that PET is increasingly expected to play for lung cancer and other tumors of the thorax.

## PET FOR DIAGNOSIS AND STAGING

PET imaging has an already well-established role in the initial diagnosis and staging of thoracic malignancies. The data and rationale for its use have previously been reported in detail and are beyond the scope of this report. Current National Comprehensive Cancer Network (http://www.nccn.org) guidelines now recommend PET imaging across thoracic malignancies for initial diagnosis or staging. Their specific recommendations are to obtain a PET scan for all patients with esophageal cancer without evidence of distant metastatic disease; all patients with mesothelioma without clinical stage IV disease and sarcomatoid histology; all patients with non–small cell lung cancer (NSCLC), although patients with extensive extrathoracic disease may forgo PET; all patients with small cell lung cancer suspected of having limited-stage disease (clinical stage I–III); optional in patients with malignant thymomas and thymic carcinomas; considered in patients with well-differentiated thyroid cancers; and recommended for all patients with anaplastic thyroid cancer. PET has also demonstrated great value in the identification of primary tumors in patients with carcinoma of unknown primary.[11]

> **Box 1**
> **Uses of fluorodeoxyglucose PET in thoracic radiation oncology**
>
> *Established roles*
> - Identify tumor to establish the initial cancer diagnosis
> - Evaluate the extent of disease and clinical stage
> - Assess prognosis
> - Aid in radiation therapy target volume delineation
> - Monitor treatment response
> - Evaluate for and detect tumor recurrence following treatment
>
> *Emerging roles*
> - Better assess prognosis
> - Evaluate for radiation-induced toxicities
> - Verify radiation dose delivery

The authors' group previously demonstrated the importance of PET staging for limited-stage small cell lung cancer. Among 54 consecutive patients with limited-stage disease treated with concurrent chemoradiation, patients who underwent PET staging had improved disease control and better overall survival than patients staged solely based on CT and MR imaging, likely because of improved staging accuracy and better identification of intrathoracic disease in patients who underwent PET staging.[12] Similarly, PET can help identify extensive-stage small cell lung cancer. In a systematic review and meta-analysis assessing the accuracy of PET or PET/CT in staging small cell lung cancer, the sensitivity and specificity for detecting extensive-stage disease were 97.5% and 98.2%, respectively.[13]

PET imaging has an even more well-established and long-seeded role in staging NSCLC (**Fig. 1**). Most recently, PET/CT imaging has been investigated as a potential replacement for pathologic nodal staging. In a multicenter prospective study of 200 patients, the negative predictive value of PET/CT to accurately identify nodal metastases was 91%.[14] A meta-analysis assessing the value of PET and CT for stage T1-2N0 NSCLC demonstrated a negative predictive value for mediastinal metastases of 94% with PET/CT in T1 disease and 89% in T2 disease, suggesting limited benefit from performing invasive staging procedures beyond what can be identified based solely on imaging with PET/CT.[15]

PET imaging may also be contributing to an increase in early stage NSCLC. Currently, approximately 15% of patients with NSCLC have early stage localized diseased at the time of diagnosis.[16] That proportion is expected to continue to increase with the increasing life expectancy in elderly patients, increased use of diagnostic CT scans, initiation of low-dose CT lung cancer screening programs following the publication of the National Lung Screening Trial,[17] and newer investigations of circulating tumor products[18] and other means to achieve early detection of lung cancer. Furthermore, PET may be an optimal modality for lung cancer screening. In a recent meta-analysis assessing the role of PET for lung cancer screening, PET demonstrated a high sensitivity (83%) and specificity (91%) as a selective screening modality.[19] Although further investigation is needed into the role of PET/CT as a screening test for lung cancer, this modality may lead to the detect of a higher proportion of early stage lung cancers that have higher cure rates with surgery or radiation therapy or even the detection of CT-occult bronchogenic NSCLCs

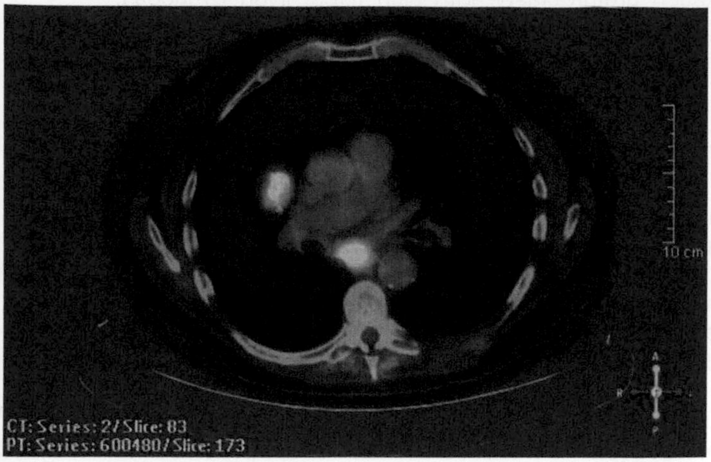


**Fig. 1.** PET for initial lung cancer staging. PET/CT scan revealing an FDG-avid mass in the paramediastinal right middle lobe measuring 30 × 27 mm with maximum standardized uptake value (SUVmax) of 8.8 suspicious for primary bronchogenic malignancy and 30 × 23 mm avid subcarinal lymph node with SUVmax of 11.1. The PET/CT scan was used to guide endobronchial biopsies, which subsequently revealed adenocarcinoma in the subcarinal lymph node.

that may be amenable to cures with less invasive modalities like photodynamic therapy.[20,21]

## THORACIC RADIATION THERAPY TREATMENT TECHNIQUES

In patients with early stage or locally advanced lung cancer, the standard of care had previously been to treat the primary tumor and regional nodes. Such nodal irradiation included the intentional targeting of all lymph nodes known pathologically or thought based on imaging to be involved with disease as well as the prophylactic targeting of regional lymph nodes not known or thought to be involved but that are at risk of harboring subclinical metastatic disease. This practice, termed *elective nodal irradiation*, resulted in significant radiation dose to critical centrally located normal structures, including the esophagus, heart, great vessels, trachea, and proximal bronchial tree; it also led to higher radiation doses to the lung. Therefore, morbidity was high and the total dose that could be delivered to the tumor was limited by normal tissue irradiation tolerances.

In an attempt to improve tumor control, several groups investigated treating to higher total or biological equivalent radiation doses to tumor. However, when treating to these higher doses, so as not to prohibitively increase treatment toxicities, elective nodal irradiation was abandoned. Specifically, in early stage NSCLC, investigators used hypofractionation (daily fraction sizes greater than the standard of 1.8–2.0 Gy) to increase the biological equivalent dose of radiotherapy without prophylactic irradiation to nodal regions and found superior rates of local control and overall survival compared with conventionally fractionated radiotherapy.[22,23] These findings largely led to the widespread utilization of stereotactic body radiation therapy (SBRT), also termed *stereotactic ablative radiotherapy*, for medically inoperative patients[24] with stage I NSCLC; SBRT is now increasingly being considered for patients with stage I NSCLC who are medically operable[25,26] and patients with stage I small cell lung cancer.[27] Similarly, for patients with locally advanced NSCLC, both nonrandomized[28] and prospective randomized[29] data suggest that the omission of elective nodal irradiation is associated with few nodal failures and that targeting only known disease may be an effective strategy to reduce radiation-induced treatment toxicities or allow for radiation dose escalation to gross disease.

The abandonment of thoracic elective nodal irradiation led to an increasing utilization of conformal radiation therapy techniques, such as IMRT and proton therapy, modalities for which precise target delineation is necessary and the use of PET imaging to more accurately identify disease has becoming more critically important in thoracic radiation oncology. Although uninvolved nodal regions still receive significant incidental prophylactic irradiation with less conformal irradiation techniques like 3-dimensional (3D) conformal radiotherapy, the dose of incidental radiation is significantly less with more conformal thoracic radiation therapy techniques like IMRT and proton therapy. With IMRT, the radiation dose can conform more precisely to the 3D shape of the tumor by modulating the intensity of the radiation beam in multiple small volumes.[30] Proton therapy further allows for improved dose localization for thoracic tumors.[31–33] With proton therapy, energy is deposited at a specific depth known as the Bragg peak, such that after the Bragg peak, there is a rapid energy falloff. This falloff allows normal tissues beyond or more distal to the target depth to receive little or no radiation dose.[34] Therefore, proton therapy may be an ideal radiotherapy modality for thoracic tumors to reduce normal tissue toxicity.[35]

## PET/COMPUTED TOMOGRAPHY FOR RADIATION THERAPY TARGET DELINEATION

Despite these benefits in protecting adjacent normal tissues with IMRT and proton therapy, these modalities may be more subject to geographic misses and local or regional failures if the tumor is not adequately contoured.[36] Therefore, the use of additional information beyond a traditional CT simulation to contour the tumor, most notably data from a PET/CT scan and pathologic staging of the mediastinum, has become much more critically important to the thoracic radiation oncologist. This point also applies for advances in radiation oncology treatment delivery imaging,[37,38] which is widely used in patients treated for lung and other thoracic cancers and further serves to make radiotherapy treatments more conformal and reduce treatment margins, but further underscores the need to have accurate target delineation based on advanced imaging modalities like PET. Nearly all radiation oncologists use advanced imaging to inform their target volume delineation, and FDG-PET is the most commonly used advanced imaging modality. In fact, its use is highest among radiation oncologists treating thoracic malignancies, in which 89% of providers use PET.[39]

The easiest and perhaps most accurate use of PET to inform treatment planning and target delineation is through the use of a PET/CT simulation. In order to devise a radiotherapy treatment plan, patients undergo a simulation in which they are immobilized in the treatment position, and then imaging with CT is acquired. During simulation, an isocenter is placed, which is a 3D reference point on the planning CT that is used to align patients for daily treatments. A diagnostic PET scan can be registered and fused to the CT simulation to help inform target delineation. When this occurs, it is important that patients undergo the diagnostic PET scan in the radiotherapy treatment position as closely as possible. Many centers are increasingly having the ability to plan their patients based on a dedicated PET/CT simulator, and the PET scan can be performed in conjunction with a diagnostic PET scan or as a limited PET examination of the thorax. In such cases, patients undergo a CT simulation just before the PET/CT scan to allow for an isocenter to be identified and custom immobilization to be created.[40]

A rapidly growing body of clinical literature has supported PET imaging to improve radiation therapy target volume delineation (**Fig. 2**). Among its many benefits, PET can lead to more accurate tumor volume delineation while reducing normal tissue coverage in the lung.[41,42] PET can also increase the concordance index of identifying target volume and lead to less variation in lung cancer contouring and uncertainties at the tumor/mediastinal interface.[43] PET can also help define the background intensity of the lung, which can further aid in tumor delineation.[44]

Although these benefits in delineation are somewhat intuitive for locally advanced lung cancer that can present with large or invasive masses in which it can be difficult to differentiate chest wall or mediastinum from tumor, the benefits for target delineation also extend to patients with stage I NSCLC treated with SBRT. Coregistration of 4-dimensional (4D) PET data to 4DCT data can help to inform target volume delineation, particularly for centrally located stage I NSCLC, and lead to less interobserver variability and reduce the risk of geographic misses with SBRT.[45] Radiation oncologists treating early stage lung cancer should, however, be cautious of strictly using PET-derived tumor volumes for SBRT; they should take into account intrafractional tumor motion by using 4DPET or 4DCT information.[46,47] A recent consensus report by the International Atomic Energy Agency on using PET/CT for target volume delineation when delivering curative-intent radiation therapy for NSCLC helps to inform this topic further.[48]

In addition to assisting with target volume delineation, PET imaging may allow for safe implementation of adaptive planning for thoracic tumors. Adaptive planning is the modification of a radiation therapy treatment plan during the course of treatment to account for interfractional tumor or normal tissue anatomic changes that, if not accounted for, can lead to overtreatment of normal tissues or undertreatment of tumor.[49] Investigators at Shandong Cancer Hospital in China initiated a clinical protocol in which patients with stage III NSCLC underwent PET/CT imaging before the start of radiotherapy and again after 40 Gy of radiotherapy was delivered.[50] Patients then received a boost of radiation for an additional 19.6 to 39.2 Gy to the shrunken target volume seen at the time of repeat PET/CT. Among 87 consecutive patients treated in this manner, the investigators found a mean reduction in tumor volume of 38% at the time of repeat PET/CT, which allowed for a smaller target volume to be irradiated during the boost radiotherapy delivery and, as a result, the ability to both dose escalate and protect normal adjacent tissues.[51] This concept of PET-based adaptive planning during the course of treatment of locally

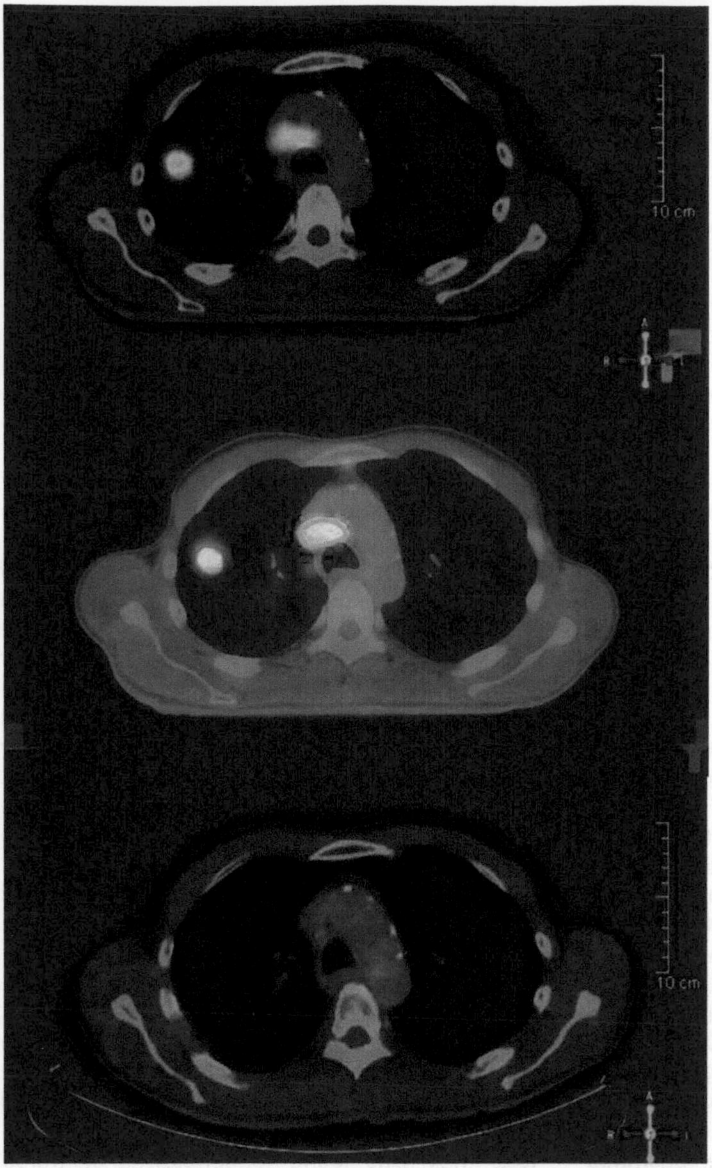


**Fig. 2.** PET to monitor response to treatment. (*Top*) Pretreatment PET/CT scan demonstrating an intensively avid 2.5-cm irregular right upper lobe mass (maximum standardized uptake value [SUVmax] 14.2) and avid right paratracheal node (SUV 15.0) concerning for malignancy and metastasis, respectively. Subsequent biopsy confirmed adenocarcinoma of lung origin. (*Middle*) Radiation therapy treatment planning PET/CT blended between the PET images and the CT images. The primary tumor is contoured in red, whereas the right paratracheal node is contoured in green. (*Bottom*) Posttreatment PET/CT scan obtained 3 months after the completion of concurrent chemoradiation with cisplatin, etoposide, and proton therapy. The patient was found to have a metabolic complete response to therapy.

advanced NSCLC is currently the subject of investigation in the cooperative group setting (Radiation Therapy Oncology Group [RTOG] 1106).

Given that the inadequate sterilization of all disease at the primary tumor site is a leading cause of recurrence in locally advanced NSCLC, investigators at Maastricht University Medical Center in the Netherlands similarly performed a randomized phase II dose escalation trial in which patients were selected to have their PET-avid primary disease boosted to a dose higher than their involved lymph nodes. Such PET-based planning allowed for successful dose escalation while maintaining limited radiation doses to normal structures.[52]

PET scans can also more precisely target nodal metastasis and avoid potentially futile irradiation. The authors' group[53] and others[54] have previously shown that performing a treatment planning PET/CT simulation or diagnostic PET/CT used for planning can identify disease not known to exist before the simulation scan, which can allow for potentially new areas of nodal metastasis to be adequately targeted that otherwise would be not intentionally be targeted and, thus, inadequately treated. Therefore, PET/CT can be used to change management and regions being target for radiotherapy.[55] Similarly, if new distant metastatic disease is identified at the time of PET/CT simulation or a diagnostic PET/CT scan obtained around the time of CT simulation in patients who are thought to have locally advanced NSCLC, definitively irradiation that may have proven futile can be avoided in lieu of initiating patients on systemic therapy alone.[56]

## PRETREATMENT PET FOR PROGNOSIS AND TO PREDICT TREATMENT RESPONSE

A rapidly growing body of literature has demonstrated that a pretreatment PET scan is prognostic and can predict for recurrences and survival following SBRT. Although the local control rate following SBRT is excellent, local failures as well as posttreatment nodal and distant metastases do occur. An early report of 50 patients treated with SBRT for stage I NSCLC failed to identify PET measures associated with clinical outcomes.[57] Subsequent reports have shown positive correlations between PET and clinical outcomes, including a report of 95 patients treated with SBRT for peripheral stage I NSCLC showing that the maximum standardized uptake value (SUVmax) as a continuous variable was significantly correlated with progression-free survival ($P = .008$) and suggested utility in predicting local control ($P = .057$).[58]

Among 163 patients with 180 stage I NSCLC lesions treated definitively with conventionally fractionated radiotherapy or SBRT, a pretreatment SUVmax of 7 or less correlated with improved progression-free survival (67% vs 51%, $P = .0096$) and lower risk of regional or distant metastases.[59] These finding may be useful in designing future clinical trials that could include adjuvant therapy for patients with high pretreatment SUVmax values who are at higher risk of recurrence.

Japanese investigators similarly demonstrated that SUVmax correlated with disease-free survival ($P<.01$) and overall survival ($P = .04$) on multivariate analysis among 152 patients with stage I NSCLC treated with SBRT.[60] In a pulled analysis of 1526 patients from 12 studies that included mostly patients with early stage NSCLC, the combined univariate hazard ratio (HR) for overall survival of SUVmax was 1.43 (95% confidence interval [CI], 1.22–1.66). When controlling for age, stage, tumor size, and resection status, the multivariate HR for SUVmax was 1.58 (95% CI, 1.27–1.96).[61]

Preradiotherapy PET information has similarly been demonstrated to be prognostic for survival and risk of recurrence among patients with locally advanced NSCLC in most but not all[62] studies. An early such report among 105 patients treated with radiotherapy, including approximately half with locally advanced NSCLC, revealed that pretreatment PET whole-body total lesion glycolysis (TLG), whole-body metabolic tumor volume (MTV), lung TLG, lung MTV, and SUVmax were all significant prognostic factors for progression-free survival on univariate analysis (all $P<.01$), with TLG maintaining significance on multivariate analysis (HR 2.92; 95% CI 1.62, 5.26; $P<.01$).[63]

Among 28 patients with stage III NSCLC treated with concurrent chemoradiation, MTV less than 60 mL was associated with improved progression-free survival (median 14.3 months vs 9.7 months, $P = .039$), suggesting a potential to initiate treatment intensification strategies for patients with high-risk lesions with high MTV.[64] Similarly, high uptake regions on PET based on SUVmax may serve as a biological target volume for escalated radiation dose.[65] Among 91 mixed early stage and locally advanced patients, higher pretreatment SUVmax was associated with higher rates of local extension ($P = .016$), distant metastases ($P = .046$), and nodal metastasis ($P = .002$).[66]

The most notable trial assessing pretreatment PET metrics for locally advanced NSCLC was ACRIN 6668/RTOG 0235, a prospective study in which patients underwent PET scans before and after concurrent chemoradiation. Among 214 analyzable patients, multivariable analysis incorporating pretreatment clinical and imaging data revealed that MTV was an independent predictor of overall survival ($P<.001$) and locoregional failure ($P<.001$) at 6 months (HR = 1.05 per 10-cm$^3$ increase, 95% CI 1.02–1.07, $P<.001$) but not at 12 months or later time points.[67] Similarly, among 161 patients with locally advanced NSCLC treated with neoadjuvant concurrent chemoradiation followed by surgical resection, a higher pretreatment total MTV was found to correlate with worse disease-free survival (HR 1.82; $P = .036$) and overall survival (HR 2.97; $P = .012$) on multivariable analysis.[68]

PET has also been demonstrated to be valuable in identifying occult mediastinal lymph node involvement. Among 201 patients who underwent pretreatment PET imaging, increased primary tumor SUV predicted for increased risk of mediastinal nodal metastasis.[69]

In addition to volumetric measures to assess tumor on PET like MTV and TLG, which may be more prognostic than semiquantitative measures like SUVmax and SUVmean, alternative tracers for PET imaging are being investigated and may also be prognostic. PET/CT with 3'-deoxy-3'-(18)F-fluorothymidine may be a more sensitive tracer of early treatment response to chemoradiation than

(18)F-FDG PET/CT for lung cancer and may hold future promise in assessing prognosis.[70]

## POSTTREATMENT PET FOR PROGNOSIS AND TO PREDICT TREATMENT RESPONSE

Posttreatment PET imaging has also been widely used in thoracic oncology to monitor response to treatment, assess prognosis, and detect recurrences. Successive small studies have suggested that PET information obtained after SBRT can monitor treatment response, predict outcomes, identify local failures,[71] and detect regional progression even when conventional CT scans might not.[72] PET scans can also differentiate local failures from fibrosis (**Fig. 3**). In fact, in a 59-patient study,[73] an SUVmax greater than 4.5 after SBRT was associated with a high predictive value for local recurrence (sensitivity and specificity both 100%).

A larger study of 128 patients with stage I or recurrent/secondary lung lesions treated with SBRT similarly demonstrated that PET can distinguish SBRT-induced consolidation from local failure and that an SUVmax cutoff of 5.0 after SBRT has a 100% sensitivity, 91% sensitivity, 50% positive predictive value, and 100% negative predictive value for predicting local recurrence.[74] Another study of 132 patients with stage I NSCLC treated with SBRT demonstrated that an SUVmax of 5.0 or greater obtained 12 weeks after SBRT was associated with an increased risk of local failure (20.0% vs 2.3%, $P = .019$).[75]

PET may similarly have a role in assessing response and prognosis following SBRT for patients with oligometastatic lung cancer. Thoracic radiation therapy is increasingly playing a role in the treatment of patients with oligometastatic disease or oligoprogression, and its use may be associated with an improvement in survival in well-selected patients.[76,77] Most reported factors predicting for clinical outcomes in oligometastatic patients are related to timing of metastasis development,[78] location of extrathoracic metastases, number of metastases,[79] or presence of nodal metastases.[80] Less is known about how metabolic data correlate with prognosis in this patient population. However, in a study of 31 patients enrolled on a prospective dose escalation trial in which SBRT was delivered to all sites of known metastatic disease, patients underwent pretreatment and posttreatment PET scans. PET response to SBRT allowed for the characterization of treatment response in tumors nonmeasurable by CT.[81] This finding is in keeping with PET response being correlated with overall survival after chemotherapy in metastatic NSCLC.[82] More investigation is needed to assess the role of posttreatment PET for oligometastatic or oligoprogressive lung cancer.

The bulk of existing literature on PET imaging obtained after radiotherapy start has been for locally advanced NSCLC. PET imaging during the course of radiation therapy has been shown in smaller single-institution studies[83] and prospective analyses[84] to correlate with treatment response and overall survival and that a decrease in MTV or SUV during treatment correlates with long-term survival. Therefore, the use of PET imaging during treatment is currently being investigated in RTOG 1106.

However, most studies to date have obtained PET scans 1 to 3 months after radiotherapy completion (see **Fig. 2**). In a small randomized trial

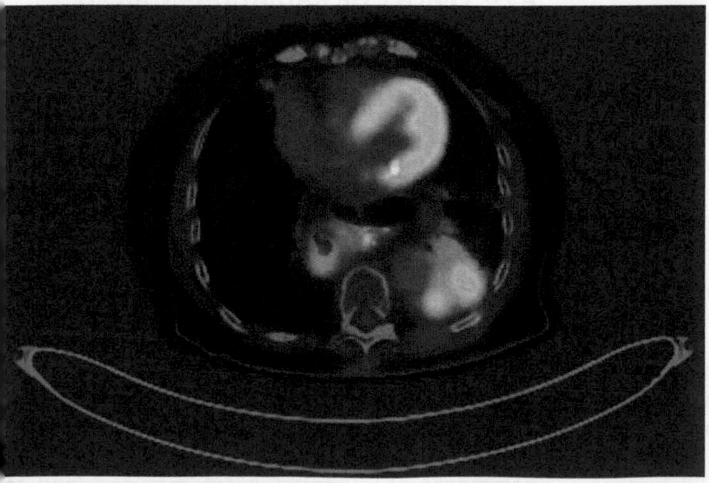

**Fig. 3.** PET to differentiate radiation fibrosis from recurrence. Axial slice of a PET/CT scan of a patient who had stereotactic body radiotherapy 14 months earlier for a cT2aN0M0 4.2-cm left lower lobe lung cancer that was centered just posterolateral to the descending aorta. Images reveal postradiation changes within the left lower lobe, with increased atelectasis of the left lower lobe but a focal area of increased FDG uptake with SUVmax 7.3 concerning for recurrence. Recurrence could not be assessed on an early CT chest because of the radiation changes in the region. Based on the uptake on the PET/CT scan, the patient was referred for biopsy, where recurrent malignancy was identified histologically.

of 2 interventions for patients with locally advanced NSCLC, PET/CT was able to distinguish responders from nonresponders early after chemoradiation completion.[85] Posttreatment PET scans may allow for an early assessment of tumor control probability that could be used to guide additional radiation dose or used to initiate early salvage therapies.[86] PET as surveillance for NSCLC was further found to correlate with response in 26 patients treated with chemoradiation.[87]

In a study of 49 patients with stage III NSCLC who underwent PET scans before and up to 3.5 months after chemoradiation, postradiotherapy SUVmax correlated with overall survival (HR 1.27, *P*<.0001 for the primary tumor; HR 1.32, *P* = .004 for lymph nodes) and disease-free survival (HR 1.16, *P* = .004 for the primary tumor; HR 1.32, *P* = .001 for lymph nodes). Furthermore, that study found that the greater the decrease in SUVmax, the longer the overall survival (HR 0.06, *P* = .002), disease-free survival (HR 0.03, *P* = .001), local-regional control (HR 0.04, *P* = .002), and distant metastasis-free survival (HR 0.07, *P* = .028).[88]

In other analyses in which patients with lung cancer underwent both preradiotherapy and post-radiotherapy PET scans, posttreatment SUV has been shown to predict for local recurrence-free survival; both pretreatment and posttreatment SUV have been shown to predict for distant metastasis-free survival, progression-free survival, and overall survival in a study of 84 patients with stage III NSCLC.[89] In a meta-analysis of 13 studies on the use of PET in patients with NSCLC treated with radiotherapy, both pretreatment (HR 1.05; 95% CI, 1.02–1.08) and posttreatment (HR 1.3; 95% CI, 1.15–1.512) SUVmax were found to predict for overall survival. Similarly, pretreatment (HR 1.26; 95% CI, 1.05–1.52) and posttreatment (HR 2.01; 95% CI, 1.16–3.46) SUVmax predicted for local control.[90] In a study of 44 patients with NSCLC, most of whom had locally advanced disease, both qualitative visual assessments and semiquantitative measurements of PET demonstrated predictive classification for survival.[91]

As with pretreatment PET assessments, the largest prospective trial reporting on posttreatment PET metrics for locally advanced NSCLC was ACRIN 6668/RTOG 0235. In that study, higher posttreatment SUVpeak and SUVmax were associated with worse survival for patients with stage III NSCLC. In fact, of the 173 patients with analyzable posttreatment PET scans, posttreatment SUVpeak was associated with survival in a continuous variable model (HR 1.087, *P* = .020). Furthermore, in an exploratory analysis, SUVpeak cutoffs of 5.0 (*P* = .041) and 7.0 (*P*<.001) both correlated with overall survival, as did cutoffs for SUVmax.[92,93] In another large study of 119 patients with stage III NSCLC treated with definitive chemoradiation, PET/CT performed 2 to 4 weeks after radiotherapy completion correlated with local control and overall survival.[94]

PET may also allow for early detection of recurrence following radiation therapy for locally advanced NSCLC.[95] In the Navelbine and Radiotherapy in Locally Advanced Lung Cancer (NARLAL) prospective trial, 92 patients with stage IIB to IIIB NSCLC treated with concurrent chemoradiation were followed with or without PET/CT imaging 9 months after the start of radiotherapy. The addition of PET imaging for surveillance was found to increase the likelihood of early detection of disease progression.[96]

In additional to its established roles in detection and staging disease and aiding in radiation oncology target delineation for small cell lung cancer, PET may have a role in prognosis or monitoring response to radiotherapy for small cell lung cancer. In a retrospective study of 50 patients with limited-stage small cell lung cancer treated with chemoradiation, although pretreatment SUV was not significantly associated with locoregional control or overall survival, patients with residual SUVmax less than the median of 5.5 had numerically higher rates of 3-year locoregional control (65% vs 36%) and overall survival (69% vs 34%).[97] A second analysis of 41 patients with limited-stage small cell lung cancer treated with chemoradiation demonstrated that differences between pretreatment and posttreatment SUV correlated with relapse-free survival (HR 0.3, *P* = .004) and overall survival (HR 0.2, *P* = .014).[98]

## ASSESSMENT OF RADIATION-INDUCED TOXICITY

PET imaging may also aid in the assessment and prediction of radiation-related complications. The adverse effects on normal tissues of radiation therapy most often manifest as inflammatory changes. Such inflammatory changes induced by radiation therapy have been shown to be FDG avid and, thus, detectable by FDG-PET/CT.[99] By reducing the doses to normal structures, proton therapy may allow for less radiation-induced inflammation and toxicity of adjacent organs at risk compared with other radiotherapy modalities. The authors' group has recently reported in detail in this journal on the use of PET to predict radiation-induced toxicities.[100]

Radiation-induced lung inflammation is a commonly encountered event that can lead to acute radiation pneumonitis, a potentially fatal complication of therapy occurring within weeks to 6 months of finishing radiation therapy, and late pulmonary fibrosis, which can limit patients' quality of life. Radiation pneumonitis is a clinical diagnosis; this diagnosis is often challenging because of other confounding medical factors like underlying malignancy, pulmonary edema, thromboembolic disease, and infection. PET may help aid in this diagnosis and also serves as a predictive tool to identify patients at highest risk of developing radiation pneumonitis.[101,102]

The authors' group has recently demonstrated that quantification of the global lung parenchymal FDG uptake after radiotherapy for patients with locally advanced NSCLC can be achieved by subtracting the tumor uptake from the total lung FDG uptake via volume-based quantitative FDG-PET/CT parameters. In doing so, significant increases in global lung uptake parameters can be identified in the irradiated lung, suggesting that volumetric PET parameters may be able to serve as potential biomarkers for assessing lung inflammation after radiotherapy.[103]

Cardiac toxicity is increasingly being recognized as a complication from thoracic radiation therapy, particularly when treating centrally located tumors or mediastinal lymph nodes, as is done for locally advanced NSCLC.[104] A wide spectrum of radiation-induced cardiovascular diseases has been reported, including pericarditis, cardiomyopathy, coronary artery disease, valvular disease, conduction system abnormalities, autonomic dysfunction, and vascular changes.[105] Myocardial effects from thoracic radiation therapy may be identified on PET.[106–108] PET may also serve as a surrogate for radiation-induced vascular inflammation and atherosclerosis following thoracic irradiation.[109]

Radiation esophagitis is another commonly encountered acute toxicity from thoracic radiation therapy. Late esophageal toxicities occurring in the months to years after radiation therapy, including ulceration, fistula, and stricture, are less common but can significantly limit quality of life. PET may similarly aid in the detection of radiation-induced esophageal toxicity, as PET uptake has been correlated with radiation esophagitis.[110,111]

## FUTURE DIRECTIONS AND SUMMARY

FDG-PET has become an indispensable component of diagnosing and staging thoracic tumors. PET is having an increasing role in radiation oncology target volume delineation during treatment planning. This role of PET has become more critical with the advent of involved field irradiation and the increasing use of IMRT and proton therapy to treat thoracic tumors. A rapidly growing body of literature for both early stage and locally advanced NSCLC has supported the use of pretreatment PET scans to assess for prognosis and of posttreatment PET scans to assess for prognosis and to monitor treatment response and evaluate for recurrences. Most of these analyses have focused on semiquantitative measures like SUVmax. Emerging evidence suggests that volumetric PET parameters like MTV and TLG may be more optimal measures for assessing outcomes and prognosis in NSCLC. Additional investigations, including already-underway secondary analyses of ACRIN 6668/RTOG 0235 assessing MTV and TLG, are needed to determine if volumetric parameters should supersede SUVmax. With the increasing use of SBRT for early stage NSCLC and now stage I small cell lung cancer, and the difficulties in differentiating radiation-induced fibrosis from residual or recurrent disease after SBRT, PET will play a greater role in the surveillance of patients with early stage lung cancer in the future, as it has for locally advanced NSCLC. Furthermore, emerging data suggest that PET may help to diagnosis complications or predict who will develop radiation-induced toxicities following thoracic radiation therapy. With the rapid proliferation of proton therapy centers in the United States and abroad, increasing interest in investigating the use of PET/CT for treatment verification[112] after proton delivery is expected.

## REFERENCES


1. Siegel RL, Miller KD, Jemal A. Cancer statistics, 2016. CA Cancer J Clin 2016;66(1):7–30.
2. Torre LA, Bray F, Siegel RL, et al. Global cancer statistics, 2012. CA Cancer J Clin 2015;65(2):87–108.
3. Simone CB 2nd, Jones JA. Palliative care for patients with locally advanced and metastatic non-small cell lung cancer. Ann Palliat Med 2013;2(4):178–88.
4. Jones JA, Simone CB 2nd. Palliative radiotherapy for advanced malignancies in a changing oncologic landscape: guiding principles and practice implementation. Ann Palliat Med 2014;3(3):192–202.
5. Hayman JA, Abrahamse PH, Lakhani I, et al. The use of palliative radiotherapy among patients with metastatic non-small cell lung cancer. Int J Radiat Oncol Biol Phys 2007;69:1001–7.
6. Speirs CK, Grigsby PW, Huang J, et al. PET-based radiation therapy planning. PET Clin 2015;10(1):27–44.

7. Truong MT, Kovalchuk N. Radiotherapy planning. PET Clin 2015;10(2):279–96.
8. De Ruysscher D, Nestle U, Jeraj R, et al. PET scans in radiotherapy planning of lung cancer. Lung Cancer 2012;75(2):141–5.
9. Mac Manus MP, Hicks RJ. The role of positron emission tomography/computed tomography in radiation therapy planning for patients with lung cancer. Semin Nucl Med 2012;42(5):308–19.
10. Scripes PG, Yaparpalvi R. Technical aspects of positron emission tomography/computed tomography in radiotherapy treatment planning. Semin Nucl Med 2012;42(5):283–8.
11. Han A, Xue J, Hu M, et al. Clinical value of 18F-FDG PET-CT in detecting primary tumor for patients with carcinoma of unknown primary. Cancer Epidemiol 2012;36(5):470–5.
12. Xanthopoulos EP, Corradetti MN, Mitra N, et al. Impact of PET staging in limited-stage small-cell lung cancer. J Thorac Oncol 2013;8(7):899–905.
13. Lu YY, Chen JH, Liang JA, et al. 18F-FDG PET or PET/CT for detecting extensive disease in small-cell lung cancer: a systematic review and meta-analysis. Nucl Med Commun 2014;35(7):697–703.
14. Li X, Zhang H, Xing L, et al. Mediastinal lymph nodes staging by 18F-FDG PET/CT for early stage non-small cell lung cancer: a multicenter study. Radiother Oncol 2012;102(2):246–50.
15. Wang J, Welch K, Wang L, et al. Negative predictive value of positron emission tomography and computed tomography for stage T1-2N0 non-small-cell lung cancer: a meta-analysis. Clin Lung Cancer 2012;13(2):81–9.
16. Groome PA, Bolejack V, Crowley JJ, et al, IASLC International Staging Committee, Cancer Research and Biostatistics, Observers to the Committee, Participating Institutions. The IASLC Lung Cancer Staging Project: validation of the proposals for revision of the T, N, and M descriptors and consequent stage groupings in the forthcoming (seventh) edition of the TNM classification of malignant tumours. J Thorac Oncol 2007;2(8):694–705.
17. National Lung Screening Trial Research Team, Aberle DR, Adams AM, et al. Reduced lung-cancer mortality with low-dose computed tomographic screening. N Engl J Med 2011;365(5):395–409.
18. Dorsey JF, Kao GD, MacArthur KM, et al. Tracking viable circulating tumor cells (CTCs) in the peripheral blood of non-small cell lung cancer (NSCLC) patients undergoing definitive radiation therapy: pilot study results. Cancer 2015;121(1):139–49.
19. Chien CR, Liang JA, Chen JH, et al. [(18)F]Fluorodeoxyglucose-positron emission tomography screening for lung cancer: a systematic review and meta-analysis. Cancer Imaging 2013;13(4):458–65.
20. Simone CB 2nd, Friedberg JS, Glatstein E, et al. Photodynamic therapy for the treatment of non-small cell lung cancer. J Thorac Dis 2012;4(1):63–75.
21. Simone CB 2nd, Cengel KA. Photodynamic therapy for lung cancer and malignant pleural mesothelioma. Semin Oncol 2014;41(6):820–30.
22. Slotman BJ, Antonisse IE, Njo KH. Limited field irradiation in early stage (T1-2N0) non-small cell lung cancer. Radiother Oncol 1996;41(1):41–4.
23. Bogart JA, Hodgson L, Seagren SL, et al. Phase I study of accelerated conformal radiotherapy for stage I non-small-cell lung cancer in patients with pulmonary dysfunction: CALGB 39904. J Clin Oncol 2010;28(2):202–6.
24. Simone CB 2nd, Wildt B, Haas AR, et al. Stereotactic body radiation therapy for lung cancer. Chest 2013;143(6):1784–90.
25. Chang JY, Senan S, Paul MA, et al. Stereotactic ablative radiotherapy versus lobectomy for operable stage I non-small-cell lung cancer: a pooled analysis of two randomised trials. Lancet Oncol 2015;16(6):630–7.
26. Simone CB 2nd, Dorsey JF. Additional data in the debate on stage I non-small cell lung cancer: surgery versus stereotactic ablative radiotherapy. Ann Transl Med 2015;3(13):172.
27. Verma V, Simone CB 2nd, Zhen W. Stereotactic radiotherapy for stage I small cell lung cancer. Oncologist 2016;21(2):131–3.
28. Rosenzweig KE, Sura S, Jackson A, et al. Involved-field radiation therapy for inoperable non small-cell lung cancer. J Clin Oncol 2007;25(35):5557–61.
29. Yuan S, Sun X, Li M, et al. A randomized study of involved-field irradiation versus elective nodal irradiation in combination with concurrent chemotherapy for inoperable stage III nonsmall cell lung cancer. Am J Clin Oncol 2007;30(3):239–44.
30. Galvin JM, Ezzell G, Eisbrauch A, et al, American Society for Therapeutic Radiology and Oncology, American Association of Physicists in Medicine. Implementing IMRT in clinical practice: a joint document of the American Society for Therapeutic Radiology and Oncology and the American Association of Physicists in Medicine. Int J Radiat Oncol Biol Phys 2004;58(5):1616–34.
31. Wink KC, Roelofs E, Solberg T, et al. Particle therapy for non-small cell lung tumors: where do we stand? A systematic review of the literature. Front Oncol 2014;4:292.
32. Simone CB 2nd, Rengan R. The use of proton therapy in the treatment of lung cancers. Cancer J 2014;20(6):427–32.
33. Vogel J, Berman AT, Lin L, et al. Prospective study of proton beam radiation therapy for adjuvant and definitive treatment of thymoma and thymic

carcinoma: early response and toxicity assessment. Radiother Oncol 2016;118(3):504–9.
34. Gerweck LE, Kozin SV. Relative biological effectiveness of proton beams in clinical therapy. Radiother Oncol 1999;50(2):135–42.
35. Lin L, Kang M, Huang S, et al. Beam-specific planning target volumes incorporating 4D CT for pencil beam scanning proton therapy of thoracic tumors. J Appl Clin Med Phys 2015;16(6):5678.
36. Kesarwala AH, Ko CJ, Ning H, et al. Intensity-modulated proton therapy for elective nodal irradiation and involved-field radiation in the definitive treatment of locally advanced non-small-cell lung cancer: a dosimetric study. Clin Lung Cancer 2015;16(3):237–44.
37. Simpson DR, Lawson JD, Nath SK, et al. A survey of image-guided radiation therapy use in the United States. Cancer 2010;116(16):3953–60.
38. Corradetti MN, Mitra N, Bonner Millar LP, et al. A moving target: image guidance for stereotactic body radiation therapy for early-stage non-small cell lung cancer. Pract Radiat Oncol 2013;3(4):307–15.
39. Simpson DR, Lawson JD, Nath SK, et al. Utilization of advanced imaging technologies for target delineation in radiation oncology. J Am Coll Radiol 2009;6(12):876–83.
40. Thomas CM, Pike LC, Hartill CE, et al. Specific recommendations for accurate and direct use of PET-CT in PET guided radiotherapy for head and neck sites. Med Phys 2014;41(4):041710.
41. Jani SS, Lamb JM, White BM, et al. Assessing margin expansions of internal target volumes in 3D and 4D PET: a phantom study. Ann Nucl Med 2015;29(1):100–9.
42. Wang YC, Tseng HL, Lin YH, et al. Improvement of internal tumor volumes of non-small cell lung cancer patients for radiation treatment planning using interpolated average CT in PET/CT. PLoS One 2013;8(5):e64665.
43. Morarji K, Fowler A, Vinod SK, et al. Impact of FDG-PET on lung cancer delineation for radiotherapy. J Med Imaging Radiat Oncol 2012;56(2):195–203.
44. Chen GH, Yao ZF, Fan XW, et al. Variation in background intensity affects PET-based gross tumor volume delineation in non-small-cell lung cancer: the need for individualized information. Radiother Oncol 2013;109(1):71–6.
45. Chirindel A, Adebahr S, Schuster D, et al. Impact of 4D-(18)FDG-PET/CT imaging on target volume delineation in SBRT patients with central versus peripheral lung tumors. Multi-reader comparative study. Radiother Oncol 2015;115(3):335–41.
46. Hanna GG, van Sörnsen de Koste JR, Dahele MR, et al. Defining target volumes for stereotactic ablative radiotherapy of early-stage lung tumours: a comparison of three-dimensional 18F-fluorodeoxyglucose positron emission tomography and four-dimensional computed tomography. Clin Oncol (R Coll Radiol) 2012;24(6):e71–80.
47. Wijsman R, Grootjans W, Troost EG, et al. Evaluating the use of optimally respiratory gated 18F-FDG-PET in target volume delineation and its influence on radiation doses to the organs at risk in non-small-cell lung cancer patients. Nucl Med Commun 2016;37(1):66–73.
48. Konert T, Vogel W, MacManus MP, et al. PET/CT imaging for target volume delineation in curative intent radiotherapy of non-small cell lung cancer: IAEA consensus report 2014. Radiother Oncol 2015;116(1):27–34.
49. Simone CB 2nd, Ly D, Dan TD, et al. Comparison of intensity-modulated radiotherapy, adaptive radiotherapy, proton radiotherapy, and adaptive proton radiotherapy for treatment of locally advanced head and neck cancer. Radiother Oncol 2011;101(3):376–82.
50. Ding XP, Zhang J, Li BS, et al. Feasibility of shrinking field radiation therapy through 18F-FDG PET/CT after 40 Gy for stage III non-small cell lung cancers. Asian Pac J Cancer Prev 2012;13(1):319–23.
51. Ding X, Li H, Wang Z, et al. A clinical study of shrinking field radiation therapy based on (18)F-FDG PET/CT for stage III non-small cell lung cancer. Technol Cancer Res Treat 2013;12(3):251–7.
52. van Elmpt W, De Ruysscher D, van der Salm A, et al. The PET-boost randomised phase II dose-escalation trial in non-small cell lung cancer. Radiother Oncol 2012;104(1):67–71.
53. Geiger GA, Kim MB, Xanthopoulos EP, et al. Stage migration in planning PET/CT scans in patients due to receive radiotherapy for non-small-cell lung cancer. Clin Lung Cancer 2014;15(1):79–85.
54. Gregory DL, Hicks RJ, Hogg A, et al. Effect of PET/CT on management of patients with non-small cell lung cancer: results of a prospective study with 5-year survival data. J Nucl Med 2012;53(7):1007–15.
55. Mac Manus MP, Everitt S, Bayne M, et al. The use of fused PET/CT images for patient selection and radical radiotherapy target volume definition in patients with non-small cell lung cancer: results of a prospective study with mature survival data. Radiother Oncol 2013;106(3):292–8.
56. Abramyuk A, Appold S, Zöphel K, et al. Quantitative modifications of TNM staging, clinical staging and therapeutic intent by FDG-PET/CT in patients with non small cell lung cancer scheduled for radiotherapy–a retrospective study. Lung Cancer 2012;78(2):148–52.
57. Vu CC, Matthews R, Kim B, et al. Prognostic value of metabolic tumor volume and total lesion glycolysis from $^{18}$F-FDG PET/CT in patients undergoing

stereotactic body radiation therapy for stage I non-small-cell lung cancer. Nucl Med Commun 2013; 34(10):959–63.
58. Horne ZD, Clump DA, Vargo JA, et al. Pretreatment SUVmax predicts progression-free survival in early-stage non-small cell lung cancer treated with stereotactic body radiation therapy. Radiat Oncol 2014;9:41.
59. Nair VJ, MacRae R, Sirisegaram A, et al. Pretreatment [18F]-fluoro-2-deoxy-glucose positron emission tomography maximum standardized uptake value as predictor of distant metastasis in early-stage non-small cell lung cancer treated with definitive radiation therapy: rethinking the role of positron emission tomography in personalizing treatment based on risk status. Int J Radiat Oncol Biol Phys 2014;88(2):312–8.
60. Takeda A, Sanuki N, Fujii H, et al. Maximum standardized uptake value on FDG-PET is a strong predictor of overall and disease-free survival for non-small cell lung cancer patients after stereotactic body radiotherapy. J Thorac Oncol 2014; 9(1):65–73.
61. Paesmans M, Garcia C, Wong CY, et al. Primary tumour standardised uptake value is prognostic in nonsmall cell lung cancer: a multivariate pooled analysis of individual data. Eur Respir J 2015;46(6): 1751–61.
62. Lin MY, Wu M, Brennan S, et al. Absence of a relationship between tumor $^{18}$F-fluorodeoxyglucose standardized uptake value and survival in patients treated with definitive radiotherapy for non-small-cell lung cancer. J Thorac Oncol 2014;9(3):377–82.
63. Chen HH, Chiu NT, Su WC, et al. Prognostic value of whole-body total lesion glycolysis at pretreatment FDG PET/CT in non-small cell lung cancer. Radiology 2012;264(2):559–66.
64. Ohri N, Piperdi B, Garg MK, et al. Pre-treatment FDG-PET predicts the site of in-field progression following concurrent chemoradiotherapy for stage III non-small cell lung cancer. Lung Cancer 2015; 87(1):23–7.
65. Shusharina N, Cho J, Sharp GC, et al. Correlation of (18)F-FDG avid volumes on pre-radiation therapy and post-radiation therapy FDG PET scans in recurrent lung cancer. Int J Radiat Oncol Biol Phys 2014;89(1):137–44.
66. Zhu SH, Zhang Y, Yu YH, et al. FDG PET-CT in non-small cell lung cancer: relationship between primary tumor FDG uptake and extensional or metastatic potential. Asian Pac J Cancer Prev 2013; 14(5):2925–9.
67. Ohri N, Duan F, Machtay M, et al. Pretreatment FDG-PET metrics in stage III non-small cell lung cancer: ACRIN 6668/RTOG 0235. J Natl Cancer Inst 2015;107(4) [pii:djv004].
68. Hyun SH, Ahn HK, Ahn MJ, et al. Volume-based assessment with 18F-FDG PET/CT improves outcome prediction for patients with stage IIIA-N2 non-small cell lung cancer. AJR Am J Roentgenol 2015;205(3):623–8.
69. Trister AD, Pryma DA, Xanthopoulos E, et al. Prognostic value of primary tumor FDG uptake for occult mediastinal lymph node involvement in clinically N2/N3 node-negative non-small cell lung cancer. Am J Clin Oncol 2014;37(2): 135–9.
70. Everitt SJ, Ball DL, Hicks RJ, et al. Differential (18) F-FDG and (18)F-FLT uptake on serial PET/CT imaging before and during definitive chemoradiation for non-small cell lung cancer. J Nucl Med 2014; 55(7):1069–74.
71. Gill BS, Rivandi AH, Sandhu SP, et al. The role of positron emission tomography following radiosurgical treatment of malignant lung lesions. Nucl Med Commun 2012;33(6):607–12.
72. Ebright MI, Russo GA, Gupta A, et al. Positron emission tomography combined with diagnostic chest computed tomography enhances detection of regional recurrence after stereotactic body radiation therapy for early stage non-small cell lung cancer. J Thorac Cardiovasc Surg 2013;145(3): 709–15.
73. Nakajima N, Sugawara Y, Kataoka M, et al. Differentiation of tumor recurrence from radiation-induced pulmonary fibrosis after stereotactic ablative radiotherapy for lung cancer: characterization of 18F-FDG PET/CT findings. Ann Nucl Med 2013;27(3):261–70.
74. Zhang X, Liu H, Balter P, et al. Positron emission tomography for assessing local failure after stereotactic body radiotherapy for non-small-cell lung cancer. Int J Radiat Oncol Biol Phys 2012;83(5): 1558–65.
75. Bollineni VR, Widder J, Pruim J, et al. Residual $^{18}$F-FDG-PET uptake 12 weeks after stereotactic ablative radiotherapy for stage I non-small-cell lung cancer predicts local control. Int J Radiat Oncol Biol Phys 2012;83(4):e551–5.
76. Xanthopoulos EP, Handorf E, Simone CB 2nd, et al. Definitive dose thoracic radiation therapy in oligometastatic non-small cell lung cancer: a hypothesis-generating study. Pract Radiat Oncol 2015;5(4):e355–63.
77. Simone CB 2nd, Burri SH, Heinzerling JH. Novel radiotherapy approaches for lung cancer: combining radiation therapy with targeted and immunotherapies. Transl Lung Cancer Res 2015; 4(5):545–52.
78. Cheruvu P, Metcalfe SK, Metcalfe J, et al. Comparison of outcomes in patients with stage III versus limited stage IV non-small cell lung cancer. Radiat Oncol 2011;6:80.

79. Albain KS, Crowley JJ, LeBlanc M, et al. Survival determinants in extensive-stage non-small-cell lung cancer: the Southwest Oncology Group experience. J Clin Oncol 1991;9(9):1618–26.
80. De Rose F, Cozzi L, Navarria P, et al. Clinical outcome of stereotactic ablative body radiotherapy for lung metastatic lesions in non-small cell lung cancer oligometastatic patients. Clin Oncol (R Coll Radiol) 2016;28(1):13–20.
81. Solanki AA, Weichselbaum RR, Appelbaum D, et al. The utility of FDG-PET for assessing outcomes in oligometastatic cancer patients treated with stereotactic body radiotherapy: a cohort study. Radiat Oncol 2012;7:216.
82. Ordu C, Selcuk NA, Erdogan E, et al. Does early PET/CT assessment of response to chemotherapy predicts survival in patients with advanced stage non-small-cell lung cancer? Medicine (Baltimore) 2014;93(28):e299.
83. van Elmpt W, Ollers M, Dingemans AM, et al. Response assessment using 18F-FDG PET early in the course of radiotherapy correlates with survival in advanced-stage non-small cell lung cancer. J Nucl Med 2012;53(10):1514–20.
84. Huang W, Fan M, Liu B, et al. Value of metabolic tumor volume on repeated 18F-FDG PET/CT for early prediction of survival in locally advanced non-small cell lung cancer treated with concurrent chemoradiotherapy. J Nucl Med 2014;55(10):1584–90.
85. Roy S, Pathy S, Kumar R, et al. Efficacy of 18F-fluorodeoxyglucose positron emission tomography/computed tomography as a predictor of response in locally advanced non-small-cell carcinoma of the lung. Nucl Med Commun 2016;37(2):129–38.
86. Choi NC, Chun TT, Niemierko A, et al. Potential of 18F-FDG PET toward personalized radiotherapy or chemoradiotherapy in lung cancer. Eur J Nucl Med Mol Imaging 2013;40(6):832–41.
87. Toma-Dasu I, Uhrdin J, Lazzeroni M, et al. Evaluating tumor response of non-small cell lung cancer patients with $^{18}$F-fludeoxyglucose positron emission tomography: potential for treatment individualization. Int J Radiat Oncol Biol Phys 2015;91(2):376–84.
88. Lopez Guerra JL, Gladish G, Komaki R, et al. Large decreases in standardized uptake values after definitive radiation are associated with better survival of patients with locally advanced non-small cell lung cancer. J Nucl Med 2012b;53(2):225–33.
89. Xiang ZL, Erasmus J, Komaki R, et al. FDG uptake correlates with recurrence and survival after treatment of unresectable stage III non-small cell lung cancer with high-dose proton therapy and chemotherapy. Radiat Oncol 2012;28(7):144.
90. Na F, Wang J, Li C, et al. Primary tumor standardized uptake value measured on F18-fluorodeoxyglucose positron emission tomography is of prediction value for survival and local control in non-small-cell lung cancer receiving radiotherapy: meta-analysis. J Thorac Oncol 2014;9(6):834–42.
91. Wang J, Wong KK, Piert M, et al. Metabolic response assessment with (18)F-FDG PET/CT: inter-method comparison and prognostic significance for patients with non-small cell lung cancer. J Radiat Oncol 2015;4(3):249–56.
92. Machtay M, Duan F, Siegel BA, et al. Prediction of survival by [18F]fluorodeoxyglucose positron emission tomography in patients with locally advanced non-small-cell lung cancer undergoing definitive chemoradiation therapy: results of the ACRIN 6668/RTOG 0235 trial. J Clin Oncol 2013;31(30):3823–30.
93. Berman AT, Ellenberg SS, Simone CB 2nd. Predicting survival in non-small-cell lung cancer using positron emission tomography: several conclusions from multiple comparisons. J Clin Oncol 2014;32(15):1631–2.
94. Jeong JU, Chung WK, Nam TK, et al. Early metabolic response on 18F-fluorodeoxyglucose-positron-emission tomography/computed tomography after concurrent chemoradiotherapy for advanced stage III non-small cell lung cancer is correlated with local tumor control and survival. Anticancer Res 2014;34(5):2517–23.
95. Okusanya OT, Deshpande C, Barbosa EM Jr, et al. Molecular imaging to identify tumor recurrence following chemoradiation in a hostile surgical environment. Mol Imaging 2014;13.
96. Pan Y, Brink C, Schytte T, et al. Planned FDG PET-CT scan in follow-up detects disease progression in patients with locally advanced NSCLC receiving curative chemoradiotherapy earlier than standard CT. Medicine (Baltimore) 2015;94(43):e1863.
97. Gomez DR, Gladish GW, Wei X, et al. Prognostic value of positron emission tomography/computed tomography findings in limited-stage small cell lung cancer before chemoradiation therapy. Am J Clin Oncol 2014;37(1):77–80.
98. Lee J, Kim JO, Jung CK, et al. Metabolic activity on [18f]-fluorodeoxyglucose-positron emission tomography/computed tomography and glucose transporter-1 expression might predict clinical outcomes in patients with limited disease small-cell lung cancer who receive concurrent chemoradiation. Clin Lung Cancer 2014;15(2):e13–21.
99. Ulaner GA, Lyall A. Identifying and distinguishing treatment effects and complications from malignancy at FDG PET/CT. Radiographics 2013;33(6):1817–34.
100. Houshmand S, Boursi B, Salavati A, et al. Applications of fluorodeoxyglucose PET/computed tomography in the assessment and prediction of radiation therapy-related complications. PET Clin 2015;10(4):555–71.

101. Hicks RJ, Mac Manus MP, Matthews JP, et al. Early FDG-PET imaging after radical radiotherapy for non-small-cell lung cancer: inflammatory changes in normal tissues correlate with tumor response and do not confound therapeutic response evaluation. Int J Radiat Oncol Biol Phys 2004;60(2):412–8.
102. Robbins ME, Brunso-Bechtold JK, Peiffer AM, et al. Imaging radiation-induced normal tissue injury. Radiat Res 2012;177(4):449–66.
103. Abdulla S, Salavati A, Saboury B, et al. Quantitative assessment of global lung inflammation following radiation therapy using FDG PET/CT: a pilot study. Eur J Nucl Med Mol Imaging 2014;41(2):350–6.
104. Bradley JD, Paulus R, Komaki R, et al. Standard-dose versus high-dose conformal radiotherapy with concurrent and consolidation carboplatin plus paclitaxel with or without cetuximab for patients with stage IIIA or IIIB non-small-cell lung cancer (RTOG 0617): a randomised, two-by-two factorial phase 3 study. Lancet Oncol 2015;16(2):187–99.
105. Adams MJ, Hardenbergh PH, Constine LS, et al. Radiation-associated cardiovascular disease. Crit Rev Oncol Hematol 2003;45(1):55–75.
106. Unal K, Unlu M, Akdemir O, et al. 18F-FDG PET/CT findings of radiotherapy-related myocardial changes in patients with thoracic malignancies. Nucl Med Commun 2013;34(9):855–9.
107. Zöphel K, Hölzel C, Dawel M, et al. PET/CT demonstrates increased myocardial FDG uptake following irradiation therapy. Eur J Nucl Med Mol Imaging 2007;34(8):1322–3.
108. Evans JD, Gomez DR, Chang JY, et al. Cardiac $^{18}$F-fluorodeoxyglucose uptake on positron emission tomography after thoracic stereotactic body radiation therapy. Radiother Oncol 2013;109(1):82–8.
109. Wang YC, Hsieh TC, Chen SW, et al. Concurrent chemo-radiotherapy potentiates vascular inflammation: increased FDG uptake in head and neck cancer patients. JACC Cardiovasc Imaging 2013;6(4):512–4.
110. Nijkamp J, Rossi M, Lebesque J, et al. Relating acute esophagitis to radiotherapy dose using FDG-PET in concurrent chemo-radiotherapy for locally advanced non-small cell lung cancer. Radiother Oncol 2013;106(1):118–23.
111. Yuan ST, Brown RK, Zhao L, et al. Timing and intensity of changes in FDG uptake with symptomatic esophagitis during radiotherapy or chemo-radiotherapy. Radiat Oncol 2014;9(1):37.
112. Parodi K, Paganetti H, Shih HA, et al. Patient study of in vivo verification of beam delivery and range, using positron emission tomography and computed tomography imaging after proton therapy. Int J Radiat Oncol Biol Phys 2007;68(3):920–34.

# PET-Based Percutaneous Needle Biopsy

Ghassan El-Haddad, MD

**KEYWORDS**

• FDG • PET/CT • Image guidance • Percutaneous biopsy • Tissue sampling • Navigation • Fusion

**KEY POINTS**

- PET can be used to guide percutaneous needle biopsy to the most metabolic lesion, improving diagnostic yield.
- PET biopsy guidance can be performed using visual or software coregistration, electromagnetic needle tracking, cone-beam computed tomography (CT), or intraprocedural PET/CT guidance.
- PET/CT-guided biopsies allow the sampling of lesions that may not be clearly visible on anatomic imaging, or of lesions that are morphologically normal.
- PET can identify suspicious locations within complex tumors that are most likely to contain important diagnostic and prognostic information.

## INTRODUCTION

PET-based interventional applications have increased in the last decade, particularly in Interventional Oncology.[1–4] The use of morphologic or anatomic imaging in planning and assessing the effectiveness of oncologic treatments is essential and usually performed by using ultrasound (US), computed tomography (CT), or MR imaging. However, these anatomic imaging modalities are limited in the amount of information provided at a molecular level.[5] On the other hand, PET provides functional and metabolic information from lesions[6] and continues to make significant impact on the management of oncology patients, with reports on $^{18}$F-fluorodeoxyglucose (FDG) PET changing the management of patients with various forms of cancer in 30% to 40% of cases.[7] Image-guided percutaneous biopsy has been playing an essential role in the management of oncology patients, by confirming the diagnosis of cancer and staging the disease. However, in the era of personalized medicine, whereby diseases are more and more categorized and treated based on detailed molecular and genetic information, biopsy samples are required for more than just histologic diagnosis.[8]

Traditionally, image-guided percutaneous biopsies have been performed using anatomic imaging modalities for guidance such as fluoroscopy, US, CT, and MR imaging. Recently, there has been significant increase in the use of molecular information provided by PET for guiding percutaneous biopsies.

In this article, the growing role of PET in image-guided percutaneous needle biopsy, the limitations of anatomic imaging-based biopsies, the different navigation tools for image guidance, and available data on PET-based biopsies are reviewed.

## ANATOMIC IMAGING-BASED PERCUTANEOUS NEEDLE BIOPSY

Percutaneous image-guided biopsy is widely used as a minimally invasive alternative to open surgical biopsy for obtaining tissue; this is performed by either fine needle aspiration (FNA) or core needle biopsy.

Percutaneous image-guided biopsies are used to

- Obtain a diagnosis and establish whether a lesion is benign or malignant

The author has nothing to disclose.

Division of Interventional Radiology, Department of Radiology, H. Lee Moffitt Cancer Center and Research Institute, 12902 Magnolia Drive, Tampa, FL 33612-9416, USA
*E-mail address:* ghassan.elhaddad@moffitt.org

PET Clin 11 (2016) 333–349
http://dx.doi.org/10.1016/j.cpet.2016.02.009

- Obtain material for laboratory analysis (culture, molecular analysis)
- Determine response to therapy or transformation of the disease
- Predict prognosis and guide next therapy

Biopsy results may alter the future management of patients, but the clinical relevance of a biopsy must be first established, because not all radiographic findings merit a biopsy.[9] It is the interventional radiologist's role to determine whether a biopsy is warranted, and if so what would be the safest route for obtaining tissue, in order to avoid unnecessary interventions that are costly and potentially dangerous.[10] Image-guided percutaneous biopsies are usually performed using the following:

- Radiographic or fluoroscopic guidance (ie, stereotactic breast biopsy)
- US guidance for superficial soft tissue lesions (ie, Inguinal lymph nodes) or abdominal organs (ie, liver, kidney)
- CT guidance for deep lesions (ie, lung, retroperitoneum)
- MR imaging guidance for breast and prostate biopsy

In order to perform an image-guided biopsy, there are 2 essential requirements:

- Lesion visibility on an imaging modality that is usually used to guide the biopsy
- Ability to safely access the biopsy target in the patient

There is high technical success of an image-guided biopsy if both of these requirements are met. If the lesions are visible on CT scan, the diagnostic success rate for CT-guided biopsies can be as high as 90%,[11–14] with false-negative rates ranging from 3.3% in bone[15] to 6.7% in abdomen or chest.[16] Unfortunately, malignant tumors may sometimes be invisible on anatomic imaging modalities US, CT, or MR imaging. CT scan is commonly used for biopsy guidance, especially for deep lesions, but accurately targeting the area of concern can be challenging if the lesion is not easily visualized on noncontrast CT.[17] Depending on the size and location of the lesion, this may result in higher false negative biopsy results compared with lesions that can be clearly visualized on CT.[18] Even the administration of intravenous contrast media may only temporarily improve the visibility of certain lesions,[18] because tumor visibility may be temporally limited to the arterial or venous phase of contrast-enhanced imaging. In order to circumvent the different scenarios of difficult biopsies, interventional radiologists have recurred to

- Mentally registering information from preprocedural to procedural imaging modality using anatomic landmarks and estimation (**Fig. 1**)
- Using software to register different imaging modalities
- Using navigation tools whereby the position of the biopsy needle is displayed on the procedural imaging modality in real time[19–21]

## FLUORODEOXYGLUCOSE-PET AND PERCUTANEOUS NEEDLE BIOPSY

FDG remains the most widely used radiotracer for both diagnostic and PET-based interventional applications.[1] FDG-PET/CT has been shown to have a higher accuracy than anatomic imaging modalities in differentiating viable tumor from fibrosis in residual masses after therapy.[22–24] Despite the

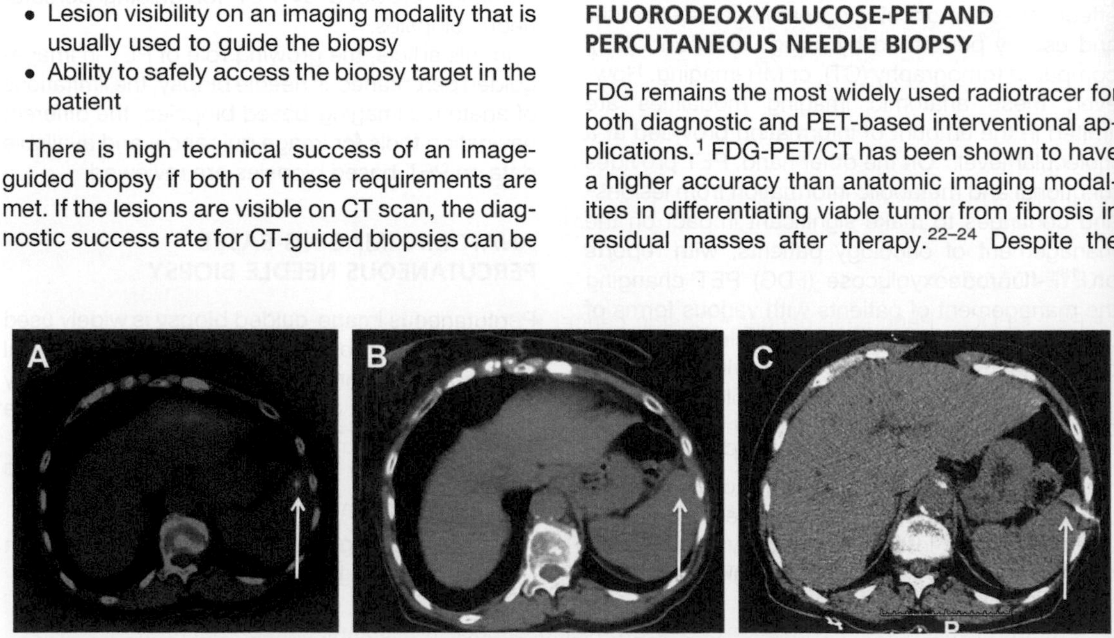


**Fig. 1.** Transaxial PET/CT image demonstrating a focus of increased FDG uptake (SUVmax 3.8) in the spleen (*A, arrow*) without any corresponding anatomic abnormality on the noncontrast CT scan (*B, arrow*). Because the patient had completed resection of a right groin melanoma with lymph node dissection and local radiation therapy 4 months before, a biopsy of that spot was warranted. Using the PET findings, a CT-guided biopsy of the spleen (*C, arrow*) accurately sampled the abnormal FDG focus yielding metastatic melanoma. This finding significantly affected the management of this patient because that was the only visible site of disease.

overall high accuracy of FDG-PET for cancer staging,[25] there are several benign tumors or inflammatory processes that can mimic cancer on FDG-PET,[26,27] and false positive results may occur in about 10% to 26 % of all patients[28–31] (**Fig. 2**). This nonspecificity of FDG-PET means that

- Diagnostic imaging is limited, and obtaining tissue diagnosis is sometimes imperative for optimal management of patients
- FDG-PET/CT offers an incremental benefit by targeting the most metabolically active portion of a lesion whether it is morphologically normal or abnormal[32]
- PET-positive but benign-appearing lesions on CT should not preclude obtaining tissue diagnosis

Because FDG concentrates in several malignant tumors and inflammatory processes, it can be used to distinguish regions of tissue viability from regions of tissue necrosis[33] (**Fig. 3**), thereby improving the diagnostic yield of biopsies[32] and avoiding futile, even potentially dangerous biopsies.[10] It is important to note that a "diagnostic" biopsy means that it leads to a definitive histopathological diagnosis, and not necessarily that the lesion has a neoplastic cause. It may not be necessary or cost-effective to obtain an FDG-PET/CT scan before each image-guided biopsy, but if a patient has had one, reviewing those images is axiomatic because it may change the biopsy site. This finding was particularly important for the biopsy of bone (66.6%) and soft tissue lesions (57.8%), and less important for lung lesions (40.7%).[32] In a patient who has multiple or complex lesions, FDG-PET can be used to aim at the area that is most likely to be informative or representative of the disease (**Fig. 4**).

Some lesions, namely large masses, may contain malignant, inflammatory areas mixed with necrotic or fibrotic regions characterized by low or absent metabolic activity.[33,34] If there are multiple lesions with variable levels of metabolic activity, then random sampling may not provide the most appropriate tissue for correct diagnosis, resulting in false negative biopsy results.

In general, the intensity of FDG uptake within malignant tumors correlates with biological activity[35] and may facilitate identification and targeting of more aggressive or genetically transformed regions of tumor (**Fig. 5**). This concept was recently proven by autoradiography that found in situ high-spatial-accuracy correlation between FDG uptake and histopathology findings on PET/CT-guided biopsy specimens.[36]

Intratumoral heterogeneity due to variations of genetic expressions[37] as well as temporal tumoral heterogeneity that can result from genomic variations within the same or metastatic tumors over time[38] can obviously cause significant challenges for choosing the adequate therapy because these changes may be hard to depict on anatomic imaging. There is increasing work on FDG-PET and radiomics[39] (conversion of digital medical images

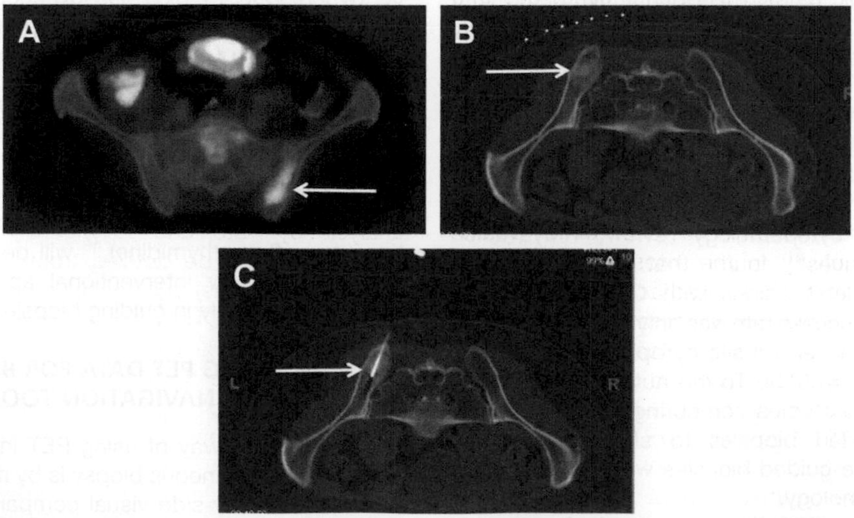


**Fig. 2.** Unilateral focal increased FDG uptake in the posterior left iliac bone marrow seen on an axial image of a PET/CT scan (*A*, *arrow*) obtained for restaging of a rectal adenocarcinoma. The patient was placed in a prone position; a radiopaque grid was placed on the skin for planning of biopsy needle entrance, and a noncontrast CT scan was obtained demonstrating focal sclerosis in the same area of increased FDG activity (*B*, *arrow*). A percutaneous CT-guided biopsy of that suspicious area (*C*, *arrow*) on PET/CT scan was negative for malignancy, an example of falsely positive PET and CT scan.

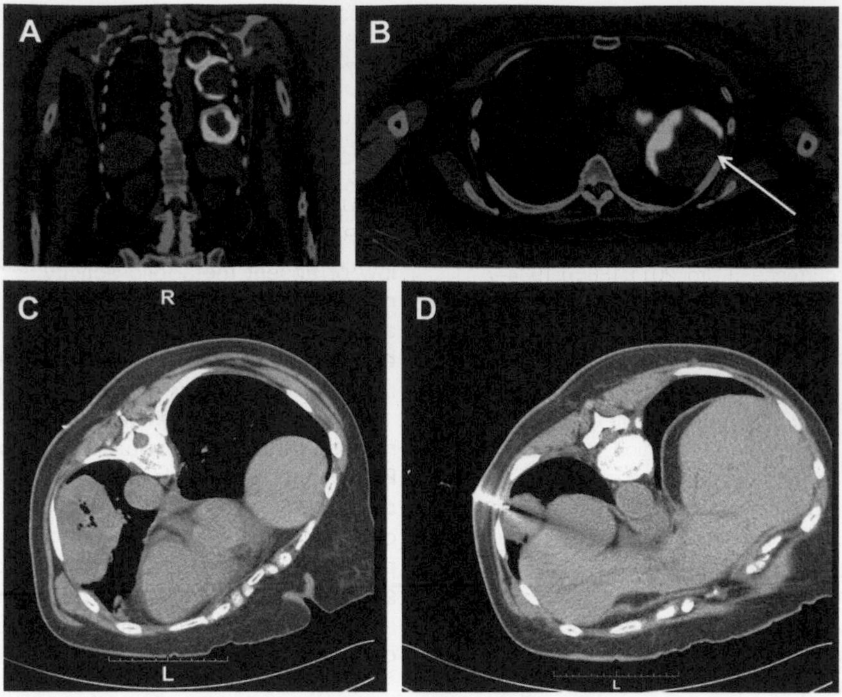


**Fig. 3.** An 85-year-old female patient with a history of endometrioid uterine adenocarcinoma status after total abdominal hysterectomy, and bilateral salpingo-oophorectomy was found 5 years later to have multiple lung masses. PET/CT scan demonstrates multiple hypermetabolic left lung masses with partial tumor necrosis that is not limited to the central part of the masses (*A*), but also involves the periphery (*B*, *arrow*). Sampling of the tumor without the PET information (*C*) by targeting the edge of the tumor at that level would have led to sampling error, and repeat biopsy increased the patient's risks. Therefore, the percutaneous needle sampling was taken from one of the most metabolic portions of the lowest tumor (*D*), yielding endometrial adenocarcinoma.

into phenotypic data and integration with large-scale biologic data). This quantitative data might lead to PET/CT-guided biopsies of biologically relevant tissue needed to determine future treatments.[40]

When a hypermetabolic focus is seen on PET without a clear anatomic correlation, PET-guided biopsies can have a tremendous impact on the management of patients[32] (**Fig. 6**). Even when using on-site cytopathology review, Virayavanich and colleagues[41] found that when biopsying musculoskeletal lesions with CT guidance, the diagnostic success rate was only 77.0% compared with 63.3% when on-site cytopathology was not available ($P$ = .015). To the author's knowledge, there are no studies comparing the accuracy of PET/CT-guided biopsies to standard percutaneous image-guided biopsies with the use of on-site cytopathology.

Of course, FDG-PET/CT-guided biopsies are limited in certain scenarios:

- Non-FDG-avid lesions (ie, well-differentiated prostate adenocarcinoma, well-differentiated neuroendocrine tumor)[42,43]
- Locations such as mediastinal lymph node, where FDG-PET/CT has low accuracy; better and safer sampling can be performed with endoscopic US[44,45]

Future clinical application of newer PET radiotracers targeting other key molecular events than metabolism (FDG), such as tissue hypoxia (ie, fluoromisonidazole), neovascularity (ie, arginine-glycine-aspartic acid peptides), and cell proliferation (deoxyfluorothymidine),[46] will definitely open the door to new interventional applications of PET/CT, especially in guiding biopsies.

## INCORPORATING PET DATA FOR BIOPSY AND THE USAGE OF NAVIGATION TOOLS

The most basic way of using PET information in guiding a percutaneous biopsy is by mental registration or side-by-side visual comparison of preprocedural PET and intraprocedural anatomic imaging, usually CT[32] (**Fig. 7**). This mental or visual integration by the interventional radiologist is

- Dependent on the use of anatomic landmarks and estimation

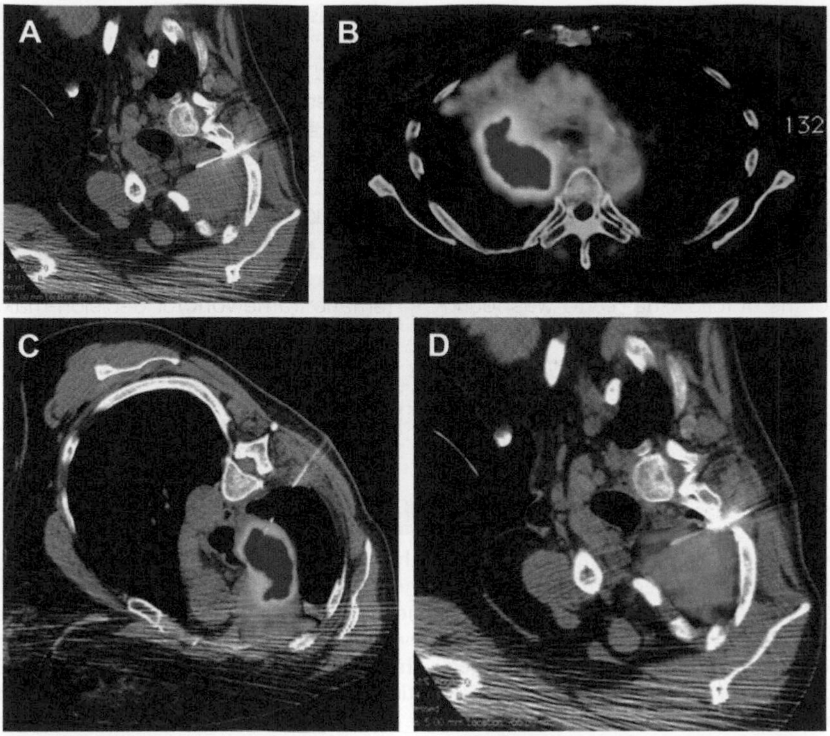


**Fig. 4.** A 60-year-old female patient with dyspnea underwent a chest radiograph followed by a noncontrast CT scan due to renal failure and was found to have a large right upper lobe lung mass, for which a percutaneous biopsy was requested. She was placed in a lateral decubitus position, and using a posterior approach, core samples were obtained from the periphery of the mass in order to avoid the central necrosis and/or large vessels (*A*). However, the biopsy revealed inflammation and no malignancy. In view of the clinical suspicion for malignancy, an FDG-PET/CT scan was performed revealing a hypermetabolic right lung hilar mass and postobstructive pneumonitis (*B*). A new biopsy was guided by the fusion of FDG-PET and biopsy CT images, with the biopsy needle positioned in the highest metabolic portion of the lung mass (*C, red area*), yielding squamous cell carcinoma. Retrospective fusion of PET with the first biopsy CT revealed that the biopsy needle was initially placed in the least metabolically active portion of the lesion within the postobstructive pneumonitis (*D, green area*).

- Highly reliant on the operator's experience and ability in spatial orientation
- Inexpensive, because no additional equipment or software is needed

In lesions that are nonvisualized on morphologic imaging, anatomic landmarks can be used to guide tissue sampling, but confirmation of accurate needle positioning can be challenging (**Fig. 8**).

Software algorithms can also be used to register the intraprocedural anatomic imaging with preprocedural PET/CT data using matched anatomic landmarks in the 2 data sets.[47–50] Rigid (linear) and nonrigid (elastic) coregistration of anatomic and molecular imaging can be used.[48,51,52] The rigid registration is easier to use, but is more prone to errors with deformable organs, particularly next to the diaphragm because of patient motion, respiration, or cardiac motion.[48] These so-called offline registration techniques do not offer real-time guidance. For patients in whom image registration is expected to be challenging and time consuming due to significant variation in position during biopsy in comparison to a preprocedural PET/CT scan, a visual side-by-side registration is more practical. The characteristics of different registration techniques are presented in **Table 1**.

More recently, PET-guided biopsy using electromagnetic (EM) tracking,[53] cone-beam CT (CBCT),[54] or intraprocedural PET/CT[55] has been described. EM tracking, which is also referred to as medical global positioning system,[56] provides real-time device (ie, biopsy needle) location in the patient using preprocedural (CT/MR imaging/PET) and intraprocedural imaging (US or CT), a field generator, field sensors (FS) (in the tracked device such as biopsy needle), skin sensors (positioned near the procedure area), and a processing computer.[21] The field generator produces a very weak magnetic field that induces currents in the FS present in the biopsy needle and skin sensors placed on the patient, allowing the determination

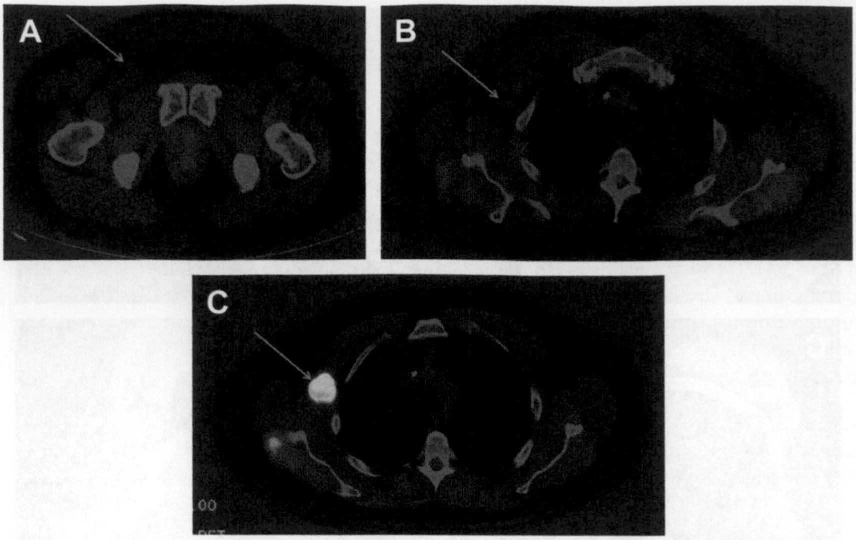


**Fig. 5.** A 48-year-old male patient initially diagnosed with follicular lymphoma. Seven years later, he underwent a PET/CT scan for palpable tender right inguinal lymph node (*A, arrow*) followed by a US-guided biopsy of this node for concern of transformation, but the biopsy was negative. On a follow-up PET/CT scan a year later, he was found to have the same low metabolic activity in the previously biopsied palpable right inguinal lymph node (*B, arrow*), but there was intense activity in an enlarged right axillary lymph node measuring 2.7 × 3.5 cm with an SUVmax of 12.1 (*C, arrow*). These results helped in directing the new US-guided biopsy, and the patient was ultimately diagnosed with transformation of the follicular lymphoma into diffuse large B-cell lymphoma.

of the needle tip position in the patient referenced to fused preprocedure and intraprocedure imaging.[21] A tracked US is optional and allows for real-time navigation. EM needle tracking offers the option of performing the entire percutaneous biopsy procedure using US, thereby limited radiation exposure.

The rotation of a CBCT C-arm generates 3-dimensional (3D) imaging data set that may be fused with live fluoroscopy and previous imaging

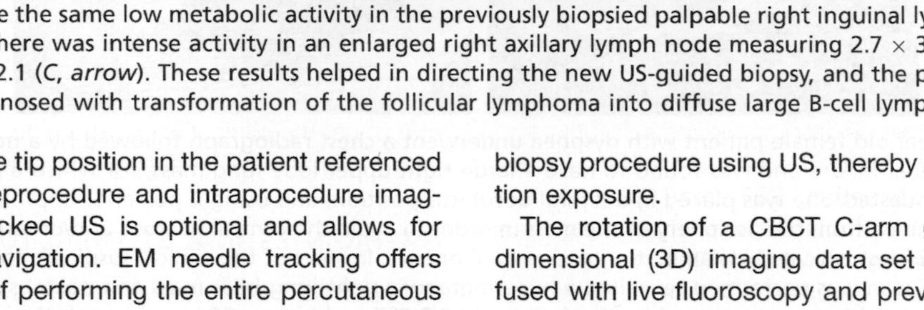

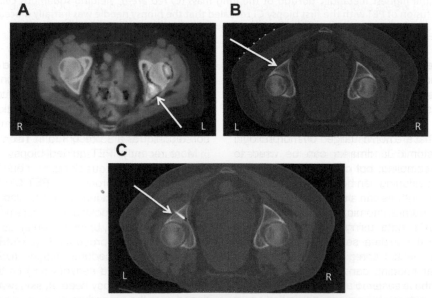


**Fig. 6.** Transaxial PET/CT images demonstrating a focal area of intense FDG uptake in the bone marrow of the left iliac bone (*A, arrow*), with no corresponding morphologic abnormalities seen on noncontrast CT scan used for biopsy guidance (*B, arrow*). The patient was placed in a prone position (*B*) with a grid on the skin to determine biopsy needle entrance and direction. A PET/CT-guided biopsy of the abnormal bone marrow focus (*C, arrow*) yielded metastatic pancreatic adenocarcinoma.

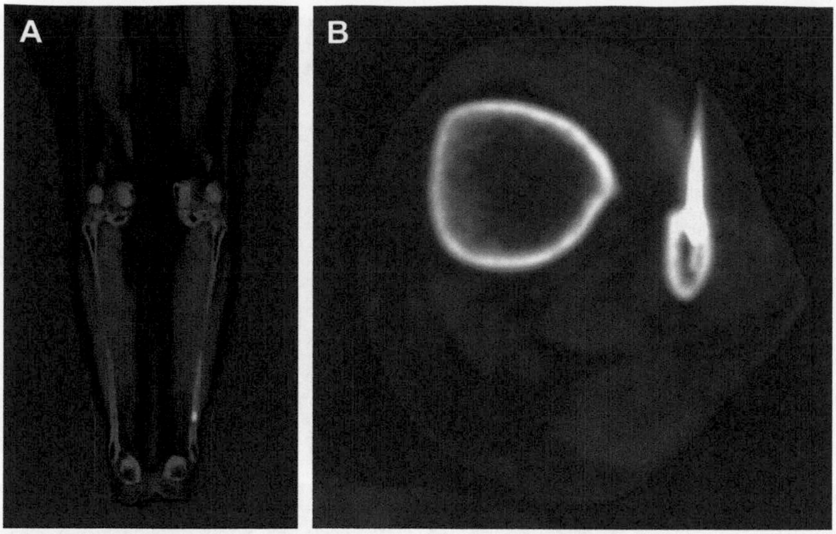


**Fig. 7.** A 75-year-old female patient with history of mantle cell lymphoma, status postchemotherapy. On follow-up, an FDG-PET/CT scan detected only a suspicious focal area of increased glucose metabolism within the distal left fibular bone marrow without any significant anatomic abnormalities (*A*). A percutaneous biopsy of this area (*B*) guided by the PET/CT findings and using anatomic landmarks revealed a relapsed mantle cell lymphoma. This area of the skeleton would not have been sampled if it were not for the PET/CT scan, and a "blind" BMB of the iliac crest may have missed the diagnosis and delayed appropriate treatment.

(ie, PET) without the need for additional hardware or disposables.[54] Although CBCT data are mostly used in the field of angiography for tracking of wires and catheters, it can also provide a visual reference for image-based tracking of percutaneous devices such as biopsy needles and ablation probes.[20] After fusing the CBCT images to preprocedural imaging (ie, PET), the interventionalist chooses on a workstation the desired percutaneous access to target the lesion. Then, the desired trajectory is projected on fluoroscopy images, which the interventionalist uses to advance the biopsy needle following the planned trajectory (**Fig. 9**).

Both EM tracking and CBCT-based needle biopsy

- Provide real-time feedback with referencing of tracked biopsy needle to PET data throughout the procedure
- Facilitate targeting lesions in difficult locations, or lesions that are not well seen on anatomic imaging
- Help target the most metabolic lesions (ie, in large tumors with heterogeneous FDG uptake)
- Allow 3D real-time multimodality image fusion of CT/US/MR imaging/PET
- Can be negatively affected with motion artifact (ie, respiratory motion), or hardware within or in the vicinity of the patient (ie, beam hardening for CBCT, electrical equipment distorting the EM field), and large body habitus

The most common benefits of PET/CT-guided biopsies, whether using coregistration, navigation tools, or intraprocedural PET/CT, are listed in **Box 1**.

The intraprocedural PET/CT-guided biopsies or "in-suite" PET/CT-guided biopsies may avoid the challenges of fusion with previously acquired PET images due to the different placement and position of the patients during the biopsy procedures. These biopsies allow a direct detection of the hypermetabolic lesions and needle placement in real time, which may improve the diagnostic yield of such biopsies.[55] In the first study on a small group of patients who underwent an intraprocedural PET/CT-guided biopsy directing the correct biopsy needle position to the center of the FDG-avid had an additional clinical impact on 50% of the patients.[57] This step-by-step technique of intraprocedural PET/CT-guided biopsy was described by Klaeser and colleagues.[57] Importantly, the complication rates of intraprocedural PET/CT-guided biopsies were found to be similar to CT-guided biopsies.[11–16,58–60] The advantages and limitations of intraprocedural PET/CT-guided biopsies are listed in **Table 2**.

## DATA ON PET-GUIDED BIOPSY BY LOCATION

The initial reports on PET-guided biopsies were limited with a relatively small number of patients studied.[49,50,53,54,57,61,62] The largest series on PET-guided biopsies are listed in **Table 3**.

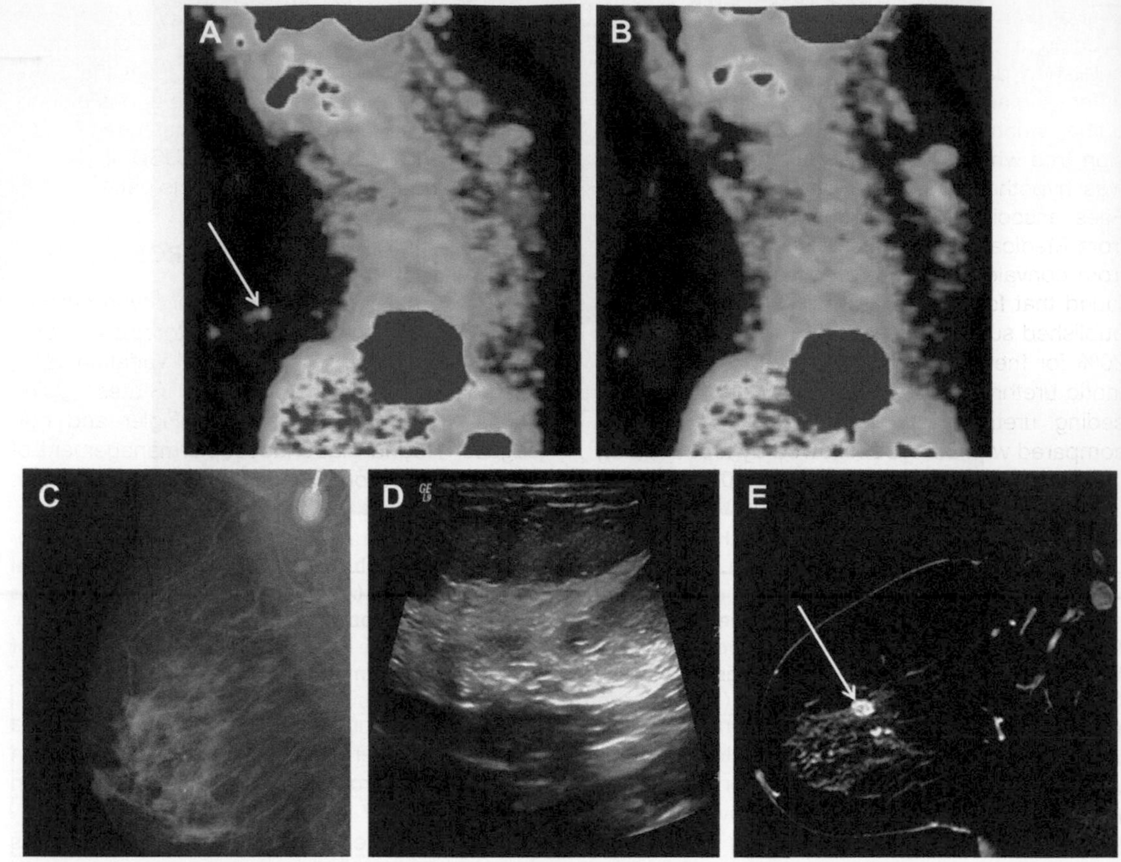


**Fig. 8.** A 69-year-old female patient with a history of colon cancer in remission who underwent an FDG-PET/CT scan that revealed a new hypermetabolic focus in the right breast as seen on the oblique view of a maximum intensity projection (*A, arrow*), not seen on the prior study that was done 8 months before (*B*). Further evaluation with mammography (*C*) and breast sonography (*D*) failed to detect any abnormalities. She then proceeded to have bilateral breast MR imaging that showed an abnormally enhancing lesion within the right breast (*E, arrow*), correlating with the area of increased FDG uptake. Using the PET/MR imaging data led to an MR imaging–guided right breast biopsy yielding an invasive ductal carcinoma.

## *Soft Tissue Lesions*

Most of the time, it is not possible to clearly distinguish benign from malignant soft tissue lesions based on morphologic imaging, and patients with suspected soft tissue sarcoma must have tissue diagnosis before treatment. Even when biopsies are performed based on morphologic imaging, there is an error in diagnostic accuracy in up to 17.8% of cases,[63] which obviously can lead to significant morbidity and mortality.[64]

In one of the initial studies by Hain and colleagues[61] evaluating the coregistration of FDG-PET with MR imaging for guiding biopsies of soft tissue tumors

- FDG-PET scan was able to guide the biopsy to the most malignant site as confirmed by histology of the surgically resected soft tissue masses
- Benign lesions had low or no FDG uptake
- There was no added benefit in registering the PET to the MR imaging for targeting

Early diagnosis of malignant transformation of benign peripheral nerve sheath tumors into malignant peripheral nerve sheath tumors (MPNST) is crucial because complete surgical resection is the only curative treatment, because MPNST is one of the most common causes of death in patients with neurofibromatosis 1 (NF1).[65,66] Despite FDG-PET/CT being the most efficient imaging modality for detection of MPNST in NF1 patients, it has a low positive predictive value (PPV) of 61.5%.[67] Therefore, obtaining a tissue sample remains necessary for patient management. Brahmi and colleagues[68] retrospectively reviewed the PET/CT-guided percutaneous biopsies performed on 26 NF1 patients with a clinical suspicion of

**Table 1**
**Characteristics of rigid and nonrigid image registration**

| | Rigid Registration | Nonrigid Registration |
|---|---|---|
| Ease of use | + | – |
| Speed | + | – |
| Accuracy with deformable organs | – | + |
| Prone to motion artifact (especially near the diaphragm) | ++ | + |
| Time consuming | – | + |
| Labor intensive | – | + |
| Requires powerful computers | – | + |

MPNST and a suspected lesion from a PET/CT scan (tumor/liver standardized uptake value [SUV]max ratio > 1.5). In this study, wherein US and CT-guided biopsies were performed based on the FDG-PET/CT findings, the diagnostic accuracy rate was 96%.[68] The only case of false negative result may have been related to the high heterogeneity of the tumor biopsied, whereby benign and malignant areas were contiguous and associated with inflammation as seen on the surgical resected specimen.[68]

Some soft tissue lesions, namely large masses, may contain malignant, inflammatory areas mixed with necrotic or fibrotic regions characterized by low or absent metabolic activity.[33,34] If there are multiple lesions with variable levels of metabolic activity, then random sampling may not provide the most appropriate tissue for correct diagnosis, resulting in false negative biopsy results.

## *Bone Lesions*

In bone marrow lesions, FDG-PET was found to accurately guide percutaneous biopsies to the most suspicious areas for lymphomatous involvement even in areas that did not demonstrate any anatomic abnormality.[62,69] Bone marrow biopsy (BMB) allows the evaluation of only a limited area and can miss unifocal or multifocal disease if present at locations other than the iliac crest. In a retrospective analysis by Wang and colleagues,[70] it was found that the discrepancy rate between the left and right iliac crest biopsies was identified in 48 specimens (11.7% of positive samples), predominantly in patients with Hodgkin disease (HD) (39% of samples), sarcoma (29% of samples), carcinoma (23% of samples), and non-Hodgkin lymphoma (NHL) (9.2% of samples).

Schaefer and colleagues[69] retrospectively studied 50 patients with HD (n = 22) or aggressive NHL (n = 28) in whom FDG-avid bone lesions were detected by FDG-PET/CT. There was no evaluation of any positive BMB with negative PET scan because only FDG-avid lesions were included. Otherwise,

- All biopsies (n = 18) of the FDG-avid bone lesions detected the presence of lymphoma
- PET/CT information regarding unifocal or multifocal bone involvement resulted in lymphoma upstaging in 21 (42%) patients compared with the combined information provided by CT and BMB
- There was no change in morphologic bone alterations on CT scan after the end of therapy
- FDG-PET was found to be superior to CT alone or in combination with unilateral BMB

These results were in line with a previous retrospective study comparing FDG-PET/CT and BMB by Cheng and colleagues[71] that showed the overall sensitivity of detecting bone marrow involvement by lymphoma being 92% and 54% ($P < .05$), respectively.

In a retrospective study of 68 subjects, Pezeshk and colleagues[72] demonstrated that FDG-PET-directed skeletal biopsies (n = 39) resulted in a higher number of true positive (TP) (n = 35) and a lower number of false positive (FP) (n = 4) biopsies than did bone scintigraphy–directed biopsies (n = 29) (21 TP, 8 FP), but the PPV was not statistically significant ($P = .10$). This finding may have been related to the small number of patients in the study.

Intraprocedural PET/CT-guided bone biopsy of 20 patients by Klaeser and colleagues[62]:

- Was technically successful in all patients
- Had definite histologic diagnosis obtained in 19 of 20 patients
- Had no complications or adverse effects
- Changed the planned treatment in overall 56% of patients

## *Lung Lesions*

In a retrospective study of 311 patients who underwent CT-guided FNA of lung nodules and FDG-PET/CT within an interval of less than 30 days, it was found that, when registering the biopsy, CT images with corresponding PET/CT scan[73]:

- There is a direct correlation between the degree of metabolism at the site of biopsy and the accuracy of FNA

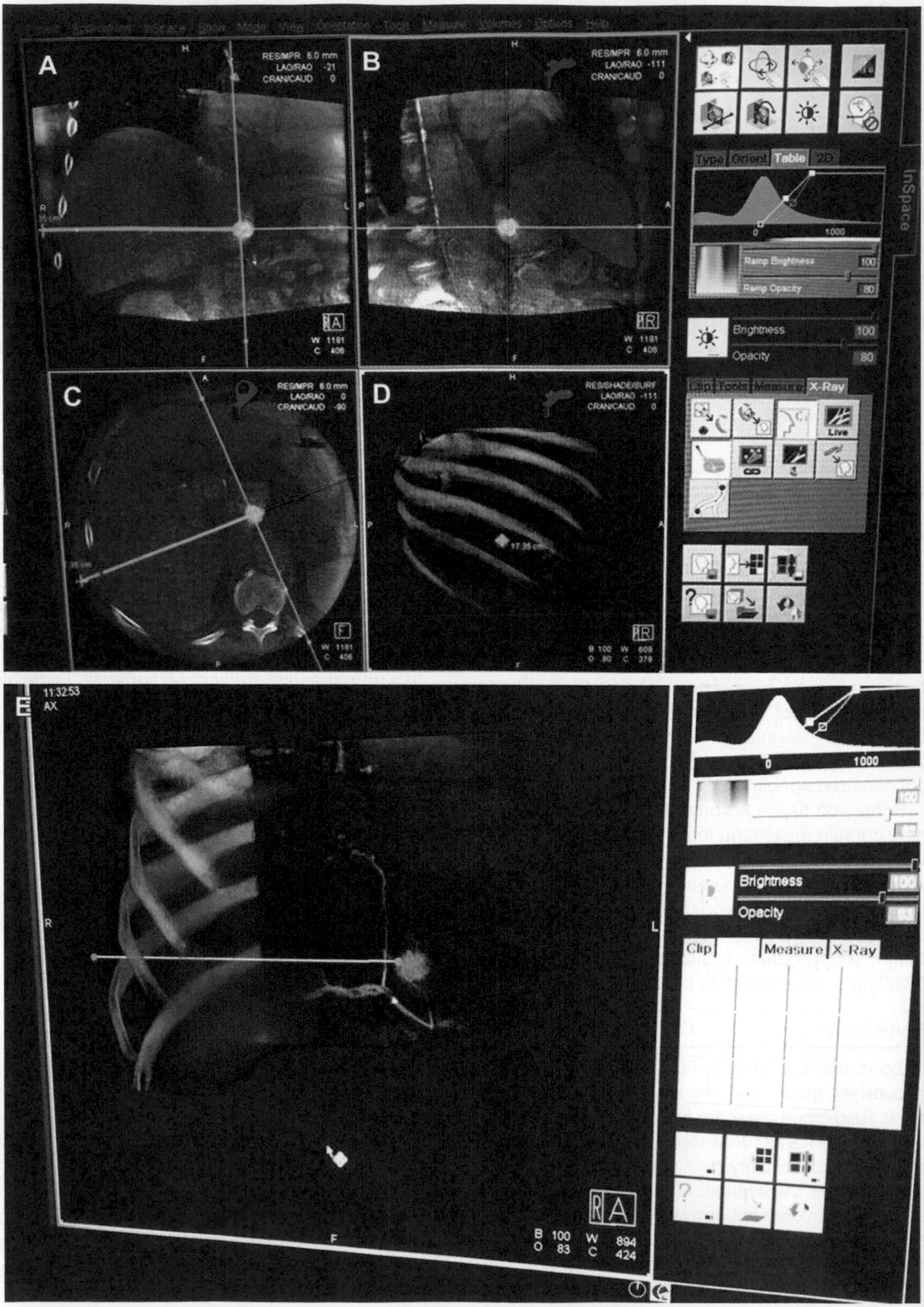


**Fig. 9.** 3D planning (*A, coronal*; *B, oblique*; and *C, axial*) for percutaneous biopsy using CBCT of the liver following intra-arterial contrast enhancement for an arterially enhancing lesion deep in the liver. After reconstruction of the images on a separate workstation, the biopsy needle entry point is determined on the 3D image (*D*), and the final trajectory of the fluoroscopically guided biopsy needle can be reviewed (*E*).

**Box 1**
**Most common benefits for PET-guided biopsies using coregistration, navigation tools, or intraprocedural PET/computed tomography**

- Lesions that are not visualized or poorly visualized on anatomic imaging
- Lesions that are seen on one phase of a multiphase contrast enhanced study (ie, liver lesion only seen on arterial phase)
- Lesions that are difficult to access (ie, liver dome lesion, renal hilum, mediastinum requiring nonorthogonal access)
- Complex lesions (ie, containing areas of necrosis)
- For patients who have a contraindication for contrast-enhanced studies
- Decreasing radiation exposure (ie, performing the biopsy using US guidance after fusing the images with previously obtained PET/CT)
- Decreasing the procedure time by quickly accessing a target lesion
- Decreasing risks related to biopsy by decreasing the number of attempts at sampling a target lesion
- Planning intervention on specific part of a lesion (ie, radiofrequency ablation of area of residual/recurrent disease, area near a heat sink)

- The distance between the needle tip and the highest SUV in the lesion was significantly greater in the false negative (FN) group (15.4 $\pm$ 14 mm) than in the TP group (5.9 $\pm$ 13.4 mm, $P<.001$)
- SUVmax at the biopsy needle tip was significantly higher in the TP group, at 6.4 $\pm$ 6.4, than in the FN group, at 4 $\pm$ 4.7 ($P<.05$)

It was not mentioned in this study how many patients received their PET/CT scan before the biopsy, and how much influence that could have had on needle position and accuracy.

Bitencourt and colleagues[74] retrospectively evaluated 64 PET/CT-guided biopsies whereby the target to be biopsied was determined after evaluating the PET/CT images side by side with noncontrast CT. In this study, wherein most of the sampled lesions were in the lungs (n = 28, 43.8%), the biopsies were positive for malignancy in 71.9% of cases (n = 46), negative in 23.4% of cases (n = 15), and inconclusive in 4.7% (n = 3) of cases. It is worth noting that the lesions with an SUV $\geq$4.0 were more likely to be malignant (85.4% vs 46.2%; $P = .006$).[74]

It is questionable whether lung lesions that are smaller than 4 cm need coregistration with PET because of the lower likelihood these lesions will show necrosis and complexity.

### *Mediastinal Lesions*

There are limited data on the effect of PET-guided percutaneous sampling of mediastinal tumors. Yokoyama and colleagues[75] retrospectively evaluated 106 patients who underwent CT-guided percutaneous biopsy of mediastinal tumors with (n = 56, group 1) or without coregistration with a prior PET/CT (n = 50, group 2). Despite a trend for a better performance for group 1, the investigators found that the difference in diagnostic accuracy between group 1 and 2 (95.8% and 91.8%) was not statistically significant ($P = .32$).

**Table 2**
**The advantages and limitations of intraprocedural PET/computed tomographic–guided biopsies**

| Intraprocedural PET/CT-guided Biopsies | |
|---|---|
| **Advantages** | **Limitations** |
| • Radiotracer (ie, FDG) remains in the targeted lesion for a longer period of time<br>• Useful for lesions not visible with anatomic imaging<br>• Guides the biopsy to most active tumor or part of a tumor<br>• No need for tracking devices or disposables<br>• Less prone to registration bias or misalignment seen with navigations tools<br>• Complication rates similar to CT-guided biopsy[55] | • Metabolic activity may not be detectable (ie, in small <5-mm lesions, or non FDG-avid tumors)[81]<br>• Increases radiation exposure<br>• No real-time navigation<br>• Can be cumbersome<br>• Costly given the occupancy of the PET-CT system<br>• May be time consuming<br>• Dedicated interventional PET/CT suites are not yet widely available<br>• Requires radiopharmaceutical handling<br>• PET acquisition time and FDG dosage are not standardized |

**Table 3**
**Summary of the largest series on PET/computed tomographic–guided biopsies**

| Author and Year | Patients N | Biopsied Lesions with PET Guidance N | Most Common Location Biopsied | Diagnostic Accuracy or PPV When Listed | Method Used to Target the Lesion: Visual vs Software Coregistration, or Intraprocedural PET/CT Biopsy |
|---|---|---|---|---|---|
| Hain et al,[61] 2003 | 20 | 20 | Soft tissue (100%) | NR | SC |
| Pezeshk et al,[72] 2006 | 68 | 39 | Bone (100%) | 89.7% PPV | VC |
| Schaefer et al,[69] 2007 | 50 | 18 | Bone (100%) | NR | VC |
| Tatli et al,[49] 2010 | 14 | 14 | Abdominal masses (liver, 43%) | NR | SC |
| Klaeser et al,[62] 2010 | 20 | 20 | Bone (100%) | NR | IP |
| Kalinyak et al,[76] 2011[a] | 19 | 24 | Breast | 66% PPV | SC |
| Bitencourt et al,[74] 2012 | 64 | 64 | Lung (44%)<br>Intra-abdominal/pelvic mass (39%)<br>Miscellaneous (17%) | NR | VC |
| Cerci et al,[78] 2013 | 126 | 130 | Lung (38.5%)<br>Liver (12.3%)<br>Soft tissue (11.5%)<br>Abdominal mass (10%)<br>Miscellaneous (27.7%) | NR | IP |
| Nguyen et al,[77] 2013 | 227 | 231 | Lymph node (31.2%)<br>Liver (16.8%)<br>Bone (11.3%)<br>Adrenal gland (11.3%)<br>Intra-abdominal/pelvic masses (10.8%)<br>Miscellaneous extrapulmonary masses (18.6%) | 72% PPV | VC |
| Purandare et al,[32] 2013 | 102 | 112 | Lung (48.2%)<br>Lymph node (24.2%)<br>Bone (10.7%)<br>Soft tissue (16.9%) | 92% | VC, SC |
| Yokoyama et al,[75] 2014 | 106 | 56 | Mediastinum (100%) | 96% | VC |
| Cornelis et al,[55] 2014 | 105 | 106 | Bone (31.1%)<br>Liver (24.5%)<br>Soft tissue (17%)<br>Lung (14.1%)<br>Abdominal mass (13.2%) | 94.3% | IP |
| Guralnik et al,[73] 2015 | 311 | 311 | Lung (100%) | 85% | SC |
| Brahmi et al,[68] 2015 | 26 | 26 | Soft tissue (100%) | 96% | VC |

*Abbreviations:* IP, intraprocedural PET/CT; NR, not reported; SC, software coregistration; VC, visual coregistration.
[a] Prospective study.

### *Breast Lesions*

The role of PET-guided biopsies in breast lesions has not been established yet, partly because FDG-PET has been limited because of the lower level of FDG uptake in some breast malignancies, and the small size of most early breast cancers. High-resolution positron emission mammography (PEM) was tested in a small prospective multicenter study designed to test the efficacy and safety of PEM biopsy guidance software in women with FDG-avid breast lesions worrisome for malignancy.[76] Nineteen patients underwent a total of 24 PEM-guided biopsies using vacuum-assisted core biopsy. In this study

- All lesions were successfully sampled
- No serious adverse events occurred
- The procedure caused only minimal to mild discomfort
- Invasive cancer was found in 13 of 24 lesions (54%)
- Four (17%) were high-risk lesions, 3 of which were upgraded to malignancy at excision
- PEM-guided biopsy has an advantage over vacuum-assisted stereotactic biopsy and MR imaging- -guided biopsy because of the ability to alter breast compression in both horizontal and vertical planes

### *Extrathoracic and Miscellaneous Lesions*

One of the first small series on PET/CT-guided abdominal mass biopsies was by Tatli and colleagues,[49] who investigated the feasibility of fusing images from a previously performed PET/CT with a CT being performed at the time of biopsy using specialized software. In this small study, 10 of 13 (76.9%) abdominal masses biopsied with previous PET/CT information were identified as malignant.[49]

A retrospective study by Nguyen and colleagues[77] found that bone and liver lesions had significantly higher likelihood to be malignant when PET was positive (96% and 90%, respectively) as compared with lymph nodes (60%) ($P<.001$). In this study,

- The most common location for FN CT scan was in bone followed by adrenals
- In FDG-avid subcentimeter lymph nodes, PPV was 38%
- More than half of biopsied PET-avid morphologically benign-appearing lesions were malignant
- PET PPV was not significantly affected by history of malignancy

When prospectively testing the technical feasibility, clinical success, and complication rates of intraprocedural PET/CT-guided biopsies on 126 patients (most common biopsy sites: lung, 38.5%; liver, 12.3%; soft tissue, 11.5%; and abdominal mass, 10.0%) in a scanner with a fluoroscopic imaging system, Cerci and colleagues[78] found that:

- 98.5% (n = 128) of PET/CT-positive lesions could be successfully sampled
- Complication rates of 11.5% were very similar to CT-guided procedures[58–60]
- Malignancy diagnosis could be obtained in 21 of 23 lesions that had a nontumoral result after conventional biopsy
- In 23 of the 130 lesions (17.7%), PET/CT was considered crucial in determining the precise biopsy location:
  - Of lesions with no corresponding anatomic abnormality on CT
  - In heterogeneous masses
  - Of lymph nodes in a chain with variable metabolism

Cornelis and colleagues[55] reported a large retrospective series of intraprocedural PET-guided biopsy on 105 patients with 106 lesions using a dedicated interventional PET/CT scanner. The lesions that were biopsied were scattered in the body as seen in **Table 3**. There were

- Comparable complication rates to CT-guided biopsies
- No FN results
- Lower FDG dose used for "in-suite" PET/CT-guided biopsy (222–259 MBq [6–7 mCi] of FDG) in an attempt to limit the cost of the procedure and the radiation exposure

In this study, contrary to what Nguyen and colleagues[77] showed, there was no significant difference in PPV of FDG-PET/CT-guided biopsy for malignancy between the different body locations.[55] This discrepancy however could be related to the major difference in baseline characteristics of the patients included in these studies, as shown in **Table 3**. The main difference was the inclusion of only extrathoracic biopsies in the study by Nguyen and colleagues,[77] whereas the study by Cornelis and colleagues[55] had 14.1% lung biopsies. In comparison, in the retrospective study of Purandare and colleagues,[32] 48.2% of patients had lung biopsies, and FDG-PET/CT-guided biopsies had

- An incremental benefit in 40.7% (22/54) of patients who underwent lung biopsies
- 44.4% (12/27) of patients who underwent lymph node biopsies
- 57.8% (11/19) of patients who underwent soft tissue biopsies

- 66.6% (8/12) of patients who underwent bone biopsies
- An overall incremental benefit seen in 47.3% (53/112 patients)
- All 9 patients who had an FDG-avid area biopsied but no histopathological diagnosis (malignant or inflammatory) was obtained, the lesions were found to be benign with spontaneous resolution of the FDG uptake on follow-up

Similar to Guralnik and colleagues,[73] the highest number of cases with incremental benefit belonged to the category in which the biopsy sample was obtained from the focal hypermetabolic portion of the lesion seen on CT.

Also, in line with Nguyen and colleagues,[77] the incremental benefit of FDG-PET/CT was highest in biopsies performed for bone lesions. The lowest incremental benefit was for lung lesions followed by lymph nodes.[32]

The lowest PPV and accuracy for FDG-PET/CT lung biopsies may be related to the fact that there is less maneuverability when inserting a biopsy needle in the lung, added to the respiratory and motion artifacts, and attempt to complete the biopsy as fast as possible in order to avoid pneumothorax and hemothorax. Avoiding pneumothorax and hemothorax is usually not an issue in bone biopsies. There is also a greater variety of infectious and inflammatory processes that can cause hypermetabolic foci in the lung as compared with the bone. Hypermetabolic lymph nodes are not very specific, which is translated into a lower PPV for PET/CT biopsies.

These results are very helpful in guiding the interventional radiologist to target the areas that potentially harbor the highest yield (ie, in patients with multiple FDG-avid lesions), keeping in mind the risk-benefits when choosing the biopsy site.

There are many limitations to the previously described studies on PET/CT-guided biopsies, including

- Most studies are retrospective in nature with a small number of patients
- Most studies exclude lesions that are either monitored or biopsied openly with surgery
- Most studies include a potential selection and verification bias

## SUMMARY

In view of the heterogeneous nature of cancer, adequate sampling using better guided biopsies can significantly affect the molecular and genomic analysis and therefore lead to a more personalized appropriate treatment.[79,80] Despite the absence of a randomized clinical trial, there is a growing body of evidence demonstrating the added value of PET/CT-guided biopsy over conventional biopsy techniques. In this era of personalized therapy, PET is going to play a bigger role in guidance of percutaneous needle biopsy due to its marked advantage in providing molecular data in comparison to the other imaging modalities. As novel therapeutic agents begin to be routinely introduced with companion biomarkers, which in turn could be coupled with specific radiotracers, it is expected that molecular biomarker testing using PET guidance will become the standard of care.

## REFERENCES


1. Shyn PB. Interventional positron emission tomography/computed tomography: state-of-the-art. Tech Vasc Interv Radiol 2013;16(3):182–90.
2. Samim M, El-Haddad GE, Molenaar IQ, et al. [18F] Fluorodeoxyglucose PET for interventional oncology in liver malignancy. PET Clin 2014;9(4):469–95, vi.
3. Ortega Lopez N. PET/computed tomography in evaluation of transarterial chemoembolization. PET Clin 2015;10(4):507–17.
4. Bonichon F, Godbert Y, Gangi A, et al. PET/computed tomography and thermoablation (radiofrequency, microwave, cryotherapy, laser interstitial thermal therapy). PET Clin 2015;10(4):519–40.
5. Antoch G, Vogt FM, Veit P, et al. Assessment of liver tissue after radiofrequency ablation: findings with different imaging procedures. J Nucl Med 2005; 46(3):520–5.
6. Basu S, Zaidi H, Salavati A, et al. FDG PET/CT methodology for evaluation of treatment response in lymphoma: from "graded visual analysis" and "semiquantitative SUVmax" to global disease burden assessment. Eur J Nucl Med Mol Imaging 2014;41(11):2158–60.
7. Hillner BE, Siegel BA, Liu D, et al. Impact of positron emission tomography/computed tomography and positron emission tomography (PET) alone on expected management of patients with cancer: initial results from the national oncologic PET registry. J Clin Oncol 2008;26(13):2155–61.
8. Marshall D, Laberge JM, Firetag B, et al. The changing face of percutaneous image-guided biopsy: molecular profiling and genomic analysis in current practice. J Vasc Interv Radiol 2013;24(8):1094–103.
9. Bota S, Piscaglia F, Marinelli S, et al. Comparison of international guidelines for noninvasive diagnosis of hepatocellular carcinoma. Liver Cancer 2012; 1(3–4):190–200.
10. Nour-Eldin NE, Alsubhi M, Naguib NN, et al. Risk factor analysis of pulmonary hemorrhage complicating CT-guided lung biopsy in coaxial and non-coaxial

core biopsy techniques in 650 patients. Eur J Radiol 2014;83(10):1945–52.

11. Huch K, Roderer G, Ulmar B, et al. CT-guided interventions in orthopedics. Arch Orthop Trauma Surg 2007;127(8):677–83.
12. Lis E, Bilsky MH, Pisinski L, et al. Percutaneous CT-guided biopsy of osseous lesion of the spine in patients with known or suspected malignancy. AJNR Am J Neuroradiol 2004;25(9):1583–8.
13. Hiraki T, Mimura H, Gobara H, et al. CT fluoroscopy-guided biopsy of 1,000 pulmonary lesions performed with 20-gauge coaxial cutting needles: diagnostic yield and risk factors for diagnostic failure. Chest 2009;136(6):1612–7.
14. Lechevallier E, Andre M, Barriol D, et al. Fine-needle percutaneous biopsy of renal masses with helical CT guidance. Radiology 2000;216(2):506–10.
15. Monfardini L, Preda L, Aurilio G, et al. CT-guided bone biopsy in cancer patients with suspected bone metastases: retrospective review of 308 procedures. Radiol Med 2014;119(11):852–60.
16. Welch TJ, Sheedy PF 2nd, Johnson CD, et al. CT-guided biopsy: prospective analysis of 1,000 procedures. Radiology 1989;171(2):493–6.
17. Shyn PB, Tatli S, Sahni VA, et al. PET/CT-guided percutaneous liver mass biopsies and ablations: targeting accuracy of a single 20 s breath-hold PET acquisition. Clin Radiol 2014;69(4):410–5.
18. Stattaus J, Kuehl H, Ladd S, et al. CT-guided biopsy of small liver lesions: visibility, artifacts, and corresponding diagnostic accuracy. Cardiovasc Intervent Radiol 2007;30(5):928–35.
19. Jung EM, Friedrich C, Hoffstetter P, et al. Volume navigation with contrast enhanced ultrasound and image fusion for percutaneous interventions: first results. PLoS One 2012;7(3):e33956.
20. Maybody M, Stevenson C, Solomon SB. Overview of navigation systems in image-guided interventions. Tech Vasc Interv Radiol 2013;16(3):136–43.
21. Abi-Jaoudeh N, Kobeiter H, Xu S, et al. Image fusion during vascular and nonvascular image-guided procedures. Tech Vasc Interv Radiol 2013;16(3): 168–76.
22. Isasi CR, Lu P, Blaufox MD. A metaanalysis of 18F-2-deoxy-2-fluoro-D-glucose positron emission tomography in the staging and restaging of patients with lymphoma. Cancer 2005;104(5):1066–74.
23. Zijlstra JM, Lindauer-van der Werf G, Hoekstra OS, et al. 18F-fluoro-deoxyglucose positron emission tomography for post-treatment evaluation of malignant lymphoma: a systematic review. Haematologica 2006;91(4):522–9.
24. Spaepen K, Stroobants S, Dupont P, et al. Prognostic value of positron emission tomography (PET) with fluorine-18 fluorodeoxyglucose ([18F] FDG) after first-line chemotherapy in non-Hodgkin's lymphoma: is [18F]FDG-PET a valid alternative to conventional diagnostic methods? J Clin Oncol 2001;19(2):414–9.
25. Margolis DJ, Hoffman JM, Herfkens RJ, et al. Molecular imaging techniques in body imaging. Radiology 2007;245(2):333–56.
26. El-Haddad G, Zhuang H, Gupta N, et al. Evolving role of positron emission tomography in the management of patients with inflammatory and other benign disorders. Semin Nucl Med 2004;34(4):313–29.
27. El-Haddad G, Alavi A, Mavi A, et al. Normal variants in [18F]-fluorodeoxyglucose PET imaging. Radiol Clin North Am 2004;42(6):1063–81, viii.
28. Antoch G, Saoudi N, Kuehl H, et al. Accuracy of whole-body dual-modality fluorine-18-2-fluoro-2-deoxy-D-glucose positron emission tomography and computed tomography (FDG-PET/CT) for tumor staging in solid tumors: comparison with CT and PET. J Clin Oncol 2004;22(21):4357–68.
29. Shin DS, Shon OJ, Byun SJ, et al. Differentiation between malignant and benign pathologic fractures with F-18-fluoro-2-deoxy-D-glucose positron emission tomography/computed tomography. Skeletal Radiol 2008;37(5):415–21.
30. Mahner S, Schirrmacher S, Brenner W, et al. Comparison between positron emission tomography using 2-[fluorine-18]fluoro-2-deoxy-D-glucose, conventional imaging and computed tomography for staging of breast cancer. Ann Oncol 2008;19(7):1249–54.
31. Cerci JJ, Trindade E, Buccheri V, et al. Consistency of FDG-PET accuracy and cost-effectiveness in initial staging of patients with Hodgkin lymphoma across jurisdictions. Clin Lymphoma Myeloma Leuk 2011;11(4):314–20.
32. Purandare NC, Kulkarni AV, Kulkarni SS, et al. 18F-FDG PET/CT-directed biopsy: does it offer incremental benefit? Nucl Med Commun 2013;34(3):203–10.
33. Adams HJ, de Klerk JM, Fijnheer R, et al. Tumor necrosis at FDG-PET is an independent predictor of outcome in diffuse large B-cell lymphoma. Eur J Radiol 2016;85(1):304–9.
34. Riad R, Omar W, Sidhom I, et al. False-positive F-18 FDG uptake in PET/CT studies in pediatric patients with abdominal Burkitt's lymphoma. Nucl Med Commun 2010;31(3):232–8.
35. Tateishi U, Yamaguchi U, Seki K, et al. Glut-1 expression and enhanced glucose metabolism are associated with tumour grade in bone and soft tissue sarcomas: a prospective evaluation by [18F]fluorodeoxyglucose positron emission tomography. Eur J Nucl Med Mol Imaging 2006;33(6):683–91.
36. Fanchon LM, Dogan S, Moreira AL, et al. Feasibility of in situ, high-resolution correlation of tracer uptake with histopathology by quantitative autoradiography of biopsy specimens obtained under 18F-FDG PET/CT guidance. J Nucl Med 2015;56(4):538–44.
37. Gerlinger M, Rowan AJ, Horswell S, et al. Intratumor heterogeneity and branched evolution revealed by

multiregion sequencing. N Engl J Med 2012; 366(10):883–92.
38. Lindstrom LS, Karlsson E, Wilking UM, et al. Clinically used breast cancer markers such as estrogen receptor, progesterone receptor, and human epidermal growth factor receptor 2 are unstable throughout tumor progression. J Clin Oncol 2012; 30(21):2601–8.
39. Leijenaar RT, Nalbantov G, Carvalho S, et al. The effect of SUV discretization in quantitative FDG-PET radiomics: the need for standardized methodology in tumor texture analysis. Sci Rep 2015;5:11075.
40. Gillies RJ, Kinahan PE, Hricak H. Radiomics: images are more than pictures, they are data. Radiology 2016;278(2):563–77.
41. Virayavanich W, Ringler MD, Chin CT, et al. CT-guided biopsy of bone and soft-tissue lesions: role of on-site immediate cytologic evaluation. J Vasc Interv Radiol 2011;22(7):1024–30.
42. Jadvar H. Imaging evaluation of prostate cancer with 18F-fluorodeoxyglucose PET/CT: utility and limitations. Eur J Nucl Med Mol Imaging 2013;40(Suppl 1):S5–10.
43. Bahri H, Laurence L, Edeline J, et al. High prognostic value of 18F-FDG PET for metastatic gastroentero-pancreatic neuroendocrine tumors: a long-term evaluation. J Nucl Med 2014;55(11):1786–90.
44. Memoli JS, El-Bayoumi E, Pastis NJ, et al. Using endobronchial ultrasound features to predict lymph node metastasis in patients with lung cancer. Chest 2011;140(6):1550–6.
45. Tournoy KG, Praet MM, Van Maele G, et al. Esophageal endoscopic ultrasound with fine-needle aspiration with an on-site cytopathologist: high accuracy for the diagnosis of mediastinal lymphadenopathy. Chest 2005;128(4):3004–9.
46. Hoffman JM, Gambhir SS. Molecular imaging: the vision and opportunity for radiology in the future. Radiology 2007;244(1):39–47.
47. Mattes D, Haynor DR, Vesselle H, et al. PET-CT image registration in the chest using free-form deformations. IEEE Trans Med Imaging 2003;22(1):120–8.
48. Slomka PJ. Software approach to merging molecular with anatomic information. J Nucl Med 2004; 45(Suppl 1):36S–45S.
49. Tatli S, Gerbaudo VH, Mamede M, et al. Abdominal masses sampled at PET/CT-guided percutaneous biopsy: initial experience with registration of prior PET/CT images. Radiology 2010;256(1):305–11.
50. Tatli S, Gerbaudo VH, Feeley CM, et al. PET/CT-guided percutaneous biopsy of abdominal masses: initial experience. J Vasc Interv Radiol 2011;22(4): 507–14.
51. Wood BJ, Locklin JK, Viswanathan A, et al. Technologies for guidance of radiofrequency ablation in the multimodality interventional suite of the future. J Vasc Interv Radiol 2007;18(1 Pt 1):9–24.
52. Shekhar R, Walimbe V, Raja S, et al. Automated 3-dimensional elastic registration of whole-body PET and CT from separate or combined scanners. J Nucl Med 2005;46(9):1488–96.
53. Venkatesan AM, Kadoury S, Abi-Jaoudeh N, et al. Real-time FDG PET guidance during biopsies and radiofrequency ablation using multimodality fusion with electromagnetic navigation. Radiology 2011; 260(3):848–56.
54. Abi-Jaoudeh N, Mielekamp P, Noordhoek N, et al. Cone-beam computed tomography fusion and navigation for real-time positron emission tomography-guided biopsies and ablations: a feasibility study. J Vasc Interv Radiol 2012;23(6):737–43.
55. Cornelis F, Silk M, Schoder H, et al. Performance of intra-procedural 18-fluorodeoxyglucose PET/CT-guided biopsies for lesions suspected of malignancy but poorly visualized with other modalities. Eur J Nucl Med Mol Imaging 2014;41(12):2265–72.
56. Wood BJ, Kruecker J, Abi-Jaoudeh N, et al. Navigation systems for ablation. J Vasc Interv Radiol 2010; 21(8 Suppl):S257–63.
57. Klaeser B, Mueller MD, Schmid RA, et al. PET-CT-guided interventions in the management of FDG-positive lesions in patients suffering from solid malignancies: initial experiences. Eur Radiol 2009; 19(7):1780–5.
58. Tomozawa Y, Inaba Y, Yamaura H, et al. Clinical value of CT-guided needle biopsy for retroperitoneal lesions. Korean J Radiol 2011;12(3):351–7.
59. Tsai IC, Tsai WL, Chen MC, et al. CT-guided core biopsy of lung lesions: a primer. AJR Am J Roentgenol 2009;193(5):1228–35.
60. Yamauchi Y, Izumi Y, Nakatsuka S, et al. Diagnostic performance of percutaneous core needle lung biopsy under multi-CT fluoroscopic guidance for ground-glass opacity pulmonary lesions. Eur J Radiol 2011;79(2):e85–9.
61. Hain SF, O'Doherty MJ, Bingham J, et al. Can FDG PET be used to successfully direct preoperative biopsy of soft tissue tumours? Nucl Med Commun 2003;24(11):1139–43.
62. Klaeser B, Wiskirchen J, Wartenberg J, et al. PET/CT-guided biopsies of metabolically active bone lesions: applications and clinical impact. Eur J Nucl Med Mol Imaging 2010;37(11):2027–36.
63. Mankin HJ, Mankin CJ, Simon MA. The hazards of the biopsy, revisited. Members of the Musculoskeletal Tumor Society. J Bone Joint Surg Am 1996; 78(5):656–63.
64. Clasby R, Tilling K, Smith MA, et al. Variable management of soft tissue sarcoma: regional audit with implications for specialist care. Br J Surg 1997; 84(12):1692–6.
65. Evans DG, Baser ME, McGaughran J, et al. Malignant peripheral nerve sheath tumours in neurofibromatosis 1. J Med Genet 2002;39(5):311–4.

66. Rasmussen SA, Yang Q, Friedman JM. Mortality in neurofibromatosis 1: an analysis using U.S. death certificates. Am J Hum Genet 2001;68(5):1110–8.
67. Combemale P, Valeyrie-Allanore L, Giammarile F, et al. Utility of 18F-FDG PET with a semi-quantitative index in the detection of sarcomatous transformation in patients with neurofibromatosis type 1. PLoS One 2014;9(2):e85954.
68. Brahmi M, Thiesse P, Ranchere D, et al. Diagnostic accuracy of PET/CT-guided percutaneous biopsies for malignant peripheral nerve sheath tumors in neurofibromatosis type 1 patients. PLoS One 2015; 10(10):e0138386.
69. Schaefer NG, Strobel K, Taverna C, et al. Bone involvement in patients with lymphoma: the role of FDG-PET/CT. Eur J Nucl Med Mol Imaging 2007; 34(1):60–7.
70. Wang J, Weiss LM, Chang KL, et al. Diagnostic utility of bilateral bone marrow examination: significance of morphologic and ancillary technique study in malignancy. Cancer 2002;94(5):1522–31.
71. Cheng G, Chen W, Chamroonrat W, et al. Biopsy versus FDG PET/CT in the initial evaluation of bone marrow involvement in pediatric lymphoma patients. Eur J Nucl Med Mol Imaging 2011;38(8):1469–76.
72. Pezeshk P, Sadow CA, Winalski CS, et al. Usefulness of 18F-FDG PET-directed skeletal biopsy for metastatic neoplasm. Acad Radiol 2006;13(8): 1011–5.
73. Guralnik L, Rozenberg R, Frenkel A, et al. Metabolic PET/CT-guided lung lesion biopsies: impact on diagnostic accuracy and rate of sampling error. J Nucl Med 2015;56(4):518–22.
74. Bitencourt AG, Tyng CJ, Pinto PN, et al. Percutaneous biopsy based on PET/CT findings in cancer patients: technique, indications, and results. Clin Nucl Med 2012;37(5):e95–97.
75. Yokoyama K, Ikeda O, Kawanaka K, et al. Comparison of CT-guided percutaneous biopsy with and without registration of prior PET/CT images to diagnose mediastinal tumors. Cardiovasc Intervent Radiol 2014;37(5):1306–11.
76. Kalinyak JE, Schilling K, Berg WA, et al. PET-guided breast biopsy. Breast J 2011;17(2):143–51.
77. Nguyen ML, Gervais DA, Blake MA, et al. Imaging-guided biopsy of (18)F-FDG-avid extrapulmonary lesions: do lesion location and morphologic features on CT affect the positive predictive value for malignancy? AJR Am J Roentgenol 2013;201(2):433–8.
78. Cerci JJ, Pereira Neto CC, Krauzer C, et al. The impact of coaxial core biopsy guided by FDG PET/CT in oncological patients. Eur J Nucl Med Mol Imaging 2013;40(1):98–103.
79. Kim ES, Herbst RS, Wistuba II, et al. The BATTLE trial: personalizing therapy for lung cancer. Cancer Discov 2011;1(1):44–53.
80. Wistuba II, Gelovani JG, Jacoby JJ, et al. Methodological and practical challenges for personalized cancer therapies. Nat Rev Clin Oncol 2011;8(3): 135–41.
81. Kobayashi K, Bhargava P, Raja S, et al. Image-guided biopsy: what the interventional radiologist needs to know about PET/CT. Radiographics 2012; 32(5):1483–501.

# PET-Based Personalized Management of Infectious and Inflammatory Disorders

Søren Hess, MD[a,b,c,*], Abass Alavi, MD[d], Sandip Basu, DRM, DNB, MNAMS[e]

**KEYWORDS**

• FDG • PET/CT • Infection • Inflammation • Infectious disease • Inflammatory disorders

**KEY POINTS**

- PET/computed tomography (CT) is increasingly acknowledged and used in infectious and inflammatory diseases despite the generally rather limited and heterogeneous literature.
- Accurate diagnoses are paramount to tailor treatment toward a more timely, ecological, cost-effective, and specific use of antibiotic and antiinflammatory treatment strategies.
- The most well-established indications include systemic infection/inflammation, chronic bone infections, vascular graft infections, and large vessel vasculitis.
- Less well-established indications include sarcoidosis, inflammatory bowel disease, tuberculosis, diabetic foot, and general response evaluation.
- Potential new applications include chronic obstructive pulmonary disorder, rheumatoid arthritis, psoriasis, venous thromboembolism, and other vasculitides than large vessels, and atherosclerosis.

## INTRODUCTION

The use of PET/computed tomography (CT) for infectious and inflammatory disorders is increasing internationally. These diseases are characterized by being highly heterogeneous and they are managed by several different medical specialties, which makes consensus on the diagnostic pathways all the more challenging. At present, the evidence is rather limited and PET/CT is only scarcely mentioned in clinical guidelines. Nonetheless, the role of PET/CT is increasingly important in the clinical handling of these diseases, which are often characterized by nonspecific symptoms and findings that often lead to a multitude of examinations, tests, and imaging in the diagnostic workup. The key is the nonspecific traits of fluorodeoxyglucose (FDG), which leads to high sensitivity for both infectious and inflammatory foci; thus, FDG-PET/CT may be the lead-in investigation that provides guidance for further, more or less specific evaluation. Conversely, the high negative predictive value is of great clinical importance to

Disclosure Statement: The authors have nothing to disclose.

[a] Department of Nuclear Medicine, Odense University Hospital, Sdr. Boulevard 29, Odense 5000, Denmark; [b] Division of Nuclear Medicine, Department of Radiology and Nuclear Medicine, Hospital of South West Jutland, Finsensgade 10, Esbjerg 6700, Denmark; [c] Department of Clinical Research, Faculty of Health Sciences, University of Southern Denmark, Winsløwparken 19, 3, Odense 5000, Denmark; [d] Division of Nuclear Medicine, Department of Radiology, Hospital of the University of Pennsylvania, University of Pennsylvania Perelman School of Medicine, 3400 Civic Center Boulevard, Building 421, Philadelphia, PA 19104, USA; [e] Radiation Medicine Center (BARC), Tata Memorial Hospital Annexe, E. Borges Marg, Parel, Mumbai-400012, India
* Corresponding author. Department of Nuclear Medicine, Odense University Hospital, Sdr. Boulevard 29, Odense, Denmark.
*E-mail address:* Soeren.hess@rsyd.dk

PET Clin 11 (2016) 351–361
http://dx.doi.org/10.1016/j.cpet.2016.02.008

rule out disease in settings of suspected infectious, inflammatory, or malignant disease.[1–3]

In general, the available literature is as heterogeneous as the diseases themselves and is dominated by small series and only few systematic reviews and metaanalyses. The evidence is still being mounted at this point, and several unclarified issues remain. In this paper, we outline contemporary use and potential future applications of FDG-PET/CT in the infectious and inflammatory realm with a focus on personalized medicine aspects. The aim of this paper is not to provide exhaustive evidence for the diagnosis of infections and inflammation, but rather to outline overall results from the current literature.

## DIAGNOSIS

On might argue that mere diagnosis of infectious and inflammatory diseases is not personalized enough to constitute the concept. On the other hand, the therapeutic strategies in early stages of infection are usually relatively empirically and comprise a rather broad-spectrum regimen. Accurate diagnosis is paramount for tailoring treatment toward earlier institution of more specific regimens.

### *Systemic Infections*

The clinical entity fever of unknown origin constitutes a heterogeneous multitude of very different disorders, although they can generally be divided according to etiologic origin into malignancies, infections, and inflammatory disorders, all of which are characterized by some degree of FDG avidity (**Fig. 1**). Conversely, the sensitivity also gives rise to potentially high negative predictive value, which may be equally important in different settings of fever, for example, suspected recurrence of tuberculosis (**Fig. 2**).

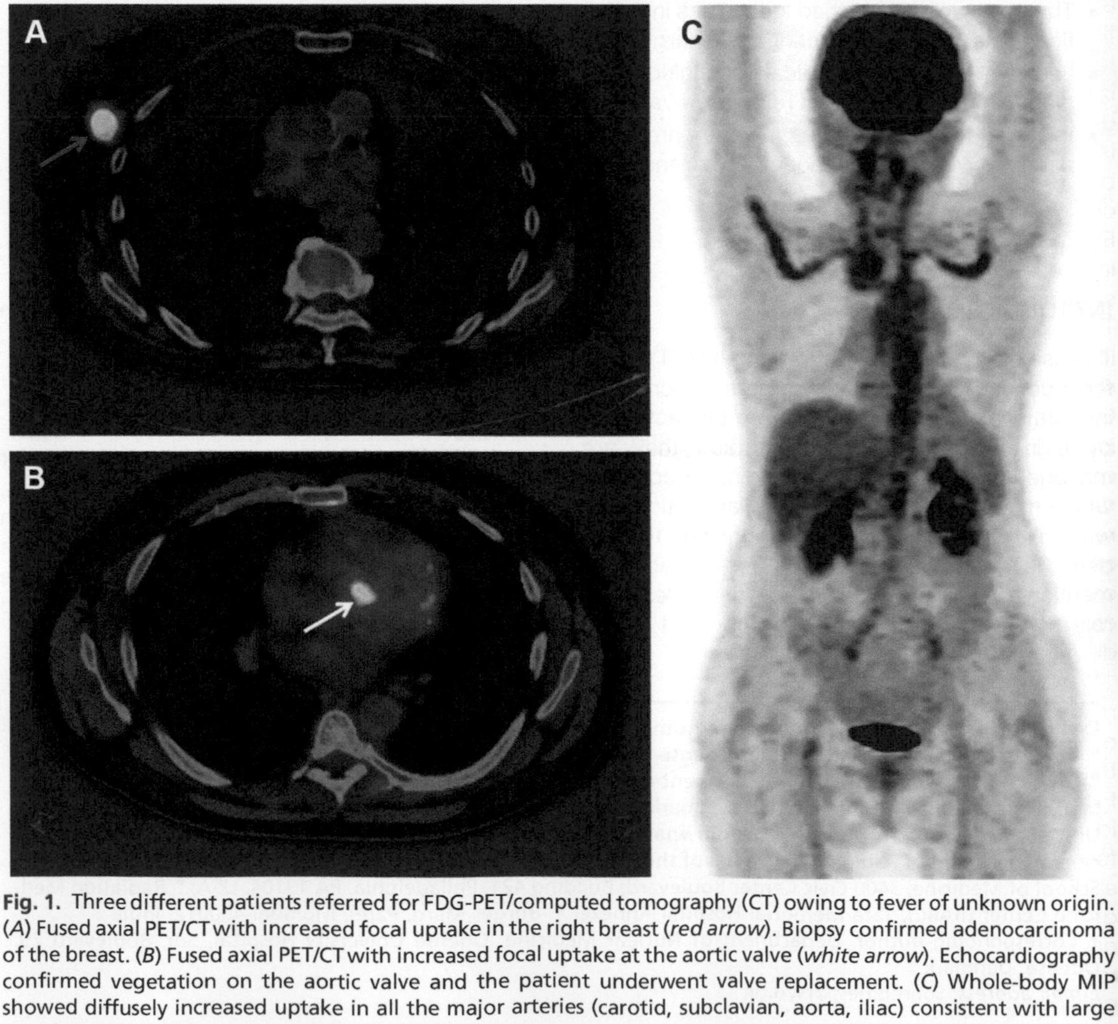


**Fig. 1.** Three different patients referred for FDG-PET/computed tomography (CT) owing to fever of unknown origin. (*A*) Fused axial PET/CT with increased focal uptake in the right breast (*red arrow*). Biopsy confirmed adenocarcinoma of the breast. (*B*) Fused axial PET/CT with increased focal uptake at the aortic valve (*white arrow*). Echocardiography confirmed vegetation on the aortic valve and the patient underwent valve replacement. (*C*) Whole-body MIP showed diffusely increased uptake in all the major arteries (carotid, subclavian, aorta, iliac) consistent with large vessel vasculitis. MIP, maximum intensity projection.

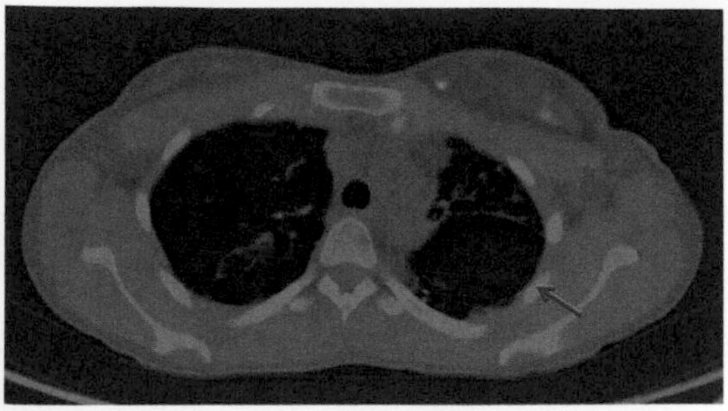

**Fig. 2.** Patient with fever and general malaise. She was treated for tuberculosis (TB) 6 years prior and recurrence was suspected. Fused axial PET/computed tomography scan revealed a chronic cavernous lung lesion but no pathologic FDG-uptake (*red arrow*), and recurrent TB was ruled out. There was diffuse uptake in her breast owing to lactation. The patient recovered spontaneously.

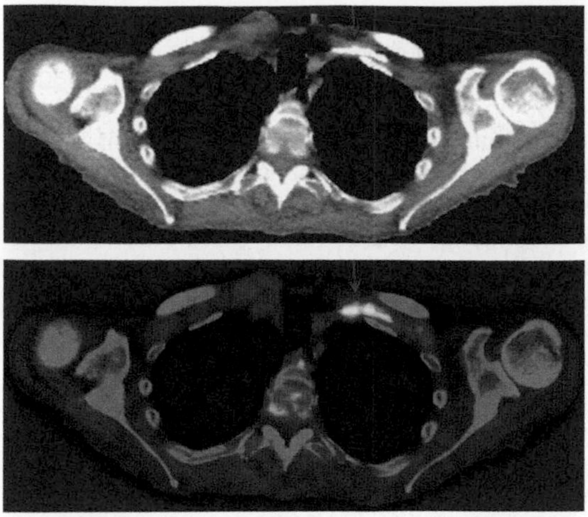

**Fig. 3.** Patient with bacteremia of unknown origin. Axial computed tomography (CT; *upper*) and fused axial PET/CT (*lower*) revealed increased uptake along the pace electrode (*red arrows*). The electrode was replaced and microbiologic culture was positive for *Staphylococcus aureus*.

Currently, the diagnostic pathways for each patient is highly influenced by their entrance in the health care system and as such often characterized by a heterogeneous, extensive, and to some degree arbitrary diagnostic workup. The literature is mounting, although still relatively sparse and based on smaller series with high variable methodologies. However, overall results show that FDG-PET/CT contributes with clinically relevant information in 42% to 92% of cases, which is substantially higher than any other modality.[2–4] Two metaanalyses have evaluated the available literature (including older techniques such as stand-alone PET as well as contemporary PET/CT) and have found pooled sensitivities for locating the underlying disease in 86% to 98% of cases.[5,6] Thus, although there are no randomized, prospective studies, it seems reasonable based on current evidence to conclude that a final diagnosis can be reached earlier and with a more limited diagnostic process for any given patient if FDG-PET/CT is introduced early.

In bacteremia of unknown origin/suspected metastatic infection (**Fig. 3**), only a few case reports and smaller series are available, but they have all shown high clinical impact of FDG-PET/CT findings (eg, change of therapy or identification of clinically relevant additional foci) in about one-half of the patients initially evaluated by conventional diagnostics.[3,7,8] One group has also shown that early FDG-PET/CT can actually be cost effective owing to lower recurrence rate and lower mortality because targeted therapy can be instituted earlier.[9] The diagnostic yield of FDG-PET/CT has also been found favorable in more specialized settings such as immunocompromised patients with human immunodeficiency virus infection, febrile neutropenia, or critically ill intensive care patients.[3]

The use of FDG and PET/CT in endocarditis is controversial and many aspects are still unclarified including the issue of physiologic FDG uptake in the heart. The literature is characterized by many case reports and studies with suboptimal methodology, including the lack of stringent reference standard. Generally, FDG-PET/CT can be considered an important adjunct in equivocal cases based on clinical findings and echocardiography especially in patients with valve prostheses and other cardiac devices. The strength of FDG-PET/CT is especially related to extracardiac disease, because septic emboli and metastatic infection tend to change patient management toward a more aggressive approach, and in this regard the potential of response evaluation as well as the high negative predictive value has been highlighted.[2,10]

## *Bone-Related Infections*

FDG-PET/CT has no significant place in acute osteomyelitis, although FDG has a sensitivity of greater than 95% and specificity of 75% to 99%, there is only limited added value compared with conventional imaging.[11] For chronic osteomyelitis, however, FDG-PET/CT has been found with consistently robust sensitivity and specificity; that is, in a metaanalysis sensitivity and specificity were 96% and 91%, respectively, which was clearly superior to MR imaging (84% and 60%, respectively), and with the highest accuracy.[12] Similarly, a more recent metaanalysis found pooled sensitivity and specificity of 92%, which was also significantly better than conventional radioisotope methods, that is, bone scintigraphy (83% and 45%, respectively), and leukocyte scintigraphy (74% and 88%, respectively).[13]

In the subset of spondylodiscitis, FDG-PET/CT should probably be the method of choice with superior sensitivity compared with MR imaging (>90% vs 50%) and comparable specificity (~90%); One metaanalysis has found pooled sensitivity and specificity of 97% and 88%, respectively. Furthermore, FDG-PET/CT is best for distinguishing degenerative changes from disc infection in patients presenting with back pain, and the results of FDG-PET/CT is not as influenced by metallic implants as other modalities, especially in more chronic settings apart from the immediate postoperative period.[11,14]

The choice of radioisotope imaging for suspected infection of prosthetic joints remains controversial, but recent years have pointed toward FDG-PET/CT as possible first choice. In general, sensitivity is good, whereas specificity is more moderate; the greatest sensitivity is found in knee prostheses, whereas the highest specificity is found in hip prostheses. Thus, the diagnostic accuracy ranges from 78% to 100% in knee prostheses and 68% to 100% in hip prostheses, and 2 metaanalyses have found pooled sensitivities and specificities of 86%.[11,15,16]

### *Vascular Infections*

Infections in vascular prostheses are relatively rare, but potentially severe diagnoses that carry substantial morbidity and mortality. In the early postoperative phase, CT is probably the first choice with both sensitivity and specificity of greater than 95% in patients with high clinical suspicion. However, in late, chronic, or low-grade infections, the sensitivity of CT is much less convincing (~55%), whereas PET demonstrates higher sensitivity than CT. The first study comparing stand-alone PET with CT found sensitivity and specificity of 91% and 64% for PET versus 64% and 86%, respectively, for CT. Combined PET/CT has provided better results with overall sensitivity and specificity of 78% to 100% and 70% to 93%, respectively, although only in smaller series.[17] Improved diagnostic criteria can probably further enhance the diagnostic value; thus, one study accomplished a positive predictive value of 97% and an overall accuracy of greater than 95% in three-quarters of nonacute cases with low-grade infections.[18]

### *Inflammatory Disorders*

Large vessel vasculitis is the most well-established indication among the inflammatory disorders with overall sensitivity and specificity of 77% to 92% and 89% to 100%, respectively, in treatment-naïve patients with increased inflammatory markers. A recent metaanalysis found pooled sensitivity and specificity for giant cell arteritis of 90% and 98%, respectively. PET/CT is generally more sensitive than MR imaging for early diagnosis, evaluation of disease extent, and assessment of treatment response.[2,17,19]

## POTENTIAL NOVEL APPLICATIONS

The multitude of inflammatory disorders has given rise to a multitude of potential applications for FDG and PET. These indications may be divided into those with some evidence, whereas some are more speculative, and some are even still theoretic. Hence, the literature on inflammatory diseases is limited and as heterogeneous as the diseases, but some results have been promising and warrant further investigations. However, as with infectious disease, the results are still limited with regard to personalized settings outside the realm of mere diagnosis, and so, this discussion is not an exhaustive account of indications and evidence, but an overview of those indications closest to the concept of personalized medicine.

One such indication is sarcoidosis (**Fig. 4**): PET/CT finds more disease foci than CT, and although this may not in itself be that important, it may delineate alternative, more easily accessible biopsy sites in the initial workup so the patient may be spared more invasive procedures, like bronchoscopy. Some studies have also suggested a place in response evaluation as the usual markers for active sarcoidosis may be normal in up to 75% of patients with active sarcoidosis demonstrated by PET. In one study of disease activity, there was only concordance between CT and PET/CT in one-half of the patients, and FDG-PET/CT impacted patient management in 95% of discordant cases. Also, in more specialized settings may FDG and PET/CT impact patient management significantly, for

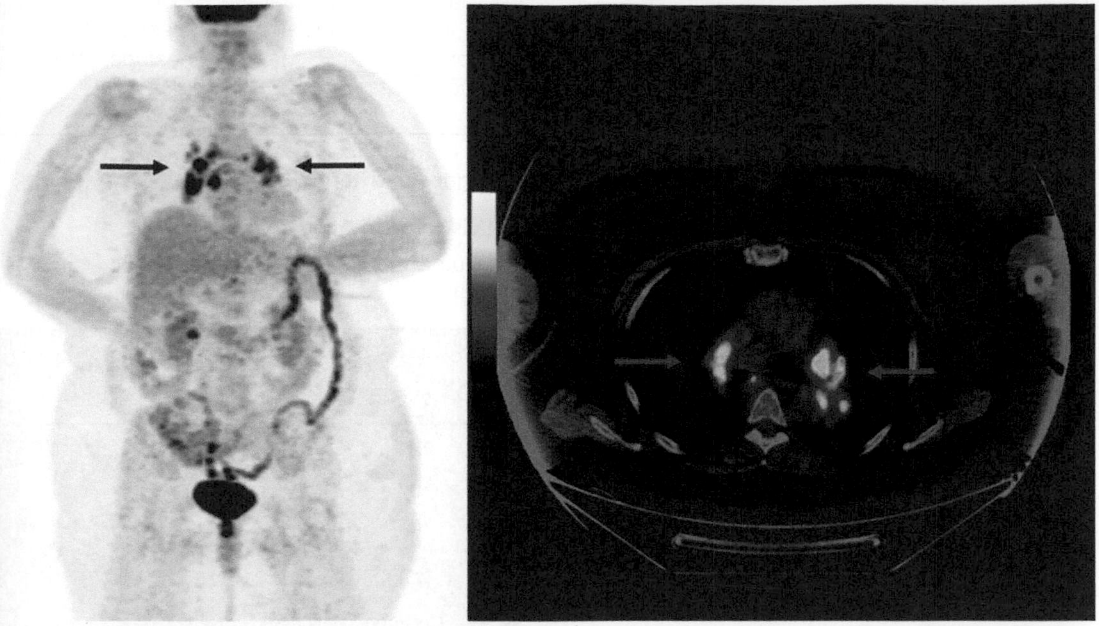

Fig. 4. Sarcoidosis. MIP PET image (*left*) and fused axial PET/computed tomography image (*right*) show intense FDG uptake in mediastinal and hilar lymph nodes bilaterally (*arrows*). Subsequent biopsy confirmed granulomatous inflammation consistent with sarcoidosis, and the patient responded clinically to relevant treatment. MIP, maximum intensity projection. (*From* Hess S, Hansson SH, Pedersen KT, et al. FDG-PET/CT in infectious and inflammatory diseases. PET Clin 2014;9(4):508; with permission.)

example, cardiac sarcoidosis, a potentially life-threatening condition that may be severely underdiagnosed. Thus, a recent metaanalysis found pooled sensitivity and specificity of FDG-PET/CT for cardiac sarcoidosis of 89% and 78%, respectively, whereas the corresponding numbers for the usual clinical criteria (the current gold standard) were 33% and 97%, respectively.[2,20–22]

Similar indications are found in inflammatory bowel disease, that is, Crohn's disease and ulcerative colitis (**Fig. 5**). The diagnostic mainstay is endoscopy, but especially in children, less invasive strategies are desirable, not the least because general anesthesia may be necessary in this setting. Again, FDG and PET have been able to delineate disease extent to help differentiate the two disease entities in indeterminate cases, and help to monitor response to treatment. The latter is especially important because the antiinflammatory drugs used may have widespread systemic side effects not least in children, and the novel biologic treatments are furthermore very expensive. Thus, recognizing treatment failure at the earliest possible is paramount for patient morbidity and health economics. A special challenge is the differentiation of stenotic bowl lesions in Crohn's disease; they may be either inflammatory or fibrostenotic, and the treatment strategy is profoundly different because the former should be managed by optimized antiinflammatory treatment, whereas the latter requires surgery. Two recent meta-analyses found overall pooled sensitivity and specificity of FDG-PET of 84% to 85% and 86% to 87%, respectively, on per-segment–based analyses.[23–26]

Proper response evaluation is not only prudent in inflammatory disorders, but also in some infectious diseases, especially those that require long-term treatment (eg, spondylitis) (**Figs. 6** and **7**), and those with systemic propagation (eg, tuberculosis). This is not only important for the individual patients' treatment regime but also on a more global scale to combat the increasing drug resistance problems. In spondylitis, there is little doubt that FDG and PET/CT is superior to MR imaging for early assessment of response. This may have significant impact on patient management since intravenous therapy that require expensive in-patient care may be substituted with oral antibiotics in a much cheaper out-patient setting at an earlier time if there is a proper early response. However, at

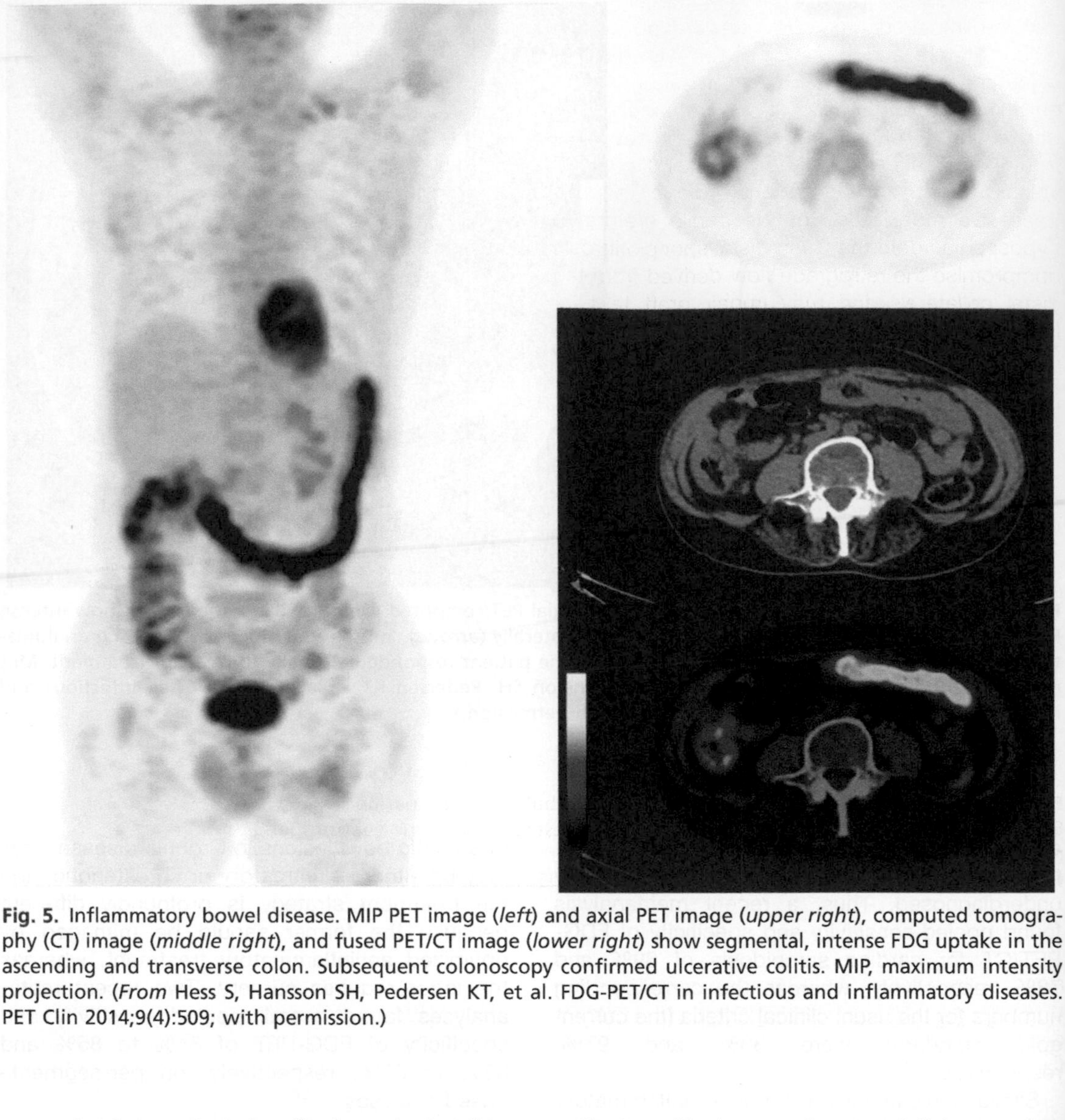

**Fig. 5.** Inflammatory bowel disease. MIP PET image (*left*) and axial PET image (*upper right*), computed tomography (CT) image (*middle right*), and fused PET/CT image (*lower right*) show segmental, intense FDG uptake in the ascending and transverse colon. Subsequent colonoscopy confirmed ulcerative colitis. MIP, maximum intensity projection. (*From* Hess S, Hansson SH, Pedersen KT, et al. FDG-PET/CT in infectious and inflammatory diseases. PET Clin 2014;9(4):509; with permission.)

present only one study has firmly evaluated this; Nanni and colleagues found changes in maximum standardized uptake values from baseline scan to interim scans to be a significantly better marker for response than changes in C-reactive protein. Similar results have been presented in skeletal tuberculosis, with significant decreases in maximum standardized uptake values or clearly decreased uptake visually between baseline scans and sequential scans during and after treatment, although again only in case reports and smaller series.[27–30] The application for response assessment in tuberculosis has been especially suggested for extrapulmonary tuberculosis,[30,31] but has also been extended to more specialized setting such as tuberculous pericarditis,[32] patients with human immunodeficiency virus and tuberculosis,[33,34] and for the evaluation of novel drugs for multidrug-resistant tuberculosis.[35]

In addition to the indications discussed, which are all to some extent supported by evidence and implemented in clinical practice, the use of FDG and PET/CT in a whole array of inflammatory diseases is currently under scrutiny and the final role of FDG in these settings remains to be seen. Nonetheless, the investigations generate some interesting insights into the diseases and may point toward future applications.

For instance, in chronic obstructive pulmonary disorder, FDG uptake patterns may enhance our pathophysiologic understanding as different

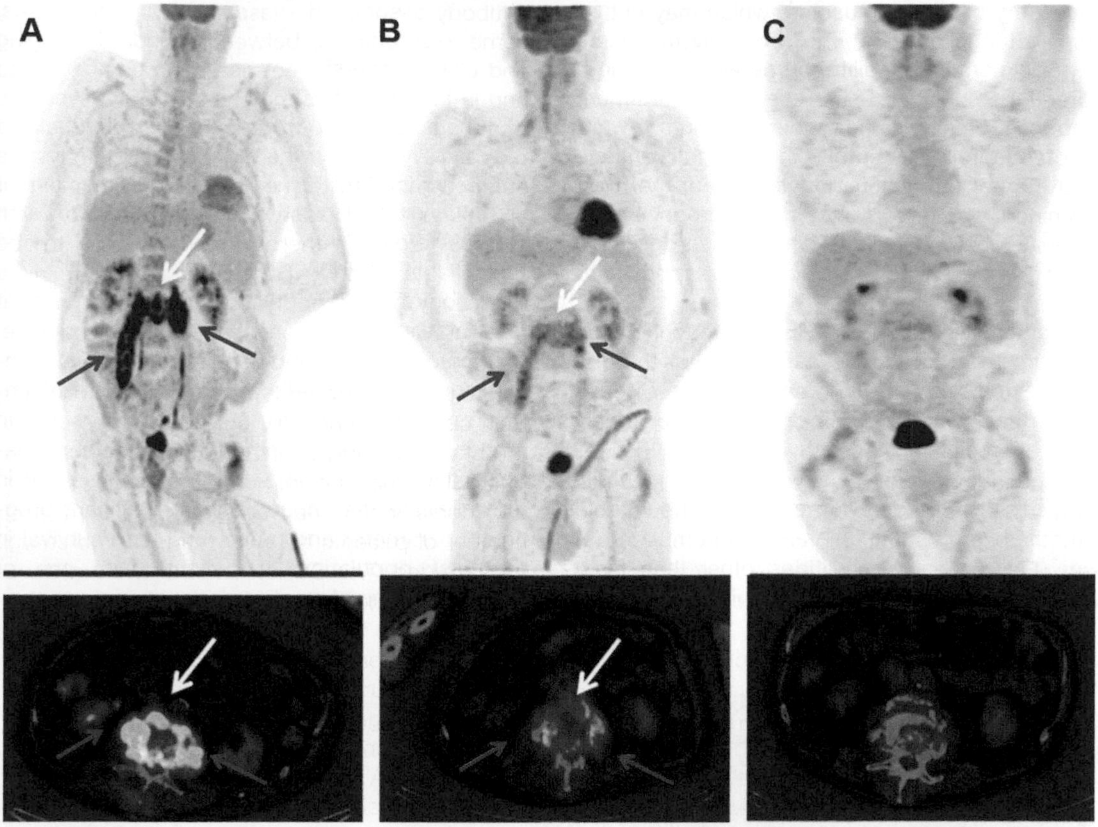


**Fig. 6.** Response evaluation of spondylitis at baseline (*A*), after 3 weeks of intravenous antibiotics (*B*), and 6 months after baseline (*C*). Whole body maximum intensity projection (*upper*) and fused axial PET/CT (*lower*) revealed severely increased uptake in the 3rd lumbar vertebra (*white arrows*) and both psoas muscles (*red arrows*) with significant decrease after 3 weeks and almost normalized uptake after 6 months.

regional patterns in different phenotypes have been suggested. Thus, FDG may be able to distinguish inflammatory phenotypes from noninflammatory ones, which could have profound impact on future patient selection and management, for example, lung volume reduction or antiinflammatory regimes. This may also be the case with the assessment of FDG uptake in

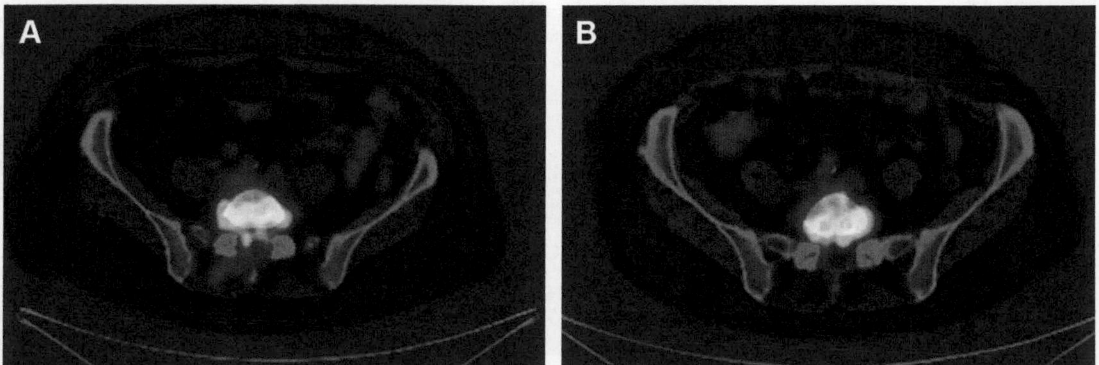


**Fig. 7.** Response evaluation of spondylitis at baseline (*A*), and after 3 weeks of intravenous antibiotics (*B*). Fused axial PET/computed tomography revealed severely increased uptake in the fifth lumbar vertebra with no significant changes after 3 weeks.

accessory breathing muscles, which may in turn help to triage patients who are likely to benefit from pulmonary rehabilitation as well as being a potential surrogate marker for treatment response. Finally, some evidence points toward a potential for FDG uptake in the right ventricle as a marker for cor pulmonale, one of the most prominent predictors of poor prognosis in chronic obstructive pulmonary disorder, and again a possibility to monitor response to treatment.[36,37]

In other disorders, FDG-PET/CT may increase our knowledge of the disease course or the disease extent by showing evidence of disease earlier than usual or areas of disease not otherwise appreciated. As such, FDG and PET/CT may provide the only way of assessing whole body disease burden, for example, rheumatoid arthritis, psoriasis (**Fig. 8**), venous thromboembolism (**Fig. 9**), and vasculitides other than large vessel ones (eg, antineutrophil cytoplasmic antibody-associated vasculitis). In all cases, some discordance between standard imaging and clinical assessment has been demonstrated and in the future this may help to direct systemic treatment strategy toward more individualized regimens.[2,17,38] Furthermore, there may be another important issue in many (if not most or all) inflammatory disorders; the association with atherosclerosis. Atherosclerosis seems to be quantifiable with FDG-PET not only in a cardiology-based population,[39–42] but it has at present also has been shown in, for instance, rheumatoid arthritis and psoriasis.[43–45] Early identification of increased systemic vascular inflammation may lead to a paradigm shift in preventive strategies aimed against atherosclerosis in these clinical settings, and this may in turn alleviate the impact of this significant prognostic parameter and better long-term survival in the vast population of patients with one or another inflammatory disorder.

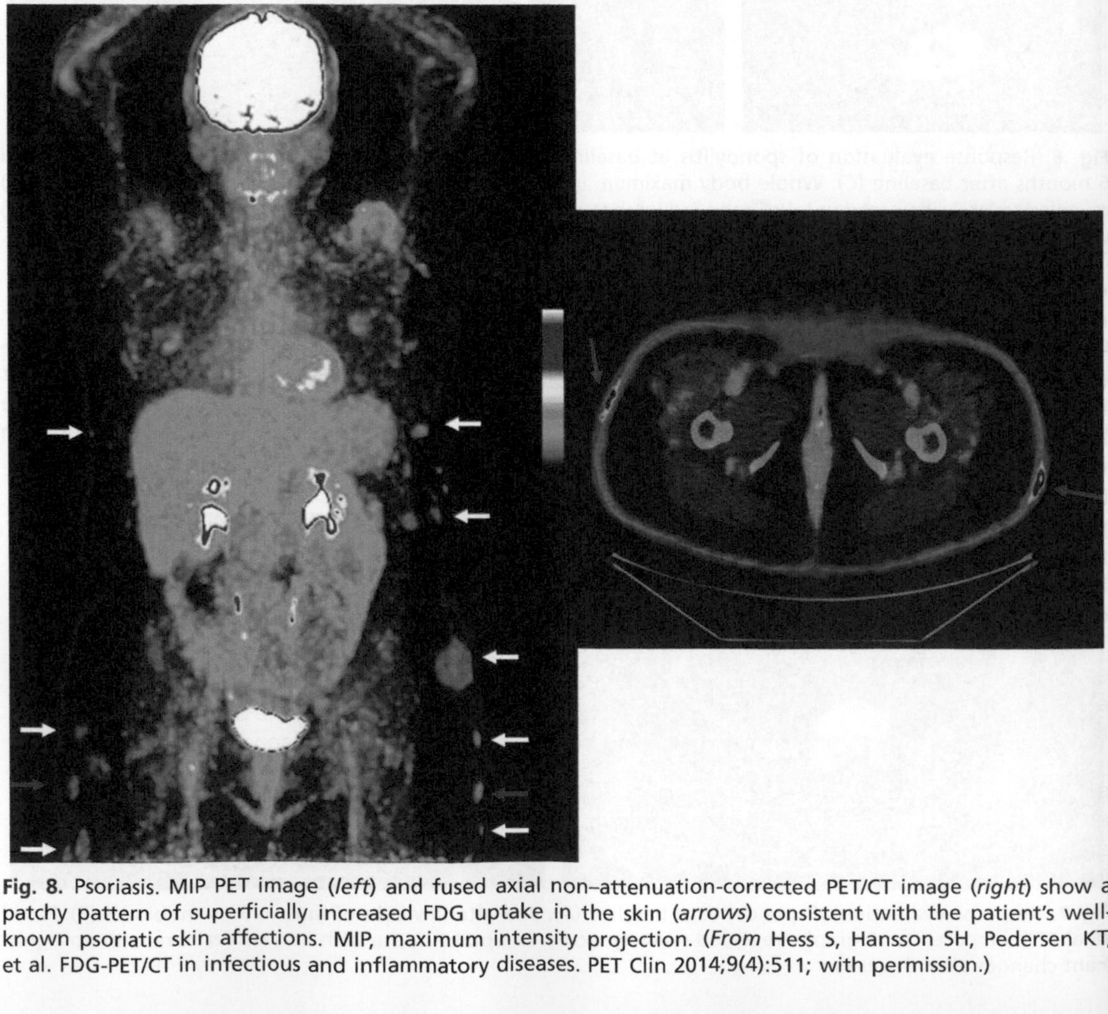

**Fig. 8.** Psoriasis. MIP PET image (*left*) and fused axial non–attenuation-corrected PET/CT image (*right*) show a patchy pattern of superficially increased FDG uptake in the skin (*arrows*) consistent with the patient's well-known psoriatic skin affections. MIP, maximum intensity projection. (*From* Hess S, Hansson SH, Pedersen KT, et al. FDG-PET/CT in infectious and inflammatory diseases. PET Clin 2014;9(4):511; with permission.)

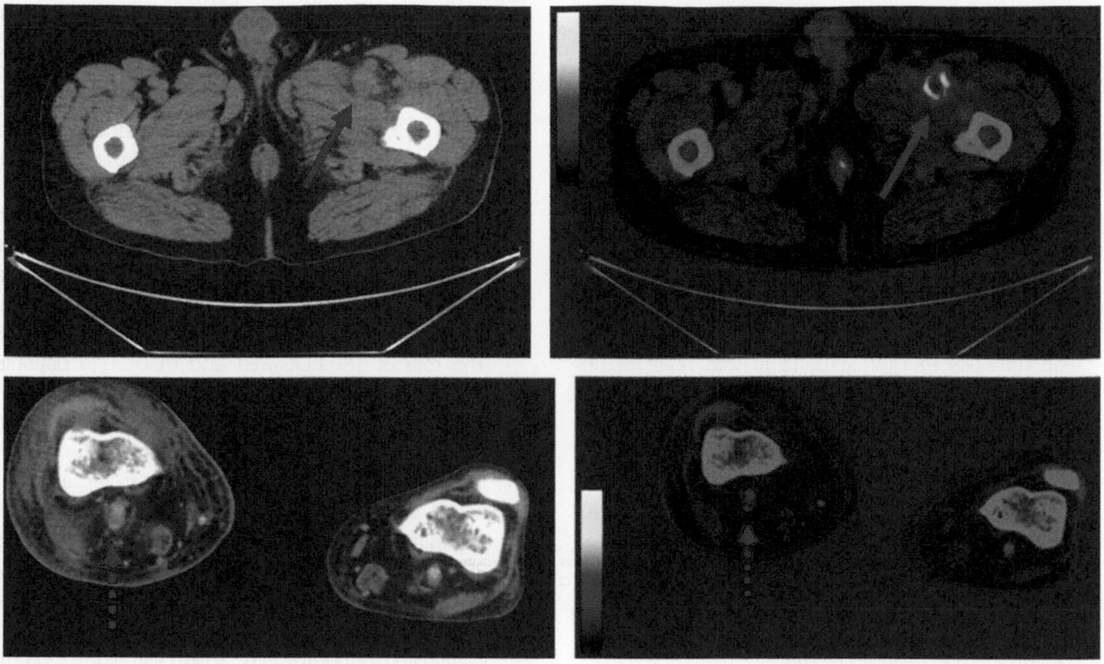

**Fig. 9.** Venous thromboembolism. Upper row shows axial computed tomography (CT) image (*left*) and fused axial PET/CT image (*right*) in a patient with confirmed acute deep venous thrombosis (DVT) with a short history. There is increased FDG uptake circumferentially in the dilated left femoral vein (*solid arrows*) consistent with acute, active inflammation. Lower row shows axial CT image (*left*) and fused axial PET/CT image (*right*) in a patient with a history of prior DVT but no current symptoms. There is no FDG uptake in the dilated right popliteal vein (*dotted arrows*) but stranding on CT consistent with prior (old) DVT without active inflammation. (*From* Hess S, Hansson SH, Pedersen KT, et al. FDG-PET/CT in infectious and inflammatory diseases. PET Clin 2014;9(4):513; with permission.)

## SUMMARY

The diagnoses of infectious and inflammatory diseases are challenging owing to the relative nonspecific symptoms and the often systemic disease patterns. Imaging plays an integral role and FDG-PET/CT is now being increasingly used in these settings owing to its highly sensitive, whole body approach. The initial treatment strategy in infectious diseases is often based on relatively broad spectrum drugs and a culprit lesion is pivotal in ensuring a more specific personalized treatment. This is not only important from the patient perspective, but also from an ecologic point of view in a world of increasing drug resistance. This is also true for the assessment of treatment success, an early realization of therapeutic failure enables the switch to alternative treatments to the benefit of patient and society alike.

Molecular imaging holds great promise in these settings owing to its sensitivity and whole body approach—culprit lesions, systemic components, and even hitherto unrecognized relations and findings can be accurately and timely assessed in a single scan. At present the literature is still relatively sparse, but evidence for the efficacy of FDG-PET/CT is mounting in several domains, such as the search for culprit lesions in systemic infections and inflammations (eg, fever or bacteremia of unknown origin and tuberculosis), the diagnosis and extent of vascular inflammation, and therapy monitoring in bone infections. In several other clinical settings, for example, sarcoidosis, inflammatory bowel disease, and rheumatoid arthritis, FDG-PET/CT has generated interesting results with potential for clinical implementation and is currently being investigated further. The preceding decades have seen tremendous developments in the use of molecular imaging in oncology, but we expect the coming decade to be centered on inflammation and we expect FDG and PET/CT to become the first-line modality in a multitude of infectious and inflammatory diseases.

## REFERENCES

1. Hess S, Blomberg BA, Zhu HJ, et al. The pivotal role of FDG-PET/CT in modern medicine. Acad Radiol 2014;21(2):232–49.
2. Hess S, Hansson SH, Pedersen KT, et al. FDG-PET/CT in infectious and inflammatory diseases. PET Clin 2014;9(4):497–519, vi–vii.

3. Hess S, Brøndserud MB, Jakobsen NM. FDG-PET/CT for systemic infections. Curr Mol Imaging 2015; 3(3):182–90.
4. Bleeker-Rovers CP, Vos FJ, de Kleijn EM, et al. A prospective multicenter study on fever of unknown origin: the yield of a structured diagnostic protocol. Medicine (Baltimore) 2007;86(1):26–38.
5. Dong MJ, Zhao K, Liu ZF, et al. A meta-analysis of the value of fluorodeoxyglucose-PET/PET-CT in the evaluation of fever of unknown origin. Eur J Radiol 2011;80(3):834–44.
6. Hao R, Yuan L, Kan Y, et al. Diagnostic performance of 18F-FDG PET/CT in patients with fever of unknown origin: a meta-analysis. Nucl Med Commun 2013;34(7):682–8.
7. Hess S, Vind SH, Skarphédinsson S. Clinical value of PET/CT in bacteraemia of unknown origin. Results from an observational pilot study. Eur J Nucl Med Mol Imaging 2010;37(Suppl 2):1.
8. Brøndserud MB, Hess S, Petersen C. The clinical value of FDG-PET/CT in bacteraemia of unknown origin: a retrospective study. Eur J Nucl Med Mol Imaging 2015;42(Suppl 1):S789.
9. Vos FJ, Bleeker-Rovers CP, Kullberg BJ, et al. Cost-effectiveness of routine (18)F-FDG PET/CT in high-risk patients with gram-positive bacteremia. J Nucl Med 2011;52(11):1673–8.
10. Rewers KI, Scholtens AM, Thomassen A. The role of 18F-FDG-PET/CT in infective endocarditis and cardiac device infection. Curr Mol Imaging 2015;3(3): 216–24.
11. Basu S, Kwee TC, Hess S. FDG-PET/CT imaging of infected bones and prosthetic joints. Curr Mol Imaging 2014;3(3):225–9.
12. Termaat MF, Raijmakers PG, Scholten HJ, et al. The accuracy of diagnostic imaging for the assessment of chronic osteomyelitis: a systematic review and meta-analysis. J Bone Joint Surg Am 2005;87(11):2464–71.
13. Wang GL, Zhao K, Liu ZF, et al. A meta-analysis of fluorodeoxyglucose-positron emission tomography versus scintigraphy in the evaluation of suspected osteomyelitis. Nucl Med Commun 2011;32(12): 1134–42.
14. Prodromou ML, Ziakas PD, Poulou LS, et al. FDG PET is a robust tool for the diagnosis of spondylodiscitis: a meta-analysis of diagnostic data. Clin Nucl Med 2014;39(4):330–5.
15. Jin H, Yuan L, Li C, et al. Diagnostic performance of FDG PET or PET/CT in prosthetic infection after arthroplasty: a meta-analysis. Q J Nucl Med Mol Imaging 2014;58(1):85–93.
16. Kwee TC, Kwee RM, Alavi A, et al. FDG-PET for diagnosing prosthetic joint infection: systematic review and metaanalysis. Eur J Nucl Med Mol Imaging 2008;35(11):2122–32.
17. Gholami S, Fardin S, Houshmand S. Applications of FDG-PET/CT in assessment of vascular infection and inflammation. Curr Mol Imaging 2014;3(3): 230–9.
18. Spacek M, Belohlavek O, Votrubova J, et al. Diagnostics of "non-acute" vascular prosthesis infection using 18F-FDG PET/CT: our experience with 96 prostheses. Eur J Nucl Med Mol Imaging 2009; 36(5):850–8.
19. Soussan M, Nicolas P, Schramm C, et al. Management of large-vessel vasculitis with FDG-PET: a systematic literature review and meta-analysis. Medicine (Baltimore) 2015;94(14):e622.
20. Treglia G, Annunziata S, Sobic-Saranovic D, et al. The role of 18F-FDG-PET and PET/CT in patients with sarcoidosis: an updated evidence-based review. Acad Radiol 2014;21(5):675–84.
21. Youssef G, Leung E, Mylonas I, et al. The use of 18F-FDG PET in the diagnosis of cardiac sarcoidosis: a systematic review and metaanalysis including the Ontario experience. J Nucl Med 2012;53(2):241–8.
22. Basu S, Asopa RV, Baghel NS, et al. Early documentation of therapeutic response at 6 weeks following corticosteroid therapy in extensive sarcoidosis: promise of FDG-PET. Clin Nucl Med 2009;34(10):689–90.
23. Christlieb SB, Hess S, Høilund-Carlsen PF. Feasibility of FDG PET in inflammatory bowel disease. Curr Mol Imaging 2014;3(3):195–205.
24. Malham M, Hess S, Nielsen RG, et al. PET/CT in the diagnosis of inflammatory bowel disease in pediatric patients: a review. Am J Nucl Med Mol Imaging 2014;4(3):225–30.
25. Zhang J, Li LF, Zhu YJ, et al. Diagnostic performance of 18F-FDG-PET versus scintigraphy in patients with inflammatory bowel disease: a meta-analysis of prospective literature. Nucl Med Commun 2014;35(12):1233–46.
26. Treglia G, Quartuccio N, Sadeghi R, et al. Diagnostic performance of Fluorine-18-Fluorodeoxyglucose positron emission tomography in patients with chronic inflammatory bowel disease: a systematic review and a meta-analysis. J Crohns Colitis 2013; 7(5):345–54.
27. Hu N, Tan Y, Cheng Z, et al. FDG PET/CT in monitoring antituberculosis therapy in patient with widespread skeletal tuberculosis. Clin Nucl Med 2015; 40(11):919–21.
28. Ozmen O, Gökçek A, Tatcı E, et al. Integration of PET/CT in current diagnostic and response evaluation methods in patients with tuberculosis. Nucl Med Mol Imaging 2014;48(1):75–8.
29. Dureja S, Sen IB, Acharya S, et al. Potential role of F18 FDG PET-CT as an imaging biomarker for the noninvasive evaluation in uncomplicated skeletal tuberculosis: a prospective clinical observational study. Eur Spine J 2014;23(11):2449–54.
30. Martinez V, Castilla-Lievre MA, Guillet-Caruba C, et al. (18)F-FDG PET/CT in tuberculosis: an early

non-invasive marker of therapeutic response. Int J Tuberc Lung Dis 2012;16(9):1180–5.

31. Yadla M, Sivakumar V, Kalawat T. Assessment of early response to treatment in extrapulmonary tuberculosis: role of FDG-PET. Indian J Nucl Med 2012; 27(2):136–7.
32. Ozmen O, Koksal D, Ozcan A, et al. Decreased metabolic uptake in tuberculous pericarditis indicating response to antituberculosis therapy on FDG PET/CT. Clin Nucl Med 2014;39(10):917–9.
33. Sathekge M, Maes A, Kgomo M, et al. Use of 18F-FDG PET to predict response to first-line tuberculostatics in HIV-associated tuberculosis. J Nucl Med 2011;52(6):880–5.
34. Sathekge M. FDG-PET imaging in HIV infection and tuberculosis. Semin Nucl Med 2013;43(5):349–66.
35. Coleman MT, Chen RY, Lee M, et al. PET/CT imaging reveals a therapeutic response to oxazolidinones in macaques and humans with tuberculosis. Sci Transl Med 2014;6(265):265ra167.
36. Hess S, Madsen PH. Potential applications of FDG-PET/CT in COPD: a review of the literature. Curr Mol Imaging 2015;3(3):191–4.
37. Madsen PH, Hess S, Høilund-Carlsen PF, et al. Positron emission tomography in chronic obstructive pulmonary disease. Hell J Nucl Med 2013;16(2):121–4.
38. Kristensen SB, Hess S. FDG-PET/CT in rheumatoid arthritis: a review. Curr Mol Imaging 2015;4:1–5.
39. Blomberg BA, Akers SR, Saboury B, et al. Delayed time-point 18F-FDG PET CT imaging enhances assessment of atherosclerotic plaque inflammation. Nucl Med Commun 2013;34(9):860–7.
40. Blomberg BA, Thomassen A, Takx RA, et al. Delayed F-fluorodeoxyglucose PET/CT imaging improves quantitation of atherosclerotic plaque inflammation: results from the CAMONA study. J Nucl Cardiol 2014;21(3):588–97.
41. Blomberg BA, Hoilund-Carlsen PF. [(1)(8)F]-fluorodeoxyglucose PET imaging of atherosclerosis. PET Clin 2015;10(1):1–7.
42. Mehta NN, Torigian DA, Gelfand JM, et al. Quantification of atherosclerotic plaque activity and vascular inflammation using [18-F] fluorodeoxyglucose positron emission tomography/computed tomography (FDG-PET/CT). J Vis Exp 2012;(63):e3777.
43. Rose S, Sheth NH, Baker JF, et al. A comparison of vascular inflammation in psoriasis, rheumatoid arthritis, and healthy subjects by FDG-PET/CT: a pilot study. Am J Cardiovasc Dis 2013;3(4):273–8.
44. Yu Y, Sheth N, Krishnamoorthy P, et al. Aortic vascular inflammation in psoriasis is associated with HDL particle size and concentration: a pilot study. Am J Cardiovasc Dis 2012;2(4):285–92.
45. Mehta NN, Yu Y, Saboury B, et al. Systemic and vascular inflammation in patients with moderate to severe psoriasis as measured by [18F]-fluorodeoxyglucose positron emission tomography-computed tomography (FDG-PET/CT): a pilot study. Arch Dermatol 2011;147(9):1031–9.

Printed and bound by CPI Group (UK) Ltd, Croydon, CR0 4YY
03/10/2024
01040385-0006